D1465545

Computer and Robotic Assisted Hip and Knee Surgery

Oxford University Press makes no representation, express or implied, that the drug dosages in this book are correct. Readers must therefore always check the product information and clinical procedures with the most up to date published product information and data sheets provided by the manufacturers and the most recent codes of conduct and safety regulations. The authors and the publishers do not accept responsibility or legal liability for any errors in the text or for the misuse or misapplication of material in this work.

Computer and Robotic Assisted Hip and Knee Surgery

Edited by

Anthony M. DiGioia
Institute for Computer Assisted Orthopaedic Surgery
Pittsburgh
USA

Branislav Jaramaz
Institute for Computer Assisted Orthopaedic Surgery
Pittsburgh
USA

Frederic Picard
Pole Sante et Biotech, Ecole Centrale de Paris,
France

Lutz-Peter Nolte
Maurice Muller Institute for Biomechanics
Berne
Switzerland

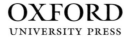

OXFORD
UNIVERSITY PRESS

OXFORD

UNIVERSITY PRESS

Great Clarendon Street, Oxford OX2 6DP

Oxford University Press is a department of the University of Oxford.
It furthers the University's objective of excellence in research, scholarship,
and education by publishing worldwide in

Oxford New York

Auckland Bangkok Buenos Aires Cape Town Chennai
Dar es Salaam Delhi Hong Kong Istanbul Karachi Kolkata
Kuala Lumpur Madrid Melbourne Mexico City Mumbai Nairobi
São Paulo Shanghai Taipei Tokyo Toronto

Oxford is a registered trade mark of Oxford University Press
in the UK and in certain other countries

Published in the United States
by Oxford University Press Inc., New York

© Oxford University Press, 2004

A catalogue record for this title is available from the British Library

ISBN 0 19 850943X (hbk)

10 9 8 7 6 5 4 3 2 1

Typeset by Newgen Imaging Systems (P) Ltd., Chennai, India
Printed in Great Britain
on acid-free paper by Biddles Ltd., King's Lynn, UK

Contents

List of Contributors

Alirezah Pashmineh Azar
Department for Trauma,
Hand and Reconstructive Surgery,
Philipps University,
Baldinger Street,
D-35033 Marburg,
Germany

Anne Z. Banks, MS
Orthopaedic Research Laboratory,
Good Samaritan Medical Center,
West Palm Beach,
Florida 33410,
USA

Scott A. Banks, PhD
Orthopaedic Research Laboratory,
Good Samaritan Medical Center,
West Palm Beach,
Florida 33410,
USA

André Bauer, MD
Marbella High Care,
Marbella,
Spain

Sorin Blendea, MD
1 Rue du Champ Gauthier,
77630 Barbizon,
France

Cyril Boeri, MD
Centre de Tramatologie et d'Orthopédie,
Strasbourg,
France

Yvan Bourquin
Maurice E. Müller Institute for Biomechanics,
University of Bern,
Switzerland

Frank F. Cook, MD
Orthopaedic Research Laboratory,
Good Samaritan Medical Center,
West Palm Beach,
Florida 33410,
USA

Scott L. Delp, PhD
Chair, Bioengineering Department,
Stanford University,
Clark Center, Room S-348,
318 Campus Drive,
Stanford, CA 94305-5450,
USA

Roger J. J. Devilee, MD
Department of Orthopaedics and
Tramatology,
Catharina Hospital,
Michelangelolaan 2,
5623 EJ Eindhoven,
The Netherlands

Anthony M. DiGioia III, MD
Institute for Computer Assisted
Orthopaedic Surgery (ICAOS),
The Western Pennsylvania Hospital,
4815 Liberty Avenue,
Mellon Pavilion, Suite 242,
Pittsburgh, PA 15224,
USA

Randy E. Ellis, PhD
Department of Computing and
Information Science/Department
of Surgery,
Queen's University at Kingston,
Ontario,
Canada

Freddie H. Fu, MD
David Silver Professor and Chairman,
Department of Orthopaedic Surgery,
Division of Sports Medicine,
University of Pittsburgh Medical Center,
Pittsburgh, PA,
USA

Leo Gotzen, MD
Professor for Trauma Surgery,
Direktor of the Department for Trauma,
Hand and Reconstructive Surgery,
Philipps University,
Baldinger Street,
D-35033 Marburg,
Germany

Raymon J. E. Habets, MS
Department of Orthopaedics and
Traumatology,
Catharina Hospital,
Michelangelolaan 2,
5623 EJ Eindhoven,
The Netherlands

M. M. Harrison, MD
Department of Surgery,
Queen's University at Kingston,
Ontario,
Canada

Peter F. Heeckt, MD
Director of the Surgical Academy,
Maquet AG,
Kehler Strasse 31,
76437 Rastatt,
Germany

Andreas F. Hinsche
Department of Trauma and
Orthopaedics,
St. James's University Hospital,
Leeds,
UK

Branislav Jaramaz, PhD
Scientific Director,
Institute for Computer Assisted
Orthopaedic Surgery (ICAOS),

The Western Pennsylvania Hospital,
4815 Liberty Avenue,
Mellon Pavilion, Suite 242,
Pittsburgh, PA 15224,
USA

Jean-Yves Jenny, MD
Centre de Tramatologie et
d'Orthopédie,
Strasbourg,
France

David M. Kahler, MD
Associate Professor, Director of
Orthopaedic Trauma,
University of Virginia Health System,
Box 800159,
Charlottesville, Virginia 22908-0159,
USA

Tiburtius V. S. Klos, MD
Department of Orthopaedics and
Tramatology,
Catharina Hospital,
Michelangelolaan 2,
5623 EJ Eindhoven,
The Netherlands

Rudolf Kober, PhD
Chief Technology Officer,
U.R.S.-ortho GmbH & Co. KG,
Kehler Strasse 31,
76437 Rastatt,
Germany

Kenneth A. Krackow, MD
State University of New York at
Buffalo,
Kaleida Health,
Buffalo General Hospital,
Buffalo, NY,
USA

Manuela Kunz, PhD
Maurice E. Müller Institute for Biomechanics,
University of Bern,
Switzerland

Richard LaBarca, MS
Carnegie Mellon University,
Robotics Institute,
5000 Forbes Avenue,
Pittsburgh,
PA 15213,
USA

Frank Langlotz, PhD
Maurice E. Müller Institute for Biomechanics,
University of Bern,
Switzerland

Sabine Mai, MD
Attending Surgeon,
Kassel Orthopaedic Center,
Kassel,
Germany

Vladimir Martinek, MD
Department of Orthopaedic Surgery,
Musculoskeletal Research Center,
University of Pittsburgh
Pittsburgh,
PA 15213,
USA

Philippe Merloz, MD
University of Grenoble,
France

Rolf Miehlke, MD
St. Josef-Stift,
Sendenhorst,
Germany

Amr M. Mohsen, PhD
Hull Royal Infirmary,
Hull,
UK

James E. Moody, MS
Institute for Computer Assisted Orthopaedic
Surgery (ICAOS),
The Western Pennsylvania Hospital,
4815 Liberty Avenue,
Pittsburgh,
PA 15224,
USA

Andrew B. Mor, PhD
Institute for Computer Assisted Orthopaedic
Surgery (ICAOS),
The Western Pennsylvania Hospital,
4815 Liberty Avenue,
Pittsburgh,
PA 15224,
USA

Constantinos Nikou, MS
CASurgica, Inc.,
4727 Friendship Ave.,
Pittsburgh, PA 15224,
USA

Lutz-Peter Nolte, PhD
Maurice E. Müller Institute for Biomechanics,
University of Bern,
Switzerland

Joerg Petermann, MD
Department for Trauma, Hand and
Reconstructive Surgery,
Philipps University,
Baldinger Street,
D-35033 Marburg,
Germany

Roger Phillips, PhD
Department of Computer Science,
University of Hull,
Hull, UK

Frederic Picard, MD
18 Rue du Champ Gauthier,
77630 Barbizon,
France

Anton Y. Plakseychuk, MD, PhD
Department of Orthopaedic Surgery,
University of Pittsburgh Medical Center,
Pittsburgh, PA 15213
USA

Michael A. Rauh, MD
Kaleida Health–Buffalo General Hospital,
Department of Orthopaedic Surgery,
100 High Street–Suite B2,
Buffalo, NY 14203, USA

John F. Rudan, MD
Department of Surgery,
Queen's University at Kingston,
Ontario,
Canada

Michael J. Rytel, MD
Greater Pittsburgh Orthopaedic Associates,
5820 Centre Avenue,
Pittsburgh, PA 15206,
USA

Dominique Saragaglia, MD
C.H.U. de Grenoble-Hôpital-Sud,
Grenoble cedex 09,
France

Marwan Sati, PhD
Surgical Navigation Specialists
Mississauga, Ontario, Canada, L4V 1S7

David Sell, MS
CASurgica, Inc.,
4727 Friendship Ave.,
Pittsburgh, PA 15224,
USA

Kevin Sherman, MD
Hull Royal Infirmary,
Hull,
UK

Werner Siebert, MD
Professor of Orthopaedic Surgery,
Chief Kassel Orthopaedic Center,
Wilhelmshoeher Allee 345,
34131 Kassel,
Germany

Raimond M. Smith
Department of Trauma and Orthopaedics,
St James's University Hospital,
Leeds,
UK

Hans U. Stäubli, MD
Department of Orthopaedics and
Traumatology,
Surgical Clinic, Tiefenauspital, Tiefenaustr. 112,
CH-3004, Bern,
Switzerland

S. David Stulberg, MD
Northwestern Orthopaedic Institute,
680 N. Lake Shore Drive, Suite 1028,
Chicago,
IL 60611,
USA

Norbert Suhm, MD
AO Development Institute,
Clavadelerstrasse,
CH-7270 Davos Platz,
Switzerland

Russell H. Taylor, PhD
Department of Computer Science,
Center for Computer-Integrated Surgical
Systems and Technology,
Johns Hopkins University,
3400 N. Charles Street,
Baltimore, MD 21218,
USA

Jocelyne Troccaz, PhD
Institut d'Ingénierie et d'Information de Santé,
Faculté de Médecine,
Domaine de la Merci,
38706 La Tronche cedex,
France

Warren Viant, MS
The Department of Computer Science,
University of Hull,
Hull,
UK

Chapter 1

History of computer-assisted orthopaedic surgery of hip and knee

Frederic Picard, James E. Moody, Anthony M. DiGioia III, Branislav Jaramaz, and Dominique Saragaglia

1.1 Pioneers in computer-assisted surgery

In a growing number of operating rooms around the world, orthopaedic surgeons are being assisted by computers and computer-enabled technologies. These synergistic partnerships of humans and machines benefit patients by increasing the accuracy of surgical execution and by increasing the surgically relevant information available to the physician before, during, and after surgery.

A first description of principles and devices for stereotaxis was reported in 1906 by Clarke and Horsley.[1] The term Computer Assisted Orthopedic Surgery (CAOS)[2] as well as implementation of it appeared almost 100 years after these principles were announced and refers to an expanding list of computer-enabled technologies that are known by many different names, including computer assisted surgery, medical robotics, computer integrated surgery, image guided surgery, operating room robotics, surgical navigation, computer-integrated advanced orthopaedics, stereotactic guidance, information-intensive surgery, and computer assisted medical interventions.[3–7]

Many CAOS technologies are derived from manufacturing and imaging technologies that have been developed over the past three decades.[8] These technologies have already undergone several cycles of testing, improvement and validation in other domains like industry and architecture (Fig. 1.1).[9,10]

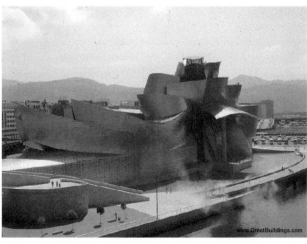

Fig. 1.1 Guggenheim bilbao museum.

The primary goals driving the adoption of Computer Assisted Surgery (CAS) technologies were optimization of surgical performance and the resulting patient's biologic response. CAS enhances progress toward these goals by increasing both the amount and the accuracy of relevant information. One of the first navigational calculations involving bone was designed in 1974 by Schlondorff and co-workers in Aachen Germany. It consisted of a radiographic centimeter scale that was held between the patient's teeth during a lateral roentgenogram. This device enabled the determination of exact distances between various anatomical points.[11] Later on, Watanabe and collaborators, working for Siemens Corporation, published in Japan one of the first versions of the neuronavigator. They used a multijointed three-dimensional digitizer to track the tip of the sensor arm by indicating its location on preoperative CT or MRI images.[12]

Neurosurgeons were the pioneers in the field of computer assisted surgery. Stereotactic neurosurgery was one of the first surgical applications of robotics and computer assisted surgery. Minimizing brain damage by avoiding vital areas during the surgical procedure is a primary goal of neurosurgery.[13,14] Kwoh *et al.* used a six axis industrial robot to replace a stereotactic frame. The robot was mounted in a known position relative to the table of the CT scanner and suitable geometric calibrations were performed. During the surgery, the patient underwent a CT scan and the desired placement for a biopsy needle probe was determined from the image data. The robot positioned a passive needle guide and the surgeon inserted the needle.

In the early 1980s, collaborative teams composed of surgeons, computer scientists, and engineers designed the first robotic systems capable of meeting various neurosurgical requirements. Several robots, such as PUMA (Pittsburgh, PA) were adapted for stereotactic guidance use in surgery in order to improve the accuracy of biopsies, trepanations, or tumor extractions.[15] Doll described the need for iterative fine adjustment in using a robotic system in neurosurgery. Doll and collaborators proposed the use of a self-adjusting component into the system, based for example on digital optical sensors. Such systems were developed in the late 1990s.

Bringing in medical images (CT scan) and Robotic arms (PUMA 200, Unimation, Danbury, CT) enabled the Memorial Medical Center in Long Beach, California to develop a neurosurgical robotic assistive system. This system was used clinically between 1980 and 1984 with the accuracy (or repeatability) of 0.05 mm.[13] In April 1985, a brain biopsy was taken from a 52 year old man using the robot system. A positive biopsy was confirmed on the first sample. In 1986, Kelly *et al.* published a paper on computer assisted stereotaxic laser resection of intra-axial brain neoplasms in the Journal of Neurosurgery in which they described a table used to reposition the patient's head relative to the focal point of a surgical microscope.

At Grenoble University Hospital in France, another computer driven robot was used for stereotactic surgery.[16] This system incorporated the CT data and magnetic resonance information to direct a robot to the target site. The system was composed of a VAX 11/780 computer, a Thomson CGR Magniscan 5000 magnetic resonance imager, a VINIX (Digital Design) processing device for reconstruction of the lesions and image processing, and an AID Universal robot controlled by an AT computer.

1.2 **From neurosurgery to spine surgery**

Robotic and computer assisted surgery evolved naturally from neurosurgery to spine surgery because most neurosurgeons performed both spine and neurosurgeries in their own practice. That was the very first time that computer assisted technology was involved in orthopaedic surgery. We will emphasize works on computer assisted 'bony structures', which generated the first basic concepts of computer assisted orthopaedic hip and knee surgery.

The first team that published on robotic assistive spine surgery was from Oklahoma State University,[17] where a passive robot (in vivo spinal kinematic instrument) was developed to evaluate surgical correction of a scoliotic spine in the operating room. According to the authors, this instrument had an accuracy of 0.3 degrees in rotation and 0.5 mm in translation. With this approach, for the first time, a computer system permitted surgeons to continuously monitor kinematic changes during the surgical procedure.

Due to significant accuracy and safety requirements of spine surgery, the spine procedures became an important topic of research and development in computer assisted surgery. Nolte and collaborators in Bern University in Switzerland developed the concept of interactive navigation of surgical instruments in spine surgery. Merloz, Lavallee and co-workers at Grenoble University in France[18–20] developed the concept of anatomically based registration using only reference anatomic structures detected with intra-operative sensors, again in spine surgery.[21] Simon in Pittsburgh, USA also implemented an anatomic registration process for bony anatomy. Similar approach was used later by Foley for pedicle screw fixations.[22,23,24]

1.3 Craniofacial surgery contribution

Because craniofacial surgery deals with bones and joints, just like orthopaedic surgery, it appeared that requirements defined by several craniofacial teams coincided with orthopaedic surgery requirements. For instance, computer assisted mandibular condyle positioning required extensive work on preoperative imaging, planning and intraoperative guidance of both bones and devices.[25,26,27] In that particular surgery, the primary goal was to implement precise computer assisted planning. According to Cutting, all simulating programs in craniofacial surgery simulation programs should have the following capabilities: (1) virtually cut the bone model; (2) virtually move the different bony segments; (3) respect regional vessels and nerves and their requirements; and (4) proceed to a cephalometric analysis afterwards. Except for the last one, these requirements are very close to those of orthopaedic surgery. In order to reach their goals, in the early 1980s several teams developed computer assisted surgical planners using modalities: computer graphics and real resin models.[28,29]

Computer graphics enabled the surgeons to create infinitely reusable preoperative 3D models that allowed simulating bone transformations. Mosges described a computer assisted 'skull' surgery system that enabled the surgeon to plan hazardous operations using computer tomography (CT) images and a three-dimensional model reconstructed from CT images.[30] Very early on, craniofacial surgeons emphasized the importance of the surgeon's involvement in decision making with data segmentation and display.[31] The 3D palpable model was adapted for measurements and permitted easier visualization and manipulation by the surgeon, for instance in determining a plate position during bone fixation in an osteotomy. The approach evolved into the computer assisted design/computer assisted manufacturing (CAD/CAM) and computer surgical template concepts in orthopaedic surgery, which would later become important fields of development in computer assisted orthopaedic surgery.[32]

General orthopaedic surgery was clearly lagging behind developments in neuro, spine and craniofacial surgeries in the field of computer assisted surgery both in concepts and in developments. It took some time for orthopaedic surgeons to become involved in the field of computer assisted surgery.

1.4 From CAD/CAM to customization

In 1979, two clinical research groups introduced methods by which CT image data were used to manufacture models of patient anatomy. Tonner[33] and co-workers recommended the use of CT to construct an actual size three-dimensional model for the conservative resection of malignant lesions of the pelvis. In a coincident effort, Burri[34] in Germany also reported a similar approach for total hemipelvectomies. The custom prostheses were then designed using the CT and three-dimensional reconstruction data.

In 1982, Nerubay reported a technique of building hemipelvic prosthesis using computed tomography. This prosthesis had to be accurately constructed to match the size and shape of the original bone. A CT scan and a three-dimensional reconstruction model were used to design and machine perfectly fitting implants.[35]

Several teams have worked on computer aided interactive surgical simulation systems. In the early 1980s, Fujioka and collaborators were among the first to introduce such a computer assisted planning system. In 1989, Fujioka *et al.* presented a CT-based three-dimensional surface reconstruction imaging system used for various procedures in orthopaedic surgery, notably for the osteotomy simulation.[36]

Murphy was one of the first to publish about computer aided simulation and design in orthopaedic surgery.[37,38] Preoperative three-dimensional reconstruction of the hip enabled Murphy and co-workers[39–41] to adjust a stem for a 28 year old woman with congenital hip dislocation. Using a three-dimensional model, the surgeon chose the parameters for an implant which was then designed and machined using a computer-controlled milling machine.

Aldinger was also a pioneer in the adoption of CAD/CAM in orthopaedic surgery. The authors described an algorithm allowing them to extract the intrafemoral canal from CT scan images and design an adapted implant that was subsequently machined. In 1984, Woolson and co-workers described three-dimensional image processing from computerized tomography, and emphasized the accuracy of the 3D model relative to the normal anatomy. This work was useful for further pursuing 3D reconstruction models using CAD/CAM technology.[42]

In 1986, Bechtold did an overview of the role of computer graphics in the design of custom orthopaedic implants. He reported the preliminary work of Giliberty *et al.* about the first attempts to use the CAD/CAM techniques to custom design a femoral stem.[43] Garg and Walker, the Muller Institute for Biomechanics in Bern (Switzerland), the Hospital for Special Surgery in New York all had developed CAD/CAM systems for joint implant or model design.

Simon [106] described a method of producing a design of anatomic knee prosthesis in three standard sizes, based on computer analysis of tibia and femur data. At the end of the 1980s, numerous teams worked in this field including Herman, Vannier, Brand, and Rhodes.[44–51] Some commercial firms also used CAD/CAM for prosthesis design, especially for implant sizing and quality control.

In an article on computer and orthopaedic surgery written in 1986, Sutherland concluded that 'real time operative rehearsal, precision surgical planning and execution, and interactive teaching programs will be widely used once the costs associated with this technology come within the reach of clinical and teaching budgets'.[52] While these capabilities have been developed for many orthopaedic surgical applications, only in recent years are they becoming more widely explored.[53] Thanks to the increasing power and decreasing prices of computers, researchers have also started using this technology as a measurement tool, for example in gait analysis[54] and spinal deformity evaluation.[55,56]

In 1990 Pho[57] wrote an overview on computer applications in orthopaedics. He described four main application areas: computerized medical information retrieval, application in rehabilitation, applications in prosthetics and computer graphics.[58] He also explained the importance of Vannier and collaborator's work on producing 3D surface reconstructions of complex anatomical structures from CT scans.[51] Although some other teams[48,59–62] also developed computational methods for three-dimensional reconstruction, Vannier and collaborators implemented a more efficient computer program in terms of computation times and storage requirements, which could be added with modest effort to virtually any modern CT scanner. The work had already been used in craniofacial surgical planning and had also been evaluated but not developed in orthopaedic surgery applications.[63] While computed tomography (CT) was first described by Hounsfield and co-workers in 1973, 3D model building and visualization appeared almost ten years after, thanks to advanced computers and new algorithms.[64–67]

1.5 From customization to robotics

The desire to improve the fit of hip implants using CAD/CAM technology resulted not only in the concept of custom design and machining of anatomic implants, but also in the attempts to enhance the bone milling quality. The guiding idea was that the robotic machining of the bone cavity would ensure a better contact between the bone and a cementless implant and therefore enable better ingrowth and ensure the long term stability.

Mittelstadt, Paul, and collaborators[68–70] were clearly the pioneers in the introduction of active robots in surgery. They developed RoboDoc™, which in 1992 became the first robot-assisted surgical system to be used on a human. Since that time, more than 4000 Total Hip Replacement (THR) procedures have been performed with it worldwide. The system was designed to prepare bone for uncemented femoral implants and included a preoperative planner (OrthoDoc™) component and an intra-operative execution component (RoboDoc™).[71,72]

At the same time, a team from The Rizzoli Institute in Bologna, Italy developed a preoperative planner and simulator for robot assisted TKR surgery.[73–75] The system used the CT scan for planning but did not need any fiducial markers for registration, which was an improvement for an active robotic system. This team also developed CT image planning in which the surgeon was able to choose anatomical landmarks such as the center of the hip, knee, and ankle in the 3D CT-derived model, but also the size of the implants and the level of the bone resection. The authors found the accuracy between planning and final result (five patients) close to 1 degree and to 1 mm.[76] So far the system has not been in routine clinical use. In addition, Pagetti from the same team developed a technique using MRI scan images for planning in TKR.[77]

More recently (1997), the first commercial European-built orthopaedic robotic system was introduced by Orto Maquet GmbH and Co. from Rastatt, Germany.[78] It was called Computer Assisted Surgical Planning and Robotics (CASPAR) and was very similar to the RoboDoc system. The clinical applications included THR (femoral milling) and knee surgery (TKR and ACL surgery).[79]

1.6 From active to semi-active robotic assistive systems

Some other concepts essential for current computer assisted orthopaedic systems were introduced back in the 1980s. In 1986, Kaiura from the University of Washington did a Master's Thesis on Robotic Assisted Total Knee Arthroplasty.[80,81] He described the basic concept, which allowed Matsen and co-workers (including Kaiura) to design one of the first computer robotic assistive systems for total knee surgery described in the literature. Matsen, in 1993,[82] and his team were the first authors to describe a 'passive' robotic system dedicated to knee arthroplasty. The robot used in their system was a Unimation Puma 260. The surgeon indicated the desired position of the prosthetic joint surface using a transparent three-dimensional template attached to the robot. The robot positioned the saw guide in such a way as to establish the correct planes of the bone cuts required for the specific component. The power saw was held by the surgeon while the robot assistant determined the plane of the cut. They only performed the cuts on the femur side.[82] A positional reproducibility of 0.025 mm has been reported. The time of the procedure was 16.8 min longer than the usual procedure and the angular accuracy was around 2 degrees. This system can be considered as the first semi-active knee robot system, because the surgeon made the bone cuts using a traditional oscillating saw blade. The saw blade was only oriented with robotic assisted jigs. This system has not been, to date, used in the operating room.

In parallel, in 1986, another robot system was also used for assisting the surgeon by holding, clamping or manipulating a limb. McEwen and collaborators from the University of British Columbia Health Sciences Hospital in Vancouver, Canada implemented a manipulating robot, called Arthrobot. During total hip replacement surgery, this robot was used to hold the limb. The robot assisted in more than 200 operations.[83] Using the same idea of a clinical 'helper', the Vancouver team developed a robot retraction[91] system able to maintain the soft tissue open during a total hip replacement approach, more accurately and more safely than an assistant. Twenty clinical trials were successfully performed using this robot.

In the early 1990s, Kienzle, Stulberg, and co-workers also described a computer assisted robotic TKR system. As with other systems, a CT scan (75 slices) was obtained preoperatively. A 3D model allowed the implant size and position to be defined. During intra-operative preparation, the patient's leg was placed in an ankle cast with pins, and landmarks were secured in the femur and tibia. The robot was secured on the surgical table to the distal femur. The robot oriented a drill, which made a hole for pins as specified by the preoperative plan. The cutting blocks (femoral and tibial cutting blocks) were then slipped on the pins and the cut was made. The preliminary cadaver results showed accuracy within 1 mm and 1 degree. Another innovative idea was also to determine the center of the femoral head, using several points recorded from the femoral markers while the femur was put through a range of motion. These measurements described a spherical surface, and the center of the sphere (center of the femoral head) could be accurately calculated. Although the robot did not actually make the bone cuts, this robotic system is not considered to be a semi-active system[84] since the robot actively drilled the holes for pins.[85]

1.7 Semi-active robotic systems in orthopaedic surgery

It was not until the 1990s that semi-active robotic assistive systems were developed for orthopaedic surgery. Moctezuma *et al.* described in 1994[86,87] a computer and robotic aided surgery system for performing femoral osteotomies, which they also recommended for knee arthroplasty. A robotic assistive twin-blade (for reducing temperature) was set up on a handle held by a surgeon while the robot constrained the cut orientation. Cadaver experiments were performed but this system has not been used clinically.

Based on their experience in robotic prostate surgery, Davies[88,89] and his team worked on a semi-active robot for TKR. Again, a CT scan of the patient's whole leg was taken preoperatively, with slices closely spaced in the region of the knee. A detailed 3D model of the knee was then built from the scan, and the surgeon was able to choose the position of the knee prosthesis in the model. During surgery, the patient's leg was clamped to the table using orthopaedic fixators. Based on the 3D model (and associated fiducial markers), the shape and the orientation of the planned regions of resection are transferred into the robot's coordinate reference frame. A semi-active robot (ACROBOT) actively assists the surgeon during the bone cutting. The surgeon guides the robot using a handle with a force sensor attached to the robot tip, and thus uses his/her superior human senses and understanding of the overall situation to perform the surgery. The robot provides a 3D motion constraint that prevents cutting outside a predefined safe region. The error in radius was less than 0.1 mm and the cutter was easy to move along the boundary with a precise sense of feel and with low surgeon forces.[90] The robot has not been used clinically.

Gotte[91] and co-workers described, also in 1996, a semi-active robotic assistive TKR system. Permanent and rigid patient immobilization was theoretically not necessary thanks to the use of a real time vision system for intra-operative bone tracking; this was a new concept in robotic assistive surgery. Ideally, the surgeon could freely move the saw to remove bony material. He was only limited by the guiding device keeping the movement within the cutting plane. Intra-operative usage of the system starts with calibration and registration of the X-ray system. This technique relied upon five pieces of equipment, which were the CT scan for registration, a real time vision system, an image intensifier used to compare the images coming from the CT through a graphic workstation, and a robot linked to the graphic workstation. Preoperatively, a CT scan was made and no markers were used. Intra-operative procedures were: i) active markers were secured to the tibia and femur; ii) an initial self-calibration X-ray image of the femur and tibia from at least two angles was made with the image intensifier. When computing the location of the femur and tibia by correlation of the CT scan and X-rays: iii) a specific tracking of bone location with the real time vision system can be applied; and iv) in addition to the robot used to perform the cut, another type of robot was used to stabilize the knee during the surgical procedure. To our knowledge, this system has never been used in the OR.

In 1998, an Israeli team[92] proposed a new registration process using a surface matching technique which did not require marker implants. The robot itself was used as a digitizer, eliminating the need for an extra localizer.

1.8 **From the robot to navigation**

Surgical Navigation Systems (SNS) permit intra-operative tracking of tools and anatomy and provide guidance of tools. Navigation systems typically use optical or magnetic markers to track tools and the patient's bony anatomy. Benefits of this approach are that they permit surgeons to stay in control at all phases of surgery and to update plans intra-operatively. In addition, navigational tools do not require rigid fixation of bones.

Soon after the introduction of the first robotic tools, navigation systems were developed and introduced into surgical practice. In 1995, Hans Reinhart, one of the pioneers in neurosurgery navigation technology, did a ten year review and concluded that 'compared with the automobile industry, computer assisted surgery is now in about the year 1910'. Once again, neurosurgeons and craniofacial surgeons were pioneers in the field of navigation. In 1995, only two interactive image based assistive systems were known. The most advanced of these was the device of Kelly.[93]

As mentioned previously, tremendous effort has been made in the area of image processing and understanding,[8,94] in particular methods for image segmentation, filtering, 3D model building, and registration. Especially important was the basic work on three-dimensional registration to allow the surgeon to use preoperative images and associated plans intra-operatively. In 1992, Brown[95] did an excellent survey of 2D photometric image registration with application to medical image processing, which summarizes the basic problems of registration. One year later, Van den Elsen did a new survey of techniques and applications in medical image-based registration (3D photometric image). Simon reminds us in his work that registration (back in 1996) could be divided into two categories: registration for data fusion and subsequent visualization, and registration for spatial localization. Regarding the first modality, Jian (in 1992) and Woods (in 1983) were among the first to apply multimodality data visualization and detection of anatomical changes (Ettinger in 1994) in the field of medicine. The second category of registration can be used to estimate the spatial location of a portion of a patient's anatomy based on different representations of the same anatomy.

Smith, Bucholz, and Foley described[22] free-hand stereotactic computer assisted surgery in 1995. They described the primary innovation of the NeuroStation™ technology which was the use of a 3D localization method (the 'Bucholz Free-Hand™' method) that couples a 3D optical sensor with custom forceps fitted with localizing emitters, thus providing a surgical localizer that is 'transparent' to the surgeon's standard operating procedures. The authors concluded that frameless image-guided stereotactic localization and navigation methods are being developed which can easily and effectively be integrated and utilized in daily surgical procedures.

Roberts, Evan, and Colchester also described a hand-held locator probe, used with a vision-based intra-operative measurement system for surgical navigation called VISLAN [Roberts CARS 94].

Due to the accuracy requirements and potential severe complications, spine surgery was a natural field for investigating new computer assisted navigation technologies. Trauma or scoliosis surgeries are difficult essentially because of the need to implant internal fixations, such as plates and other rigid objects, usually affixed to the vertebrae by screwing in the pedicles. The primary goal of the surgical procedure was to safely and accurately place screws into the vertebrae pedicles while avoiding cord and nerve damages. Using image navigation technology, several teams developed systems for accurately guiding the anatomic placement and controlling the insertion depth of screws in the vertebrae pedicles. Foley et al. worked with the StealthStation derived from the NeuroStation. Nolte et al. described in the *Spine Journal* a laboratory setup of image guided insertion of transepicondylar screws. Lavallee et al. also published, in the *Journal of Image Guided Surgery*, a paper on computer assisted spine surgery (Fig. 1.2).

In computer assisted hip and knee reconstruction surgery, different concepts were implemented almost concurrently:

—preoperative model image-based

—intra-operative model image-based

—image-free navigation

—individual templating

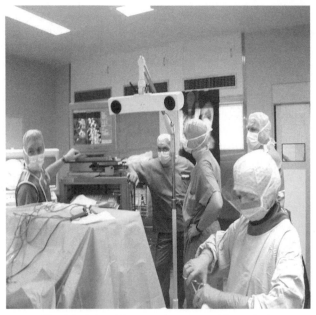

Fig. 1.2 Spine OR set up (courtesy of P. Merloz).

1.9 **Preoperative model image-based navigation systems**

The availability of optical and electromagnetic position tracking systems during the 1990s facilitated the development of surgical navigation. OptoTrak™, an optical tracking system (Northern Digital, Inc., Waterloo, Ontario) has played a special role due to its accuracy and reliability. The optical localizer with three charge coupled device (CCD) cameras in a rigid enclosure was used in the operating room to measure the position and orientation of multiple tracking markers (trackers, rigid bodies). Each tracker incorporates a set of light emitting diodes (LEDs) mounted at precise relative positions. Trackers can be affixed to tools, implants, or bones, and the position of each of these components can be continuously calculated and updated, allowing the surgeon to accurately align a tool or implant into its preplanned position.

Sati, Drouin, and de Guise developed in 1990/91, at the Ecole Polytechnique of Montreal, Canada, an image-based system for ACL reconstruction (Fig. 1.3).

In 1994, the Center for Medical Robotics and Computer Assisted Surgery group in Carnegie Mellon University in Pittsburgh (USA) began work on cup placement.[96] DiGioia and co-workers[97,98] developed the first computer assisted navigation system for cup placement in THR surgery. HipNav™ was the first image-guided surgical navigation system for total hip replacement (THR).[99] Besides the clinical application, its contributions included preoperative simulation of hip range of motion and pinless registration (Fig. 1.4). As with RoboDoc™, preoperative planning was based on CT images.

Later on, several teams followed similar principles for other applications on the hip. In Osaka, Japan an image guided navigation hip system was also developed following principles identical to those described above.

In 1994, Langlotz, Nolte *et al.* [57,86,87] (Muller Institute, Bern, Switzerland) described a system which also employed surface-based registration techniques for periacetabular osteotomy (PAO) of dysplastic

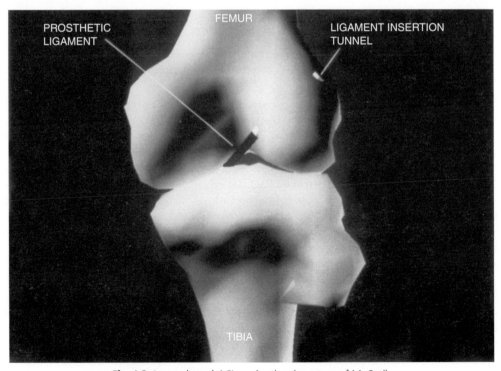

Fig. 1.3 Image based ACL navigation (courtesy of M. Sati).

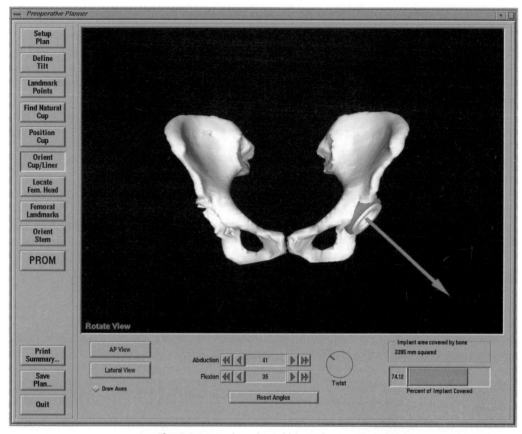

Fig. 1.4 Image based total hip replacement.

hips. This technology was used at Bern University to guide the very difficult periacetabular procedure. In this approach, the 3D anatomy of the patient and surgical plans were preoperatively generated from CT scans. Intra-operatively, pelvis and surgical tools were tracked and depicted on a monitor screen, which showed in real-time patient's CT data updated with information coming directly from the tracking system (Fig. 1.5). Numerical values of crucial angles are also displayed. The improvement in accuracy brought about by the image-guided system for PAO also enhanced the safety of the procedure. Some of the chiseling steps in the PAO procedure have to be performed with the blades of the instruments out of the surgeon's view, so there is potential for harming the hip joint and the surrounding neural and vascular structures. Safety of the conventional execution relies on the surgeon's experience and ability to navigate from visible anatomical landmarks and intra-operative two-dimensional radiographs. The use of this CAOS system has brought about an improvement in surgical techniques (Fig. 1.6).[100]

Orienting simultaneously a bone model and an acetabular fragment was new and this interesting application has 'opened the window' on computer assisted bone trauma surgery.[101,102] Several computer assisted trauma applications were developed, increasing the safety and accuracy of procedures by using image guided navigation technology. For instance, iliosacral screws are conventionally used to fixate pelvic bone fractures.[102] Percutaneous placement minimizes the surgical exposure, which, in turn, reduces muscle weakness, decreases recovery time, and diminishes complications. CAOS technologies for

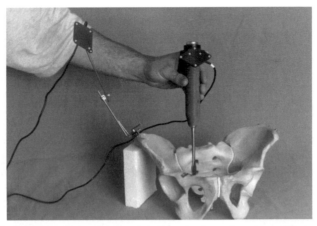

Fig. 1.5 Computer Assisted Periacetabular osteotomy (courtesy of Dr Langlotz).

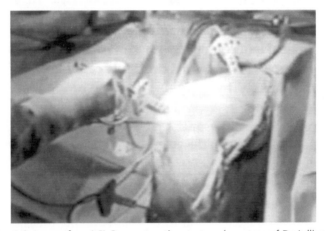

Fig. 1.6 Image free ACL Reconstruction system (courtesy of Dr Julliard).

percutaneous placement of these screws have been demonstrated recently at Grenoble University with the use of ultrasound.[103] A typical study[95] with the ViewPoint™ image-guided workstation uses preoperative CT scans and intra-operative tracking of tools and bone fragments. Fiducial screws or pins are placed prior to data collection. Helical CT data with 3 mm spacing of the entire pelvis are acquired. These raw data are transferred to the 3D image guided workstation. Screws are placed with a consistent precision in the range of 1 mm with this system, manufactured by Picker of Cleveland, Ohio.

The Stealth Station (described previously for spine applications) has also been applied to pelvic procedures, including the percutaneous internal fixation of transverse acetabular nonunions.[104] Two procedures were required for this application. In the first procedure, a two-pin external fixator was attached to the ilium. CT scans were then taken and cannulated screws were percutaneously inserted in a second procedure. In a representative operation, the total operative time required for the second procedure was only 105 minutes, and the resulting five puncture wounds were closed with single sutures. Although the nonunion had existed for 1 year without improvement prior to the operation, the patient was essentially asymptomatic 15 months after the surgery.

Femoral fracture reduction also benefited from these new concepts. Femoral fracture reduction is traditionally achieved with an intramedullary nail that needs to be locked by screws driven through the bone and through the predrilled holes in the nail. Because the holes in the nail cannot be viewed directly after the nail is placed, the locking procedure can be very difficult. Conventional methods require the use of several intra-operative fluoroscopic X-rays to localize the nail holes. A representative CAOS system called FRACAS (for FRActure Computer-Aided Surgery) was developed to reduce radiation exposure for both patient and surgeon and increases the accuracy of locking screw placement.[101] In this approach, a CT scan of the fractured bone is acquired preoperatively. A few fluoroscopic images are acquired intra-operatively to register the preoperative 3D model with the patient's anatomy on the OR table. Both the bone fragments and the drill are tracked with an optical tracking system. A custom drill guide device with four adjustable degrees of freedom is attached to the head of the nail. With image guidance, the drill is manually moved into position and locked. The surgeon's task in this maneuver is to align the drill guide with one of the holes in the nail by observing the relative positions of these two items on the monitor.

In Canada, Ellis *et al.* developed image guided technology for high tibial osteotomy (HTO). The major difficulty with HTO is in attaining an accurate correction angle. A representative CAOS for HTO[105] is similar to many other CAOS systems. Radiopaque markers were inserted into the tibia under local anesthesia before the area is CT scanned. A three-dimensional surface model of the tibia is reconstructed from the CT data. Preoperative planning was accomplished, as usual, on a graphical workstation to define the two cuts forming the wedge. The software automatically computes the resulting configuration of the new tibia shape and allows the surgeon to iterate on the plan. For this particular system, registration of the plan to the patient was performed in the operating room with a precision mechanical arm produced by FARO Technologies (Lake Mary, Florida). The arm was manually positioned so that its end point touches each of the radiopaque markers, allowing for fiducial registration. A drill was then tracked with an optical tracker to produce two holes for placement of K-wires corresponding to each resection plane. These wires are used as saw guides in the performance of the actual cutting. The bone wedge and the K-wires are removed and the fixation of the bone is carried out with staples, as is conventionally done. Laboratory results show that the accuracy of the angle of the removed lateral wedge is at least as good as the best manual jig system. The system has also been demonstrated clinically.[105] According to an experiment on five patients, the error was ±1.5 degrees which is sufficiently accurate for that particular type of surgery.

In 2000, KneeNav™, a CT-based navigation system[106,107] for TKR, was under development at the Center for Medical Robotics and Computer Assisted Surgery at Carnegie Mellon University and UPMC Shadyside Hospital in Pittsburgh, Pennsylvania. KneeNav™ relies on the same preoperative planning and intra-operative tracking principles as the HipNav™ system previously described.[108,109] Using patient data, KneeNav-TKR enables the surgeon to accurately measure cutting guide orientations during the TKR procedure and ACL as well. Moreover, a soft tissue evaluation is performed intra-operatively. During TKR, knee laxity and femorotibial gaps can be interactively appraised at any time. The innovative element is a new device called a plate-probe which is able to measure intra-operatively cutting guide positions and final cut orientations. This concept allows the system not to be specifically linked to an implant and its instrumentation.[110] This was the first time that computer assisted optical tracking of jigs was independent of the instrumentation.

1.10 Intra-operative model using-image based technology

In the middle of the 1990s,[111,112] a system was developed which allowed accurate ACL reconstruction using intra-operative fluouroscopic images in addition to conventional arthroscopy. A perfect sagittal

X-ray, obtained at the beginning of the surgical procedure, was required. Based on anatomical analyses carried out on the normal ACL position in the knee joint, the authors specified the ideal position of the graft relative to the bones. The computer places graphical overlays onto the fluoroscopic image in order to aid the surgeon in specifying the desired drilling location. The imaging system also provides the ability to project the intended path of the drill through the bones, to calculate the graft length required, and to adjust the drilling path accordingly. The claimed accuracy of the clinical was 1.1 degrees. A clinical study involving 125 patients showed a significant increase in accuracy of graft placement without an increase in operating room time.

This concept of using fluoroscopic images as a basis for navigation attracted other clinical applications, primarily in trauma, where getting intra-operative imaging is essential. One of the early applications was the locking of intramedullary nails. A system for fluoroscopic navigation consists of an optical tracking system and an air drill, nail pointer, intramedullary nail, and C-arm, each with LED targets attached. The nail pointer is used to identify the positions of the distal holes in the intramedullary nail. Its end was inserted into each hole. Then the nail was inserted into the femur in the conventional manner. The graphical monitor of the system displays the nail, with its holes, on the screen, so that the C-arm can be aligned to obtain two images: one aligned with the holes and one perpendicular to the holes. These two images are stored and displayed on the screen. The air drill can then be tracked in real time with its image continually displayed on the two orthogonal X-ray images; it can be accurately aligned and the holes for the locking screws can be drilled without further X-ray exposure. The system for this procedure was evaluated in the laboratory on plastic bones and cadaver specimens. Commercial systems using this technology are currently available. Fluoroscopic navigation is also applied to pedicle screw placement for spine surgery.[22]

1.11 **Intra-operative model image-free navigation**

An alternative concept to image-based navigation was to directly obtain patient's anatomical or kinematics information without using any form of medical imaging. In Grenoble University Orti, Dessenne, Julliard and Lavallee designed a non-image-based system for ACL surgery. This system was described first in 1993 and was used to place the graft during ACL reconstruction surgery.[25,113] At the beginning of the surgical procedure, the patient was placed in a supine position with the leg dangling. After the graft was extracted from the patellar tendon, the surgeon firmly attached two tracking markers to the femur and the tibia using two bicortical 4-mm diameter Kischner pins. Passive flexion and extension then was applied to the knee by the surgeon. From 20 to 50 knee positions ranging from maximal extension to maximal flexion, the tibial coordinates relative to the femur coordinates were computed and stored. During the arthroscopic procedure, the surgeon recorded 100 anatomical points on the knee surface using a precalibrated probe. The points were recorded on the femoral notch and roof and in the area of the natural tibial insertion of the ACL. The system would then calculate the position of the graft relative to the tibial and femoral holes (for tension of the graft) and to the roof (for impingement).[113] This was the first time that the use of intra-operatively digitized knee anatomy for surgical navigation was described (Fig. 1.6).

A similar concept was subsequently implemented at Bern University by Dessenne, Sati, *et al.*[25].

This concept of image-free navigation was later used for TKR. Picard and Leitner described the first image-free system for TKR ever used in the OR (later commercialized as Orthopilot™, Aesculap/B.Braun, Tuttlingen, Germany).[114,115] The basic principle was to determine the mechanical axes during the surgical procedure and then to orient the precalibrated cutting guides. The first step consisted in carrying out the lower limb calibration. The lower limb calibration was obtained using a kinematics technique and acquisition of several relevant anatomical points by digitizing points with a precalibrated probe. This step led to recording the femoral and tibial mechanical axes in real time. The second step consists in securing calibrated tracked jigs. A simple user interface helped the surgeon to orient the jig. An intuitive user interface, similar to those used in an airplane, represented in real time the mechanical axes and the orientation of the cutting guides. Then the surgeon secured himself the jig following the usual procedure and he cut the bone with a classical saw. This was an intra-operative procedure and the surgeon did not need an assistant to pilot the system. A footpedal is switched in order to go back and forth in the program. Moreover, this system constitutes extra-medullary instrumentation.[106,107] In a clinical study of 30 patients, in which this system was compared to the conventional procedure, this CAOS system was found to produce significantly more accurate results with fewer complications, although the duration of the surgery was longer (Fig. 1.7a).[116]

(a)
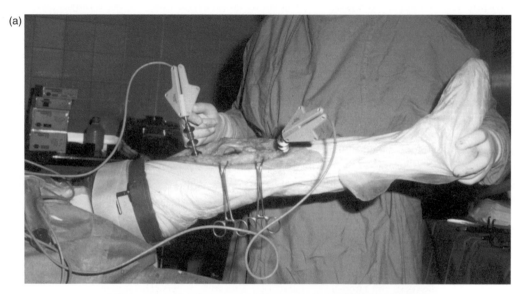

(b)
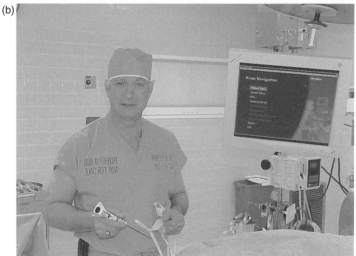

Fig. 1.7 (a) Image-free TKR orthopilot™ system (courtesy from Pr Saragaglia). (b) Image-free TKR stryker system (courtesy from Pr Krackow).

Later on, Krackow and co-workers developed a similar system (Fig 1.7b). An optoelectronic localizer was used for the surgical procedure. Two rigid bodies were fixed on the distal femur and the proximal tibia. The center of the femoral head was found after moving it around the hip joint as Kienzle suggested.[85] The main difference with the Orthopilot system was the possibility of using a cannulated intramedullary femoral rod.[117] Many systems are currently using similar concepts.[118,119]

1.12 Orthopaedic individual templates

One fairly unusual CAOS technology is the individual template method. Radermacher and co-workers described a computer assisted system used to create a bone matching template which helps to align a surgical tool.[120] This method does not use intra-operative tracking, but centers instead around custom templates produced for each operation. Each individual template is shaped on one side to exactly match the bone surface surrounding the anatomic site, thus allowing physical registration to the bone. The tool side of the template is shaped with bore holes and cutting planes to restrict the motions of the drill, saw, or mill to the preplanned trajectories. The templates themselves are milled on a desktop milling machine using surface models generated from CT scans. In this way, the procedure benefits from the accuracy and patient-specific benefits of CAOS technologies while remaining very similar in execution to conventional surgical practices.

As with most CAOS procedures, CT scanning of the surgical site occurs first. These data are transmitted to a Desktop Image-processing System for Orthopedic Surgery (DISOS). This system runs on standard PC hardware. The graphical user interface is designed specially for the nontechnical user, with intuitive color and graphics and an on-line help system. With DISOS the medical staff can perform segmentation, 3D reconstruction, and planning of the surgical procedure.

After planning is complete, data are transmitted to the CAD/CAM system via a network or floppy disk, where the individual template is manufactured on a NC milling machine. The templates are cleaned and sterilized like other surgical tools. During surgery, the surgeon places the template against the matching bone surface and then manually performs the intervention with hand-held tools resting against the back side of the template. In this way, the use of individual templates replaces the intra-operative tracking and registration procedures of typical CAOS systems with elaborate preoperative planning and machining.

The first clinical use of this technology has been for osteotomies of the pelvis at Marienhhe District Hospital, Wurselen, Germany. The templates were readily accepted by the medical staff because no unfamiliar processes or large, complicated devices or procedures were involved.

Of extremely limited use only a few years ago, multiple CAOS systems for hip and knee surgery (as well as related surgical procedures) are now in the clinical validation process or even in the commercialization phase.

1.13 CAOS technologies of the future

Many promising technologies being investigated in research laboratories are not yet used clinically.[121] Surgical training simulators that allow physicians in training to see and feel the virtual anatomical structures just as if they were actually performing a procedure are under development.[122] This field is underexploited in orthopaedic surgery and will certainly be an important field given the growing number of legal issues surrounding surgeons in training. Telesurgical systems are under development that may allow a surgeon to operate on a patient at a remote location.[123] Augmented reality devices are being investigated that will enable a surgeon to see a 3D model of the patient's internal anatomy in correct registration with the patient's external anatomy even while the patient and the surgeon have freedom of motion.[96,124,125]

Noninvasive ultrasonic sensor technologies are being adapted for use in visualizing internal bone for both registration and tracking in surgery. Finally, tissue engineering initiatives are under way that may someday provide biological implants that can be introduced through minimally invasive portals and which would be accepted by the body as well as native bone.

A list of clinical procedures to which the CAOS technologies are applied is growing, and will soon include shoulder, wrist, and ankle procedures. The next twenty years will, no doubt, generate more innovative technologies in orthopaedic surgery and will greatly modify the field.

Acknowledgements

To Brian Davies, Professor of Medical Robotics at the Imperial College of Science, Technology and Medicine of London; Justin Cobb, Orthopaedic Surgeon at the University College of London; and Simon Harris at the Imperial College of London. Ho, Hibberd, Davies, Robot Assisted Knee Surgery—A fore Control Strategy involving Active Motion Constraint. *IEEE Engineering in Medicine and Biology* Vol 14 (3) May 1995.

To Marwan Sati, Professor Jacques de Guise, and Professor Gilbert Drouin at the Ecole Polytechnique of Montreal. 'Proligs—Prosthetic and ligament information generating system' Simulated 3D knee kinematics, ligament positioning. Proceedings of SICOT July 1991.

To Professor Roger Phillips at the Department of Computer Science of the University of Hull, UK, and Professor A.M.M.A. Mohsen, Mr. W.J. Viant, Mr. K.P. Sherman. Phillips, R, Griffiths, J.G., Camplin, D.A., Marshall, S., Mohsen, A.M.M.A., 15th International Conference, IEEE Engineering in Medicine & Biology Society, San Diego, October 1993.

To Dr Andre Bauer at Marbella High Care in Spain and Martin Borner and Armin Lahmer from Frankurt University in Germany.

To Sandra Martelli, Marco Fadda (computer scientists), and Professor Maurilio Marcacci at the Biomechanics Department of Instituti Rizzoli of Bologna, Italy.

To Professor Philippe Merloz at the University of Grenoble and Professor P. Cinquin and S. Lavallee from TIMC Laboratory in Grenoble.

To Frank Langlotz, Dr Manfred Stucki, and Dr Richard Bachler at Bern University. First presentation in Zurich, Biomedizinische Technik 41:392–3: BMT-Meeting, Zurich, September, 1996. Langlotz *et al.*, The first 12 cases of Computer Assisted Periacetabular Osteotomy, *Computer Aided Surgery* 2:317–26, 1997.

To Professor Leo Joskowicz, Russ Taylor, Alan Kelvin, V. Hebrew, C.Milgkom, A. Simkin, and Z. Yaniv at the School of Computer Science in Jerusalem, Israel.

To Professor K Krackow, Clinical Director of the Department of Orthopaedic Surgery at Buffalo (New York State) and W.M. Mihalko, L. Serpe, M. Phillips, and Mary Bayers-Thering.

References

1 Clarke RH, Horsley V. On a method of investigating the deep ganglia and tracts of the central nervous system (cerbellum). *Br Med Jo* 1906;1799–800.

2 Mohsen AM, Cain TJ, Sherman KP, Karpinski MRK, Philipps R, *et al.* The CAOS projects (Computer Assisted Orthopaedic Systems). *MRCAS'94, 1st International Symposium on Medical Robotics and Computer Assisted Surgery.* 1994,vol. 1,49–56, sessions I–III. Pittsburgh, PA.

3 Cinquin P. Gestes médico-chirurgicaux assistés par ordinateur. *Société d'Edition de l'Association d'Enseignement Médical des Hôpitaux de Paris* 1993;63:386–405.

4 Cinquin P, Bainville E. Computer assisted medical intervention: passive and semi-active aids. *IEEE Eng Med Biol Mag* 1995;14:254–63.

5 DiGioia A, Jaramaz B, Blackwell M, *et al.* Image guided navigation system to measure intraoperatively acetabular implant alignment. *Clin Orthop Relat Res* 1998;355:8–22.

6 Stulberg SD, Kienzle TC. *Computer integrated surgery, technology and clinical applications*, Taylor, Lavallee, Burdea, Mosges, eds. Cambridge: MIT Press Publishers, 1995:374–80.

7 Taylor RH. Robotics in orthopedic surgery. In: Nolte LP, Ganz R, eds. *Computer assisted orthopaedic surgery* (CAOS). 35–41. 1998. Hogrefe and Huber Publishers.

8 Duncan JS, Ayache N. Medical image analysis: progress over two decades and the challenges ahead. *IEEE Trans Pattern Anal Machine Intell* 2000;22(1):85–105.

9 Guggenheim Bilbao Museum in Frank O. Gehry. *Individual imagination and cultural conservatism.* Academy Editions 1995;49–50.

10 Lemke HU. The third dimension. *CAR'85*, 628–34.

11 Schlondorff G. Computer assisted surgery: historical remarks. *Comput Aided Surg* 1998;3:150–2.

12 Watanabe K, Nakamura R, Horii E, Miura T. Biomechanical analysis of radial wedge osteotomy for the treatment of Kienbock's disease. *J Hand Surgery* 1993;18A:686–90.

13 Kwoh YS. A new CT-aided robotic sterotactiv system. 70th Scientific Assembly and Annual Meeting. Washington, DC: *Radiol Soc N Am* 1984:375–8.

14 Kwoh YS, Hou J, Jonckeere E, Hayati S. A robot with improved absolute positioning accuracy for CT guided sterotactic surgery. *IEEE Trans Biomech Eng* 1988;35(2):153–61.

15 Doll J, Schelgel W, Pastyr O, Sturm V, Maier-Borst W. The use of an industrial robot as a stereotactic guidance system. *CAR'87* 1987;314–18.

16 Benabib AL, Cinquin P, Lavallee S, Lebas JF, Demongeot J, De Rougemont J. Computer driven robot for stereotactic surgery connected to CT scan and magnetic resonance imaging. *Proceedings American Society Stereotactic Functional Neurosurgery*, Montreal, *Appl Neurophysiol* 1987;50:153–4.

17 Soni AH, Gudavalli MR, Herndon WA, Sullivan JA. Application of passive robot in spine surgery. *Proceedings of the 8th Annual Conference on IEEE/ Engineer Biology and Medical Society*, 1986, vol. 3, 1186–91.

18 Lavallee S. Registration for computer integrated surgery: methodology, state of the art. Computer integrated surgery, Technology and clinical applications. MIT Press; 1995:77–98.

19 Lavallee S, Cinquin Ph, Szeliski R, *et al.* Building a hybrid patient's model for augmented reality in surgery: a registration problem. *Comput Biol Med* 1995;25:149–64.

20 Lavallee S, Troccaz J, Sautot P, *et al.* Computer assisted spine surgery using anatomy-based registration. In: Taylor R, Lavallee S, Burdea G, Mosges R, eds. *Computer integrated surgery*. Cambridge: MIT-Press; 1996;425–9.

21 Merloz P, Tonetti J, Eid A, *et al.* Computer assisted spine surgery. *Clin Orthop* 1997;337:86–96.

22 Foley KT, Smith MM. Image guided spine surgery. *Neurosurg Clin North Am* 1996;7:171–86.

23 Simon DA, Lavallee D. Medical imaging and registration in computer assisted surgery. *Clin Orthop Rel Res* 1998;354:17–27.

24 Foley KT, Smith KR, Bucholtz RD. Frameless spinal stereotaxy. Presented at the Contemporary Update on Disorders of the Spine Conference. January 8–15. 1994. Snowbird, Utah.

25 Dessenne V, Lavallee S, Julliard R, *et al.* Computer assisted knee anterior cruciate ligament reconstruction: first clinical tests. *Image Guided Surg* 1995;1:59–64.

26 Hemmy DC, David DJ, Herman GT. Three dimensional reconstruction of craniofacial deformity using computed tomography. Technical report MIPG-81, 1983. University of Pennsylvania Department of Radiology, Medical Image Processing Group.

27 McEwen C, Robb R, Jackson I. Craniofacial surgery planning and simulation: current progress and problem areas. *CAR'89*, 398–402.

28 Lambrecht JTh, Schiel H, Jacob AL, Kreusch. CAR- CAD-CAM- CAS: 3D perspectives. *CAR'S 95*, 1364–8.

29 Tronnier U, Wolff KD, Trittmacher S. A 3-D surgical planning system and its clinical applications. *CAR'89*, 403–8.

30 Mosges R, Schlondorff G, Klimek L, Meyers- Ebrecht D, Krybus W, Adams L. CAS-computer assisted surgery. An innovative surgical technique in clinical routine. *CAR'89*, 413–15.

31 Tessier P, Hemmy D. Three dimensional imaging in medicine. A critique by surgeons. *Scand J Plastic Reconstruct Surg*, 1986;20(3):11.

32 Herman GT. *Image reconstruction from projections*. New York: Academic Press; 1980:260–76.

33 Tonner HD, Engelbrecht H. Ein neues verfahren zur herstellung alloplastischer special implantate fur denn Becken-Teilersatz, Fortschr. *Medicine* 1979;97(16):781–3.

34 Burri C, Claes L, Gerngross H, Mathys JR. Total internal hemipelvectomy. *Arch Orthop Traum Surg* 1979;94:219–26.

35 Nerubay J, Rubinstein Z, Katznelson AM. Technique of building hemipelvic prosthesis using computer tomography. Proj. *Clini Biol Res* 1981;99, Alan R Liss, Inc, NY, 147–52.

36 Fujioka M, Yokoi S, Yasuda T, Toriwaki J. Computer aided interactive surgical simulation system—its clinical application. *CAR'89*, 1989;409–12.

37 Murphy SB, Kijewski PK, Walker PS, Scott RD. Computer-assisted pre operative planning of orthopedic reconstructive surgery. *CAR'85*, 413–18.

38 Murphy SB, Kijewski PK, Simon SR, Chandler HP, Griffin PP, Reilly DT, Penenberg BL, Landy MM. Computer-aided simulation, analysis and design in orthopedic surgery. *Orthop Clin N Am*, 1986;17(4):637–49.

39 Murphy SB, Kijewski PK, Millis MB, Harless A. Simulation of osteotomy surgery about the hip joint. *CAR'89*, 371.

40 Murphy SB, Kijewski PK, Simon SR, Millis MB. Simulation of orthopaedic reconstructive surgery. *CAR'87*, 411–15.

41 Murphy SB, Kijewski PK, Millis MB, Harless A. Simulation of osteotomy surgery about the hip joint. *CAR'89*, 371.

42 Woolson ST, Dev P, Fellingham LL, Vassiliadis A. Three dimensional imaging of bone from computerized tomography. *Clin Orthop Rel Res* 1986;202:239–48.

43 Giliberty RP, Epstein HY, Faegenburg D. A prototype femoral stem using CAT and CAD/CAM. *Orthop Rev* 1983;XII-8:59–63.

44 Bechtold JE. Application of computer graphics in the design of custom orthopedic implants. *Orthop Clin N Am* 1986;17(4):605–12.

45 Brand R, Petersen D. Computer modeling of surgery and a consideration of the mechanical effects of proximal femoral osteotomies. The hip, *Proceeding of the Twelfth Open Scientific Meeting of the Hip Society,* St Louis 1984;55.

46 Essinger JR, Rhodes ML, Robertson DD, Aubaniac JM. Computer assisted prostheses selection. *CAR'89* 1989;369–70.

47 Herman GT, Liu HK. Three dimensional display of human organs from computed tomograms. *Comp Graphics Image Process* 1978;9:1–21.

48 Herman GT, Udupa JK. Display of three dimensional digital images. Computational foundations and medical applications. *IEEE Comp Graphics Appl* 1983;3(5):39–45.

49 Nelson PC, Robertson DD, Walker PS, Granholm JW. A computerized femoral intramedullary implant design package utilizing computed tomography data. *CAR'S 93*, 419–23.

50 Rhodes ML, Kuo YM, Rothman SLG. Systems integration for the manufacturing of custom prostheses and anatomic models. *CAR'87*, 416–23.

51 Vannier MW, Marsh JL, Warren JO. Three dimensional CT reconstruction images for craniofacial surgical planning and evaluation. *Radiology* 1984;150:179–84.

52 Sutherland C. Practical application of computer-generated three dimensional reconstructions in orthopedic surgery. *Orthop Clin N Am* 1986;17(4):651–6.

53 Haralson H. Current concepts review computerized information retrieval and medical education for orthopaedists. *J Bone Joint Surg* 1988;70A(4):624–9.

54 Prodomos CC, Andriacchi TP, Galante JO. A relationship between gait and clinical changes following high tibial osteotomy. *J Bone Joint Surg* 1985;67A(8):1188–94.

55 Daruwalla JS, Balasubramaniam P. Moire topography in scoliosis—its accuracy in detecting the site and size of the curve. *J Bone Joint Surg* (Br) 1985;67(2):211–13.

56 Fleiter Th, Erdtmann B, Claussen CD. High resolution 3D-CT and its applications in stereolithographic computer assisted surgical and implant planning. *CAR'93* 1993;727–31.

57 Pho RWH, Lim SYE, Pereirq BP. Computer applications in orthopaedics. *Ann Acad Med* 1990;19(5):691–7.

58 Peltier LF. The classic: computer assisted surgery. Technology and clinical application. *Clin Orthop Rel Res* 1998;354:5–7.

59 Herman GT, Reynolds TA, Udupa JK. Computer techniques for the representation of three dimensional data on a two dimensional display. *Proc SPIE* 1983;367:3–14.

60 Latamore Gb. Creating 3-D models for medical research. *Comput Graphics World'* 1983;7:31–8.

61 Schlegel W, Scharfenberg H, Doll J, Pastyr O, Sturm V, Netzebend G, Lorenz W. CT images as the basis of operation planning in stereotactic neurosurgery. Proceedings of the first international symposium on medical imaging and image interpretation. ISMIIII '82, Berlin, Oct. 1982. S172–S177.

62 Udupa JK. Display of 3D information in discreet 3D scenes produced by computerized. *Proc IEE* 1983;71:420–31.

63 Vannier M, Totty W, Stevens W. Musculoskeletal applications of three dimensional surface reconstructions. *Orthop Clin North Am* 1985;16(3):543–55.

64 Pepino A, Mosca A, Cesarelli M, Di Salle F, Bracale M. CAD techniques for the preoperative planning of intertrochanteric osteotomies. *CAR'93*, 722–6.

65 Rhodes ML. An algorithmic approach to controlling search in 3-D image data, ACM Siggraph 79. *Proceeding'79*, 134–42.

66 Rhodes ML. Towards fast edge detection for clinical 3D applications of computer tomography. Special interest group on graphics. *Proceeding'79*, 134–42.

67 Rhodes ML, Azzawi YM, Chu E, Pang AT, Glenn WV, Rothman SLG. A network solution for structure models and custom prostheses manufacturing from CT data. *CAR'85*, 403–12.

68 Mittelstadt B, Kazanzides P, Iuhars J, *et al.* Robotic Surgery: Achieving predictable results in a unpredictable environment. In *Proceedings of the Sixth International Conference on Advanced Robotics*. Tokyo, 1993 Nov 1–2, 367–72.

69 Mittelstadt B, Kazanzides P, Zuhars J, Williamson B, Cain P, Smith F, Bargar WL. The evolution of a surgical robot from prototype to human clinical use. *First International Symposium Medical Robotics and Computer Assisted Surgery, MRCAS*, 1994 vol. 1, sessions I–III, 36–41. Pittsburgh, PA.

70 Paul HA, *et al.* A surgical robot for total hip replacement surgery. *Proceedings of the 1992 IEEE International Conference on Robotics and Automation.* 1992;606–11. Nice, France.

71 Bargar W, Bauer A, Borner M. Primary and revision total hip replacement using the Robodoc system. *Clin Orthop Rel Res* 1998;354:82–91.

72 Taylor RH, Brendt D, Mittelstadt BD, Paul H, Hanson W, Kazanzides P, Williamson B, Musits B, Glassman E, Bargar W. An image directed robotic system for precise orthopaedic surgery. In: Taylor, Lavallee, Burdea, Mosges, eds. *Computer integrated surgery, technology and clinical applications.* Cambridge: MIT Press Publishers; 1995:379–91.

73 Fadda M, Bertelli D, Martelli S, Marcacci M, *et al.* Computer assisted planning for total knee arthroplasty. *First Joint Conference of CVRMed and MRCAS'94*, 1997;1:619–28.

74 Martelli S, Beltrame F, Dario P, Fadda M. A system for computer and robot assisted knee implantation. *Proceedings of the 14th IEEE Medicine and Biology Conference*, 1992, Paris.

75 Martelli S, Fadda M, Dario P, Marcassi M, Visani AM. Analysis of the accuracy of a robotic procedure for knee arthroplasty. *Proceedings of the 6th Mediterranean Conference on Medical and Biological Engineering, Medicon.* Capri; 1992:477–80.

76 Marcacci M, Buda R, Zaffagnini S, Visani A, Iacono F, Neri MP. Press-fit vs. porous-coated knee prosthesis implant. Comparison of the results with a minimum follow-up of 3 years. *Transaction of the Second Annual Conference of the European Orthopaedic Research Society.* Varese, Italy, September 1992:154.

77 Pagetti C, Ciucci T, Papa E, Allota B, Dario P. A system for computer assisted arthroscopy. CVRMed-MRCAS'97, Springer Verlag; 1997:653–62.

78 Van Ham G, Denis K, Sloten JV, Audekercke RV, Van Der Perre G, De Schutter J, *et al.* Machining and accuracy studies for a tibial knee implant using a force controlled robot. *Comput Aided Surg* 1998;3:123–33.

79 Siebert W, Mai S, Lorke C. Motivation, realization and first results of robot assisted total knee arthroplasty. *1st Annual Meeting of the International Society for Computer Assisted Orthopaedic Surgery.* February 7–10, 2001;90. Davos, Switzerland.

80 Garbini JL, Kaiura RG, Sidles JA, Larson RV, Matsen FA. Robotic instrumentation in total knee arthoplasty. *33rd Annual Meeting, Orthopaedic Research Society.* 1987,19–22 January. San Francisco.

81 Kaiura RG. Robot assisted total knee arthroplasty investigation of the feasibility and accuracy of the robotic process. Master's Thesis, Mechanical Engineering, University of Washington, 1986.

82 Matsen FA, Garbini JL, Sidles JA. Robotic assistance in orthopaedic surgery. A proof of principle using distal femoral arthroplasty. *Clin Orthop Relat Res* 1993;296:178–86.

83 McEwen C, Bussani CR, Auchinleck GF, Breault MJ. Development and initial clinical evaluation of pre robotic and robotic retraction systems for surgery. Second *Annual International Symposium Custom Orthopaedic Prosthetics.* Chicago, 1989.

84 Poyet A, Troccaz J, Cinquin Ph. Controlling the position of a robotic guiding system using external redundant sensors. *MRCAS'94, 1st International Symposium on Medical Robotics and Computer Assisted Surgery.* 1994, vol. 1, sessions I–III, 90–7. Pittsburgh, PA.

85 Kienzle TC, Stulberg SD, Peshkin M, *et al.* A computer-assisted total knee replacement surgical system using a calibrated robot. Orthopaedics. In: Taylor RH *et al.* eds. *Computer integrated surgery.* Cambridge, MA: MIT Press; 1996:409–16.

86 Moctemuza JL, Gosse F, Schulz HJ. A computer and robotic aides surgery system for accomplishing osteotomies. *MRCAS, First International Symposium on Medical Robotics and Computer Assisted Surgery.* 1994, vol. 1, sessions I–III, 31–5 Pittsburgh, PA.

87 Moctemuza JL, Schuster D. A new surgery tool for robotic aided treatment delivery. *MRCAS*; 1995:304–11.

88 Davies BL, Ho SC, Hibberd RD. The use of force control in robot assisted knee surgery. MRCAS 94, September 1994;258–62, vol. 2, session VI, 22–24, Pittsburgh, PA.

89 Davies BL, Harriss J, Lin WJ, *et al.* Active compliance in robotic surgery—the use of force control as a dynamic constraint. *J Eng Med, Proc H Institut. Mech. Eng.* (UK) 1997;211:H 4.

90 Harris SJ, Jakope M, Hibberd RD, Cobb J, and Davies BL. Interactive pre-operative selection of cutting constraints and interactive force controlled knee surgery by a surgical robot, *MRCAS'94,* 1994 vol. 1, sessions I–III, 996–1006. Pittsburgh, PA.

91 Gotte H. A new less-invasive approach to knee surgery using a vision guided manipulator. *IARP Workshop on Medical Robotics.* 1996:99–107. Vienna, Austria.

92 Glozman D, Shoham M, Fischer A. Efficient registration of 3-D objects in robotic-assisted surgery. In: *Comp Assist Orthop Surg (CAOS/USA'99),* Pittsburgh, PA: UPMC Shadyside; 1999:248–52.

93 Kelly, PJ *et al.* Computer assisted stereofaxic laser resection of intra-axial brain neoplams *J. Neurosurg.* 1986; Mar; 427–39.

94 Ayache N. Medical computer vision, virtual reality and robotics. *Image Vis Comput* 1995;13(4):295–303.

95 Brown GA, *et al.* CT image-guided surgery in complex acetabular fractures and in percutaneous placement of iliosacral screws using view point system. *Proceeding of the Third North American Program on Computer Assisted Orthopaedic Surgery,* 1999;155–61.

96 Nikou C, Jaramaz B, DiGioia. Range and motion after total hip arthroplasty. *Proceedings of Medical Image Computing and Computer Assisted Intervention.* 1998;700–9. Springer.

97 DiGioia A, Jaramaz B, Nilou C, Labarca R, Moody JE, and Colgan B. Surgical navigation for total hip replacement with the use of Hipnav. Operative techniques in orthopaedics. *Med Robot Comp-Assist Orthop Surg* 2000;10(1):3–8.

98 Jaramaz B, DiGioia A, Blackwell M, Nikou C. Computer assisted measurement of cup placement in total hip replacement. *Clin Orthop Rel Res* 1998;354:70–81.

99 Woo RYG, Morrey BF. Dislocation after total hip arthroplasty. *J Bone Joint Surg* 1982;64A:1295–306.

100 Langlotz F, Bachler R, Berlemann U, Nolte LP, Ganz R. Computer assistance for pelvic osteotomies. *Clin Orthop Rel Res* 1998;354:92–102.

101 Joskowicz L, Taylor R, Williamson B, Kane R, Kalvin-McCarthy J, Turner R. Computer integrated revision total hip replacement surgery: preliminary report. *MRCAS'95,* 1995:1–10.

102 Kahler DE, Lyttle D. Surgical interruption of the patellar blood supply by total knee arthroplasty. *Clin Orthop* 1988;221–7, 229.

103 Tonetti J, Carret L, Lavallee S, *et al.* Ultrasound-based registration for percutaneous computer assisted pelvis surgery: application to iliosacral screwing of pelvis ring fractures. *CAR'97;*11:961–6.

104 Zura RD, Kahler DM. A transverse acetabular nonunion treated with computer assisted percutaneous internal fixation. *J Bone Joint Surg* 2000;82A(2):219–24.

105 Ellis RE, Tso CY, Rudan JF, Harrison MM. A surgical planning and guidance system for high tibial osteotomy. *Comput Aided Surg* 1999;4:264–74.

106 Picard F, Leitner F, Raoult O, Saragaglia D. Computer assisted knee replacement. Location of a rotational center of the knee. Total knee arthroplasty. *International Symposium on CAOS.* 2000 February 17–19, Davos.

107 Picard F, Moody J, Jaramaz B, DiGioia A, Nikou C, LaBarca S. A classification proposal for computer assisted knee systems. Medical image computing and computer assisted intervention. MICCAI, *3rd International conference.* 2000;1145–51. Pittsburgh, PA, USA: Springer Publishers.

108 Delp SL, DiGioia, AM, Jaramaz B. Surgical navigation for THR: A report on clinical trial utilizing hipnav *MICCAI 2000, Third International Conference* 2000:1185–1194. Pittsburgh, PA: Springer Verlag.

109 DiGioia A, Jaramaz B. Computer assisted tools and interventional technologies. *Lancet* 2000;354:46.

110 Cooke TDV, Pichora D. Knee displasia: an unusual but important problem associated with progressive arthritis. *J Bone Joint Surg* (Br) 1985;67:332.

111 Banks AZ, Klos TVS, Habets RJE, Banks SA, Devilee RJJ, Cook FF. Computer assistance in arthroscopic anterior cruciate ligament reconstruction. *Clin Orthop Rel Res* 1998;354:65–9.

112 Klos TVS, Banks AZ, Banks SA, *et al.* Computer and radiographic assisted anterior cruciate ligament reconstruction of the knee. In: Nolte LP, Ganz R, eds. *Computer assisted orthopaedic surgery.* Hogrefe and Huber Publishers, 1999;184–9.

113 Julliard R, Lavallee S, Dessenne V. Computer assisted reconstruction of the anterior cruciate ligament. *Clin Orthop Rel Res* 1998;354:57–64.

114 Delp SL, Stulberg SD, Davies B, Picard F, Leitner F. Computer assisted knee replacement. *Clin Orthop Relat Res* 1998;354:49–56.

115 Leitner F, Picard F, Minfelde R, *et al.* Computer-assisted knee surgical total replacement. *First Joint Conference of CVRMed and MRCAS.* Grenoble, France: Springer; 1997:629–38.

116 Stulberg SD, Picard F, Saragaglia D. Computer assisted total knee arthroplasty. Operative techniques. In: *Orthopaedics* 2000;10(1):25–39.

117 Krackow K, Serpe L, Phillips MJ, *et al*. A new technique for determining proper mechanical axis alignment during total knee arthroplasty. *Orthopedics* 1999;22(7):698–701.

118 Fleute M, Lavallee S, Julliard R. Incorporating a statiscally-based shape model into a system for computer-assisted anterior cruciate ligament surgery. In: *Medical image analysis*, Vol.3 Oxford: Oxford University Press; 1999;209–22.

119 Kuntz M, Sati M, Nolte LP, *et al*. Computer assisted total knee arthroplasty. *International symposium on CAOS;* 2000, February 17–19, Davos.

120 Radermacher K, Staudte HW, Rau G. Computer assisted orthopaedic surgery with image-based individual templates. *Clin Orthop Rel Res* 1998;354:28–38.

121 Troccaz J. Man–machine interfaces in computer augmented surgery. In: Nolte LP, Ganz R, eds. *Computer assisted orthopaedic surgery*. Hogrefe and Huber Publishers; 1999:53–68.

122 Otoole RV, Playter RR. Virtual reality surgical simulators and trainers. *Proceedings of the Third Annual North American Program on Computer Assisted Orthopaedic Surgery*. 1999;60–1. Pittsburgh.

123 Bowersox JC. Telesurgery: transitioning from development in clinical applications. *Proceedings of Third Annual North American Program on Computer Assisted Orthopaedic Surgery*, 1999;237–8.

124 Blackwell M, Morgan F, DiGioia AM. Augmented reality and its future in orthopaedics. *Clin Orthop* 1998;354:111–22.

125 Nikou C, DiGioia A, Blackwell M, Jaramaz B, Kanade T. Augmented reality imaging technology for orthopaedic surgery. *Oper Tech Orthop*, 2000;10(1):82–6.

Chapter 2

Rationale for hip reconstructive CAOS

2.1 Issues of conventional hip reconstruction and their influence on short- and long-term outcomes

Sorin Blendea, Anthony M. DiGioia III, and Branislav Jaramaz

Recent advances in hip arthroplasty, including minimally invasive techniques, partial resurfacing, robotics and surgical navigation, need a rigorous and continuous evaluation. The increased accuracy and safety and reduced soft tissue trauma should improve the wear, stability, and functional results. To study the possible benefits of these new technologies, it is important to identify the existing challenges for total hip arthroplasty (THA).

The indications and the techniques in hip surgery changed and evolved in close interaction with technologic improvements and general social developments. Total hip replacement is an option for nearly all patients with diseases of the hip that causes chronic discomfort and functional impairment The indications for total hip replacement include patients exhibiting joint deterioration form several causes, including degenerative disease, rheumatoid arthritis, ankylosing spondilytis, avascular necrosis, post-infectious and post-surgical ankylosis, hip tumors, and hip and pelvic trauma. The main reason for performing hip replacement is to **relieve pain and disability**, when conservative treatment is failing to do so. In relative terms, arthroplasty is one of the most successful procedures in modern orthopedic surgery. However, many authors agree that research has to be done to extend the long-term durability of prosthetic joints, particularly in young and active patients. 'The challenge comes when patients between 45 and 50 years of age are to be considered for the operation, because then every advance in technical detail must be used if there is to be a reasonable chance of 20 or more years of trouble-free activity (Charnley)'.[1] Today, as mentioned by Galante,[2] 'although it is very reasonable to think in terms of 15-year lifetimes, it becomes more difficult to predict survivorship for longer periods, particularly if the patient is young and active.' The outcomes after total hip replacement can be influenced by many factors related to the surgical technique, the design of the implant or patient-related factors. Hip **stability and wear** remain important issues in hip arthroplasty.

2.1.1 Stability

Dislocation following THA remains a problem.[4] The prevalence of dislocation after total hip arthroplasty varies in different studies from 0.3% to 10% or more. Large series report prevalence rates of 2% to 3%.[3] However, more recent reports suggest that prevalence may have increased, because of 'multiple factors', like early discharge, use of modular components, and different methods of fixation.[4] The prevalence of dislocation increases after revision THA. Etienne reported 10% in a study of 530 revisions, using standard acetabular liner.[4] Some controversy exists when defining the 'early' dislocation; the first three postoperative months, for most of the authors, or the first five weeks after intervention, according to others.[5] Late dislocation should be, according to Berry,[3] related to trauma or chronic changes around the hip (laxities, decrease muscle strength, wear). Several authors attempted to identify these factors as either surgery-related factors, patient-related (clinical factors), or implant design-related factors. Just a few of them were shown to be statistically significant in the recent literature.

Instability following THA is correlated to implant alignment. Morrey[6] and others consider cup orientation as a 'critical variable', related to instability. Their studies show that a retroverted orientation predisposes to posterior instability, but excessively anteverted cup favors anterior dislocation. More recent studies[7,8] question the relationship between cup orientation and dislocation. In a matched-pair analysis,[7] there was no association between either acetabular version or abduction angle and the risk of dislocation. However, Jolles[9] recently found that dislocation risk was 6.9% higher if total anteversion was not between 40° and 60°. Ranawat[10] established a goal of achieving a good implant positioning in terms of total anteversion, recommending 25° to 45° for primary THA. Studies show also that nonunion of trochanteric osteotomy or abductor muscle malfunction caused by superior gluteal nerve injury have been associated with higher rate of dislocation.[11] The surgeon's experience is also related to the rate of dislocation, especially in Swedish studies. Hedlundh[20] reported after analysis of 4230 primary THAs that twice the number of dislocations occurred for inexperienced surgeons, compared to experienced ones. The frequency of dislocations leveled off after 30 surgeries; for every 10 primary THAs performed annually, the risk of dislocation decreased by 50%. The surgical approach also seems to influence the dislocation rates, but as with implant's orientation, authors have divergent opinions. This aspect is detailed in the next chapter.

Age over 80 years was found by Eklund[21] to be associated with a three times bigger risk of dislocation. However, Woo and Morrey[22] and Paterno[7] suggested that age does not seem to be a major risk factor for dislocation. In a recent multivariate analysis, Jolles *et al.*[9] show that the dislocation risk was 10 times higher in patients with high ASA (American Society of Anesthesiologists) scores. They considered the ASA scores to be a good variable because it is related closely to multisystem disease, increasing with age and complicating muscle recovery. Some studies also established correlations of the neuromuscular conditions, contributing to weakness in muscles, or contracture around the hip with hip dislocation.[23] Previous hip surgery, particularly a previous arthroplasty, markedly increases the incidence of instability.[22] Patients treated with THA for a diagnosis of hip fracture seem to be at high risk.[24] Despite an important number of patient-related risk factors that were more or less related to dislocation, only previous hip surgery, advanced age, and ASA scores were statistically significant risk factors.[26]

The introduction of modular implants has brought some solutions and possibly new problems for THA dislocations. The size of the head has been theoretically suspected to play a role in dislocation. In a report of Hedlundh[27] there was no difference in the rate of dislocation between the 22-mm Charnley prosthesis (2.5%) and the 32-mm Lubinus prosthesis (2.4%) at 1 year. In the same study there was however a higher rate of recurrent dislocation (2.3 times) for the 22-mm head. A more recent prospective, randomized study[28] conducted by Kelley, found that a modular 22-mm head had a significantly higher rate of dislocation than a modular 28-mm head. The authors also found an important correlation between the outer size of the cup (cementless) and dislocation. Acetabular components of 60 mm and higher increased the risk of dislocation, using a 28-mm modular femoral head, compared to cups 58 mm and smaller. The same correlation was found when using 22-mm heads and 54-mm and larger acetabular components. Other authors, like D'Lima, suggest that the head diameter shouldn't be taken into account as an isolated factor.[29] According to his study, the most important factor for the range of motion is the ratio between the head diameter and the cone diameter, called the 'head-neck ratio' (HNR). The surgeons should consider that a diminished HNR will conduct to a reduced range of motion, so to a more increased risk of dislocation. Another factor, often mentioned in the literature, is the stem's neck offset, being specific to the implant design. Modularity is used not only for the stem, but also for the acetabular component, with liners designed to cover different operative needs. Elevated rim liners (10°, 20°) have been produced to provide more stability to the prosthetic hip, preventing from dislocation, both first time and recurrent.[25]

2.1.2 Prosthetic wear

The key long-term problem in total hip replacement surgery was found to be wear and periprosthetic osteolysis.[30] Wear is affected by many factors, including design and material properties of the implants, the biological response to particles, and finally, the kinematics of the prosthetic joint. Some authors found some clinical issues of patient selectivity and activity, as an important factor of enhanced wear.[31]

The surgical technique, less studied than other issues in the context of wear and survival, has also its importance Some studies have proven the relationship between alignment of the cup and polyethylene wear.[6,32] An inclination angle greater than 50° appears to increase polyethylene wear and subsequent pelvic osteolysis. Anatomic restoration of the hip center of rotation and offset has been reported to decrease the progression of wear. Yamaguchi *et al.* have shown a relationship between increased impingement with excessive cup anteversion, small head-neck ratio, and increased linear wear rate.[33] Inadequate cementing technique has been reported to correlate with increased wear. An incomplete cement mantle around the cup, as well as unsatisfactory cementing for the femoral component, can result in increased wear and osteolysis. Other studies[31] suggest that debris generated in vivo from loose acetabular and femoral components can enter the space between femoral head and acetabular polyethylene, enhancing wear. The factors and mechanisms influencing wear are detailed in the Section 2.4, dedicated to biological aspects of the THA.

Many of these factors that influence the short-term and long-term outcomes are surgery and implant-related. The navigation and robotic tools will possibly contribute to improving postoperative results, by influencing the overall surgical accuracy and the implant selection.

References

1 Charnley J, Cupic Z. The nine and ten year results of low friction arthroplasty of the hip. *Clin Orthop* 1973;95:9.

2 Galante JO. Overview of total hip arthroplasty. In: Callaghan JJ, Rosenberg AG, Rubash HE, eds. *The adult hip*. Philadelphia: Lippincott-Raven Publishers; 1998.

3 Berry D. Unstable total hip arthroplasty: detailed overview. In: AAOS Instructional Course Lectures, vol. 50, 2001.

4 Etienne A, Cupic Z, Charnley J. Postoperative dislocation after Charnley low-friction arthroplasty. *Clin Orthop* 1978;132:19–23.

5 Joshi A, Lee CM, Markovic L, Vlatis G, Murphy J. Prognosis of dislocation after total hip arthroplasty. *J Arthroplasty*, 1998;13(1):17–21.

6 Morrey BF. Difficult complications after hip joint replacement. Dislocation. *Clin Orthop Rel Res* 1997;334:179–87.

7 Paterno SA, Lachiewicz PF, Kelly SS. The influence of patient-related factors and position of the acetabular component on the rate of dislocation after total hip replacement. *J Bone Joint Surg Am* 1997;79:1202.

8 Pollard JA, Daum WJ, Uchida T. Can simple radiographs be predictive of total hip dislocation? *J Arthroplasty* 1995;10:800–804.

9 Jolles BM, Zangger P, Leyvraz PF. Factors predisposing to dislocation after primary total hip arthroplasty. A multivariate analysis. *J Arthroplasty* 2002;17(3):282–88.

10 Ranawat CS, Maynard MJ, Deshmukh RG. Cemented primary total hip arthroplasty. In: Sledge C, ed. *Master techniques in orthopedic surgery: the hip*. Philadelphia: Lippincott-Raven; 1998.

11 Lachiewicz PF. Dislocation. In: Pelicci PM, Tria AJ, Garvin KL, eds. *Orthopedic knowledge update, 2 hip and knee reconstruction AAOS*, 2000.

20 Hedlundh U, Ahnfelt L, Hybinette CH, Weckstrom J, Fredin H. Surgical experience related to dislocation after total hip arthroplasty. *J Bone Joint Surg* 1996;78B:206–9.

21 Eklund A, Rydell N, Nilsson OS. Total hip arthroplasty in patients 80 years of age and older. *Clin Orthop* 1992;281:101.

22 Woo RYG, Morrey BF. Dislocations after total hip arthroplasty. *J Bone Joint Surg* 1982;64A:1295–1306.

23 Harkess JW. Arthroplasty of hip. In: Canale S, ed. *Campbell's operative orthopedics*, 9th edn. St. Louis: Mosby publisher; 1998.

24 Lee BP, Berry DJ, Harmsen WS, Sim FH. Total hip arthroplasty for the treatment of an acute fracture of the femoral neck: long-term results. *J Bone Joint Surg Am* 1998;80:70–75.

25 Cobb TK, Morrey BF, Ilstrup DM. The elevated–rim acetabular liner in total hip arthroplasty: relationship to postoperative dislocation. *J Bone Joint Surg* 1996;78A:80–6.

26 Gebhard JS, Amstutz HC, Zinar DM, Dorey RJ. A comparison of total hip arthroplasty for treatment of acute fractures of the femoral neck. *Clin Orthop* 1992;282:123–31.

27 Hedlundh U, Ahnfelt L, Hybinette CH, Wallinder L, Weckstrom J, Fredin H. Dislocation and the femoral head size in primary total hip arthroplasty. *Clin Orthop* 1996;333:226–33.

28 Kelley SS, Lachiewicz PF, Hickman JM, Paterno SM. Relationship of femoral head and acetabular size to the prevalence of dislocation. *Clin Orthop* 1998;355:163–70.

29 D'Lima DD, Urquart AG, Buehler KO, Walker RH, Colwell CW. The effect of orientation of the acetabular and femoral components on the range of motion of the hip at different head-neck ratios. *J Bone Joint Surg* 2000;82A(3):315–21.

30 Harris WH. Wear and periprosthetic osteolysis. The problem. *Clin Orthop* 2001;393:66–70.

31 Schmalzried TP, Callaghan JJ. Current concepts review: wear in total hip and knee replacements. *J Bone Joint Surg Am* 1999;81:115–36.

32 Kennedy JG, Rogers WB, Soffee KE, *et al*. Effect of acetabular component orientation on recurrent dislocation, pelvic osteolysis, polyethylene wear and component migration. *J Arthroplasty* 1998;13:530–34.

33 Yamaguchi M, Akisue T, Bauer TW, *et al*. The spatial location of impingement in total hip arthroplasty. *J Arthroplasty* 2000;15:305–313.

2.2 Classical surgical approaches for hip reconstruction: invasiveness, accuracy, and safety issues

Sorin Blendea and Anthony M. DiGioia III

Surgical approaches for total hip arthroplasty are an issue of actuality. As they became smaller and possibly less invasive, the new approaches are compared in the literature to the classic ones. Surgical approaches in hip surgery, in particular for reconstructive surgery, are chosen in close relation to the exposure required, quality of soft tissue (i.e., presence of scars), co-morbidity and of course, the surgeon's experience. The commonly used basic surgical approaches are the anterior, antero-lateral, direct lateral, and posterior.

The **anterior** exposure dissects the interval between the sartorius, rectus femoris and the tensor fascia lata, gluteus minimus, and medius muscles. The visualization of the superior portion of the hip and acetabulum allows open reduction of hip dysplasia, arthrotomy, arthrodesis, and fracture treatment. On one hand, it permits an excellent visualization of anterior acetabular column and wall pathology, but on the other, it offers less access to posterior acetabular column. In the **anterolateral approach**, the interval between gluteus medius and tensor fascia lata muscles is dissected. The approach can be used to perform fracture reduction, biopsy, or arthrotomy. During the exposure, the structure at risk is the superior gluteal neurovascular bundle. When it is damaged, the function of the tensor could be seriously compromised. The **direct lateral approach** can provide good exposure to the anterior hip and proximal femur. It is successfully used to perform arthrotomy, arthrodesis, arthroplasty, and revision hip surgery. It uses a dissection plane between the anterior hip abductors, the anterior third of the gluteus minimus and medius, reflected together with the anterior vastus lateralis, allowing the exposure of the anterior hip capsule. Disadvantages include limited proximal acetabular exposure, increased risk of heterotopic ossification, and slower abductor rehabilitation. The **posterolateral approach** offers a good visualization of the posterior capsule, posterior column, and acetabulum. The exposure includes splitting of the gluteus maximus, release of short external rotators and posterior capsulotomy. Some surgeons perform complete posterior capsulectomy, without reattachment of the rotators. Advantages of this procedure include preserving the abductor muscles and also relatively easy exposure, with lower heterotopic ossification rates. Important benefit is in the capsular and external rotators repair, resulting in significantly reduced dislocation rates.

In 1982, Woo and Morrey published their study on 10,500 THAs, finding a risk of dislocation of 4.3% for posterior approach, three times higher than 1.7% for anterior and 1.9% for the lateral approaches.[1] In the 1960s, Charnley always recommended that his LFA (Low-Friction Arthroplasty) should be performed by a transtrochanteric approach, with the argument of the large exposure being offered. The adopters of low-friction arthroplasty (LFA) continued to use this osteotomy, despite the high rate of nonunion of the greater trochanter. When comparing transtrochanteric approach to the Hardinge approach, Horwitz *et al.*[2] found no significant difference for range of motion, 8% trochanteric nonunion with the first one and more heterotopic ossification with the Hardinge approach. Hedlundh *et al.*[3] found in their study of 3199 LFAs four times more early dislocations using the posterior approach, than the transtrochanteric one. Mid-term dislocation rates were, however, very similar (3.3% and 3.4%). Li *et al.*[4] found 5.6% early dislocation using a posterolateral (Moore) approach and only 0.6% after a transtrochanteric one. However, the conclusion of the study was that, despite the decreased dislocation rate obtained with trochanteric osteotomy, this approach had to be abandoned because of the 6.2% nonunion rate. Simultaneously, the dislocation rate with posterolateral approach was diminishing with increasing surgeon's experience.

There are other factors that surgeons take into account when analyzing the surgical approach. The opponents of Hardinge and modified Hardinge approaches often invocate the risk of injury of the superior gluteal nerve. Another issue, observed by Webb et al.,[5] was the quality of the femoral implant positioning and cementing, related to the surgical approach. He confirmed that the Moore approach offered a better placement of the stem and better cementing than the anterolateral approach. Some of the reasons are the direct and relatively easy access to the joint and possibly diminished operating time.

The surgical technique in THA is a complex and controversial topic. Despite its richness on this subject, the literature offers no 'best' approach, with many of the authors trying to justify and scientifically argue their choice. For that reason, surgeons generally agree that the 'best' approach is the one the operator can perform successfully.

References

1 Woo RYG, Morrey BF. Dislocation after total hip arthroplasty. *J Bone Joint Surg* 1982;64-A:1295.

2 Horwitz BR, Rockowitz NL, Goll SR. A prospective randomized comparison of two surgical approaches to total hip arthroplasty. *Clin Orthop* 1993;291:154–63.

3 Hedlundh U, Hybinette CH, Fredin N. Influence of surgical approach on dislocations after Charnley hip arthroplasty. *J Arthroplasty* 1995;10(5):609–14.

4 Li E, Meding JB, Ritter M, Keating EM, Faris PM. The natural history of a posteriorly dislocated total hip replacement. *J Arthroplasty* 1995;10(6):800–4.

5 Webb JCJ, Bannister GC. Comparison of femoral component position in posterior and lateral approaches to the hip. Bristol, England: Annual European Hip Meeting; 2000.

2.3 Less and minimally invasive approaches to the hip: clinical challenges

Anthony M. DiGioia III and Sorin Blendea

During the last several years, minimally invasive surgery has influenced the techniques used in most surgical specialities. This development has not only led to the replacement of conventional procedures with minimally invasive ones, but has also stimulated surgeons to reevaluate conventional approaches with regard to perioperative parameters such as pain medication or recovery time.

There are, however, drawbacks that emerged with the introduction of these new techniques, like prolonged learning curves, increased cost due to the investment in the required equipment and the use of disposable instruments, as well as longer operating times. There is special concern about the **accuracy** of implant positioning and possible additional complications when using less and minimally invasive surgical (L/MIS) approaches. Obviously, performing hip or total knee replacement through 8–10 cm incisions is a more challenging task than the wide conventional approaches. The surgeons have to perform precise bone cuts and correctly align acetabular, femoral or tibial components, in a smaller workspace, and without the usual landmarks. Clinical research has also focused on the topic of expanding the indications for minimally invasive approaches in the elderly and in high-risk patients, to take advantage of the shorter hospital stays and reduced surgical trauma. A considerable amount of basic research has been carried out on the stress response during and after minimally invasive procedures. In hip surgery, mini-incision techniques were used mainly for percutaneous fracture fixation, after closed reduction. Some surgeons perform minimally invasive techniques for the osteoid osteoma excision under CT-scan guidance and others perform a similar technique using hip arthroscopy as guidance.[1]

More recently, successful removal of a femoral neck osteoma was reported by Eid *et al.*, using a minimally invasive technique and CT-based navigation.[2]

Conventional hip arthroplasty is typically performed through 15–30 cm incisions, required for complete visualization of the acetabulum and proximal femur. Correct orientation of the prosthetic components is obtained by identifying anatomical landmarks. Wide surgical exposure is generally necessary to achieve the goals of direct and good visualization of the soft tissue and bony structures involved. These exposures are particularly wide for revision cases. However, the extent of soft tissue trauma during surgery is directly correlated to a number of postoperative conditions. Recovery time has been found by some authors to be lengthy. Knutsson reported increased levels of pain and discomfort at 6 weeks after surgery.[3] Blood loss is also expected to correlate to the extent of surgical exposure. Perioperative complications in arthroplasty, including wound infections, hematoma, but also myocardial ischemia, respiratory failure and thromboembolic disease, occur more often in patients who required allogenic blood transfusion.[4,5] Another issue, related to the exposure extent is the heterotopic ossification. The etiology is multifactorial, and some of the important predisposing factors reported in the literature include soft tissue dissections, operative approach, and haematoma formation.[6]

Recent efforts to limit these large exposures in total hip arthroplasty are mostly done by either using posterior approaches or combined anterior and lateral (two incisions). Early results of minimally invasive hip replacement were reported by Crocket *et al.*[7] at the 1998 Annual Meeting of the American Academy of Orthopedic Surgeons. In a retrospective review the authors compared a group of forty-two patients using the minimally invasive posterior approach to a control group of conventional posterior approaches. There was no difference in operative time or complications between small and standard incision groups. The average incision length was 8.7 cm, ranging from 5.5 to 10.0 cm. Also, there was no reported postoperative misalignment on the X rays. The incision was centered over the greater trochanter, with two thirds of it distal to the tip of the trochanter and one third extending proximally. Retractors were modified, to permit the use of the incision as a 'mobile window', during the procedure.

Chimento and Sculco[8] reported a review of 1000 patients, operated with the same minimally invasive, modified posterior approach. In this series, candidates were patients with a Body Mass Index less than 30, who had not had a previous hip surgery. The external rotators with the exception of quadratus and posterior capsule, were released form the femur in a trapezoidal fashion and repaired at the end, by attachment to the greater trochanter. Two cases of neuropraxia occurred, both from direct injury of the sciatic nerve with a retractor. Dislocation rate was 1.2%, with 0.1% revision for recurrent instability. There were reported no early failures or considerable loosening at 5 years. The authors, however, recommended that 'each surgeon should use an incision that provides adequate exposure and enables him or her to perform the operation well.'

The two-incision technique uses an anterior approach passing between the sartorius muscle and tensor fascia lata and a posterior incision for the femoral stem.[9] It does not incise any muscle or tendon, but is technically challenging and requires intra-operative fluoroscopy. The overall alignment and fit were considered excellent, but there was one femoral fracture in a group of 100 patients.[9] The use of intra-operative fluoroscopy was necessary, but there is no mention of radiation dose and time. Even more than in the previously mentioned posterior approach, the authors stress that the technique 'is extremely challenging' and it should 'only be attempted with special designed instruments'. However, the authors outlined the very fast recovery times and the reduced postoperative pain.

Information about the actual anatomic data and real-time instrument's position **without a direct visual exposure** is currently available with instrument tracking and surgical navigation techniques. In a recent study, DiGioia *et al.*[2] used a hip navigation system to perform minimally invasive hip replacement. This was a prospective study, comparing a mini-incision technique and traditional posterior approach for total hip arthroplasty (THA). The author started the first mini-incision cases in 1998. To evaluate the outcome, thirty-three patients that had undergone a mini-incision THA were matched by diagnosis, sex, average age, and preoperative Harris Hip Score (HHS) to thirty-three patients that had undergone THA using a traditional posterior approach. Evaluations by an independent observer were performed preoperatively and at three, six and twelve months postoperatively. The surgical technique was a modified Moore approach, using a skin incision of two-thirds proximal and one-third distal to the tip of greater trochanter. The position of the hip was in 70° of flexion, for an optimal use of the 'mobile skin window'. Standard retractors were used during surgery. The posterior structures were repaired at the end, including short external rotators and a posterior capsule. The average length of the incision in the mini-incision group was 11.7 cm (range 7.3–13 cm). There was no difference in the average surgical time between the two groups. At three months, the HHS increased by an average of 34 points in the mini-incision group and by 27 points in the control group, a difference which was statistically significant. At 6 months, the difference was again significant, but at one year there was no more significant difference in the HHS between groups. Blood loss was significantly lower in the mini-incision group, compared to the traditional incision group. There was no heterotopic ossification, reported at one-year interval.

References

1 Khapchik V, O'Donnell RJ, Glick JM. Arthroscopically assisted excision of osteoid osteoma involving the hip. *Arthroscopy* 2001;17(1):56–61.

2 Blendea S, Eid A, Martinez T, Huberson C, Merloz P. The interest of computer-assisted surgery in the excision of osteoid osteoma. About a CT-based and fluoroscopy-based navigation in two patients. Presented at CAOS Meeting Pittsburgh, 2001.

3 Knutsson S, Endberg S. An evaluation of patient's quality of life, 6 weeks and 6 months after total hip replacement surgery. *J Adv Nursing* 1999;30:1349.

4 Bierbaum B, Hill C, Callaghan J, Galante J, Rubash H, Tooms R, Welch R. An analysis of blood management on patients having a total hip or knee arthroplasty. *J Bone Joint Surg* 1999;81A:2.

5 Borghi B, Casati A. Incidence and risk factors for allogenic blood transfusion during major joint replacement using an integrated autotransfusion regimen. *Eur J Anesthesiol* 2000;17:411.

6 Ahrengart L, Lindgren U. Heterotopic bone after hip arthroplasty: defining the patients at risk. *Clin Orthop* 1993;293:153.

7 Crockett HC, Wright JM, Bates JE, Bonner KF, Delgado SJ, Sculco TP. Mini-incision for total hip arthroplasty. New Orleans, LA: American Academy of Orthopedic Surgeons, Annual Meeting, 1998.

8 Chimento GF, Sculco TP. Minimally invasive total hip arthroplasty. *Oper techniq Orthop* 2001;11(4):270–3.

9 Berger RA. Two-incision total hip replacement: when and when not indicated. *70th Annual Meeting Proceedings*. New Orleans: AAOS, 2003, p. 113.

2.4 **Biological approach to total hip arthroplasty**

Sorin Blendea, Branislav Jaramaz, and Anthony M. DiGioia III

The last 10 years have brought a change of strategy in the orthopaedic research, with the revival of basic molecular biology research, offering in turn better understanding of disease mechanisms and healing. The main areas involved are bone regeneration, articular cartilage, and soft tissue repair. Terms like tissue engineering, cytokines, growth factors and stem cells are now becoming a part of the orthopedic surgeon's vocabulary. Currently, the directions of basic science research in joint reconstruction are cartilage regeneration, biological mechanisms of wear and biologic fixation of implants.

Factors that are determinant and others that influence these mechanisms are extensively treated in the literature. However, direct correlations between surgery-related issues and biological mechanisms are much less discussed. The principal areas of biological research regarding hip reconstruction are mechanisms of wear and periprosthetic osteolysis in hip replacement. One of the consensuses in literature concerning this area is that the wear of the polyethylene and its resulting osteolysis represent the dominant long-term problem in total hip replacement surgery. Molecular biology studies brought the answers to many unsolved problems and corrected some previous misinterpretations.

The incidence of periprosthetic osteolysis is considered in most 10 years studies to be more important than sepsis, fatal pulmonary embolization, dislocation, and other complications. The metallic, polymeric, and ceramic particles resulting from prosthetic wear are not biodegradable. They can be the stimulus for foreign body and inflammatory reactions, resulting in the production and release of inflammation mediators. These enzymes, cytokines, and other substances will eventually lead to periprosthetic osteolysis and finally to decreased stability of the implants. The effects of wear debris on macrophage and monocyte cell lines have been studied extensively. Recent studies have also shown that osteoblasts are involved in the phagocytosis of wear debris and contribute to the progression of the osteolysis. A recent study, by Vermes *et al.*,[1] pointed out that metallic particulate debris affect osteoblast functions in two ways: a direct negative effect on cellular function and an effect mediated by cytokines. Osteoblasts stimulated by particulate debris produced interleukin-6 and prostaglandin E2, leading to stimulation of osteoclast function. The addition of exogenous growth factors to the cell cultures reversed the suppressive effect of titanium particles on procollagen alpha-1 mRNA. This opens the way to an eventual pharmacologic treatment or prevention of osteolysis. Andersson showed a negative effect on osteoblast function, when the cells were exposed to synovial fluid from hips presenting aseptic loosening of implants and undergoing revision surgery.[2]

Synovial fluid can penetrate sites that are distant to the actual joint cavity and can redistribute the debris particles to other periprosthetic regions. Schmalzried *et al.* evidenced this mechanism,[3] by observing that zones of osteolysis, associated with particle-induced inflammation, occur in regions that are in contact with the synovial fluid containing the wear debris. Studies done until now suggest that these biological mechanisms are initiated by debris particles, followed by inflammatory cell accumulation, particle-cell interaction, and liberation of cytokines and enzymes. In the end the bone is responding by its own mechanisms to granulomatous inflammation and finally generating osteolysis.

It was already determined and discussed in Section 2.1 that surgery-related factors, like implant position or size, can affect the wear and osteolysis. What is even more difficult to establish is whether patients have different capacities to respond to implant wear and what are the factors contributing to that. Some studies suggest that individual immune or genetic factors can lead to differentiated response to wear debris. For example, individuals with rheumatoid arthritis have shown important immune granulomatous reactions, important lymphocyte infiltration being observed.[4] But, even these individual factors seem to be influenced by the implant design and surgical techniques associated with the implant fixation and biomechanics of the reconstructed joint.[5,6] Creating accurate models of osteolysis would possibly lead in the future to improvements in surgical techniques, to better design implants, and open the door for reliable pharmacologic and immunologic modulation of host response.

Concerning the clinical applications of cartilage regeneration, mentioned earlier, the knee is at the center of attention mainly because of the relatively easy access and the progress of arthroscopy. These aspects will be detailed in the Section 3.4. Despite recent advances, hip arthroscopy remains much more challenging than knee arthroscopy, and much less used routinely. Anatomically, the femoral head is deeply recessed in the bony acetabulum and is convex in shape, unlike the more planar surface of the knee. Volumetric distension of the hip joint is more difficult than in the knee and the relative proximity of the sciatic nerve, lateral femoral cutaneous nerve, and vascular structures, introduces more risks.[7]

References

1 Vermes C, Chandrasekaran R, Jacobs JJ, Galante JO, Roebuck KA, Glant TT. The effects of particulate wear debris, cytokines, and growth factors on the functions of MG-63 osteoblasts. *J Bone Joint Surg Am* 2001;83:201–11.

2 Anderson MK, Anissian L, Stark A, Bucht E, Fellander-Tsai L, Tsai JA. Synovial fluid from loose hip arthroplasties inhibits human osteoblasts. *Clin Orthop* 2000;378:148–54.

3 Schamalzried TP, Kwong LM, Jasty MJ, *et al*. The mechanisms of loosening of cemented acetabular components in total hip arthroplasty. *Clin Orthop* 1992;274:60–78.

4 Goldring SR, Wojno WC, Schiller AL, Scott RD. In patients with rheumatoid arthritis the tissue reaction associated with loosened total knee replacements exhibits features of rheumatoid synovium. *J Orthop Rheum* 1988;1:9–21.

5 Schamalzried TP, Guttman D, Grecula M, Amstutz HC. The relationship between the design, position and articular wear of acetabular components inserted without cement and the development of pelvic osteolysis. *J Bone Joint Surg Am* 1994;76:677–88.

6 Zicat B, Engh CA, Gokcen E. Patterns of osteolysis around total hip components inserted with and without cement. *J Bone Joint Surg Am* 1995;77:432–9.

7 Dvorak M, Duncan CP, Day B. Arthroscopic anatomy of the hip. *Arthroscopy* 1990;6:264–73.

Chapter 3

Rationale for knee reconstructive CAOS

3.1 Introduction: Computer assisted surgery in knee arthroplasty

Frederic Picard, Anthony M. DiGioia III, and Branislav Jaramaz

Since the 1970s, when prosthetic knee surgery truly began to develop, progress in this field has increased steadily. The aging of the population, coupled with technological improvements naturally led to an increase in the number of prosthetic implants.[1]

Around 10–15% of all prostheses require at length surgical revision at some point.[1,2] The increasingly strict controls on the costs of each surgical operation, the functional requirements of patients, and the pressure by insurance companies to 'guarantee the results of these operations', have led surgeons and health organizations to pay greater attention to the overall quality of the results. It is estimated that in 1997, from 1 to 2.5% of the gross domestic product of the United States, Canada, Great Britain, France and Australia was allocated to the treatment of musculo-skeletal problems![3]

Whatever the prosthetic model implanted, certain factors must be controlled to ensure an optimal anatomical and functional result. The main success factors are the careful selection of patients and their post-surgery follow-up, the appropriate choice of the material implanted, and the quality of the placement of the prosthetic device. Among these factors, two in particular must be well mastered during the surgical operation: carrying out bone cuts and the ligament balance of the knee. These two requirements of prosthetic knee surgery influence, in an extremely important way, the functional results in the short term and the survival of implants.

In spite of the improvements in mechanical instrumentation used to carry out these acts, bone cuts and ligament balance still remain largely dependent on the knowledge and experience of the operating surgeon.[4] However, even the most experienced professionals recognize their limits, but also the weaknesses of implant instrumentation.[5,6]

One of the remaining difficulties is that of regularly carrying out the bone cuts in a best possible way. Typically, during a TKR operation seven different cut orientations have to be managed: five for the femur, one for the tibia, and one for the patella (which is a lot in comparison with the low number of cuts carried out in prosthetic hip surgery). Although modern instrumentation allows cutting several parts of the bone with the same guide (for example the anterior and posterior sides of the femur) thus limiting the grossest errors, difficulties of orienting the implant remain. As the literature on the subject points out,[7,8] these difficulties concern as much the frontal/sagittal plane as the transversal plane (implant rotation).

The second difficulty is the ligament balance. All surgeons practicing prosthetic knee surgery know how delicate it is to obtain this balance, even with experience.[9,10] The improved understanding of the physiopathology of the prostheticized knee has led manufacturers to increase the complexity and the quantity of instrumentation. This is advantageous neither for the patient (for potential liberation of metallic particles during manipulation of the instrumentation), nor for society (instrumentation costs).

In order to prevent peri-operative errors, numerous authors have insisted on radiological planning of these operations. In spite of this, incorrect placement of the implant occurs daily. The main reasons for these errors are the lack of precision in the radiological angles and the difficulty of using radiographically defined reference points during the operation. These reference points end up being problematical either because they are located deep within the patient's anatomy (for example the coxofemoral joint) or because they are inconsistent and unreliable (for example the knee landmarks).

Vince[11] has shown that the majority of prosthetic loosenings occur in varus implanted knees. Bargren[2] observed a failure rate of 67% for varus implanted knees as opposed to 29% for those implanted in a neutral position. Ritter[12] has shown a shorter survival curve for knee prostheses that are not well oriented or well balanced in comparison with prostheses that are 'well oriented'. Feng and Stulberg[4] have compared the survival period of correctly oriented ($\pm 5°$) prostheses to those varus-oriented or excessively valgus-oriented, and they observed shorter survival for prostheses that were poorly oriented.

We have reviewed the majority of radiological results reported in the bibliography between 1975 and 1995, of all prostheses taken together and we have found that the mean frontal femoro-tibial angle has been estimated at 181.3° (i.e., 1.3° in valgus), with a standard deviation of 3.3°.[13] The mean alignment of all these prostheses is quite acceptable. This can partially explain why, on the whole, the results of prosthetic knee surgery are satisfying and that, for example,[3] the number of prosthetic knee replacements in the United States is greater than that of hip replacements. But most frequently these reports concern series from centers specialized in knee surgery. However, many of these surgeries (80%) are carried out by orthopedic surgeons who are not hyperspecialists in the field and who implant no more than twenty prostheses per year.[6] A recent study carried out in Canada found rates of revision ranging from 4.2% to 8%, which would correspond to between 10,000 or 20,000 prostheses per year.[1]

The majority of studies thus confirm what Insall[14] had written in 1976: 'the majority of failures can be attributed to poor ligamentary balance or incorrect alignment'. Laskin[15] confirmed in 1989 that: 'the number or radiological signs of loosening is greater in unaligned prostheses than in aligned prostheses and the difference is statistically significant'.

These results explain the necessity of increasing the precision and the regularity of means of control. Hungerford[16] wrote: 'after all, what is most important in prosthetic knee surgery are the brain and the human eye'. We now know that the machines, thanks to progress in computerization, have, in numerous fields, gone beyond what man is capable of with regard to measurement techniques and the objectivity of the results. Now, the improvements that can be made today as regards prosthetic knee replacement concern more the optimization of the technique than the implants themselves.

We must, therefore, take advantage of technological evolution in order to evaluate more objectively the surgical results of our patients. It is this impartial analysis that will allow us to identify clearly the problems and, no doubt, to solve them.

There are numerous advantages to using a computerized system for the placement of knee prostheses. We will not dwell on the interest of planning which is one advantage of it that has been developed in the other chapters. Simulation is also an extraordinary tool, only in its infancy in the field of orthopedic surgery. It is possible, as of today, to simulate the impact of an operation on tendons and muscles. It is also possible to analyze, by models of completed elements, the forces generated on the implants. We can imagine that, in the near future, it will be possible to simulate completely a surgical operation and its consequences on bones, ligaments, muscles, functioning, and therefore, to optimize all the criteria in order to obtain an ideal result.

Above all, these computerized systems allow using the totality of this information directly during the surgical operation, avoiding a priori any hesitation by the surgeon. This interactive control of the surgical act certainly increases the chances of the success of the implant. Finally, this technology creates new research and teaching tools which will modify our grasp of the remaining uncertain sectors of orthopedics and will result in reflection on the new goals to be reached in this knee surgery.

References

1 Coyte PC. Revision knee replacement in Ontario, Canada. *J Bone J Surg* 1999; 81A, n°6.

2 Bargren JH, Blaha JD, Freeman MAR. Alignment in total knee arthroplasty: correlated biomechanical and clinical observations. *Clin Orthop* 1983;173:178–83.

3 Ayers DC, Dennis DA, Johanson NA, *et al.* Common complications of total knee arthroplasty. *J Bone J Surg* 1997;2(79A):278–311.

4 Feng EL, Stulberg SD, Wixson RL. Progressive subluxation and polyethylene wear in total knee replacements with flat articular surfaces. *Clin Orthop Relat Res* 1994;299:60–71.

5 Freeman MAR, Mac Leod HC, Levai JP. Cementless fixation of prosthetic components in total arthroplasty of the hip and knee. *Clin Orthop* 1983;176:88–94.

6 Laskin RS. Alignment of the total knee components. *Orthopaedics* 1984;7:62.

7 Berger RA, Crosset LS, Jacobs JJ. Malrotation causing patellofemoral complications after total knee arthroplasty. *Clin Orthop Relat Res* 1998;356:144–53.

8 Dejour H, Deschamps G. Technique opératoire de la prothèse totale à glissement du genou. Les prothèses totales du genou. *Cahier d'Enseignement de la SOFCOT* n°35 1989;13–24.

9 Dejour H, Neyret Ph. Les gonarthroses. *7è Journée Lyonnaise de Chirurgie du genou* 1994; 97–114.

10 Krackow K, Serpe L, Phillips MJ, *et al.* A new technique for determining proper mechanical axis alignment during total knee arthroplasty. *Orthopedics* 1999;22(7):698–701.

11 Vince KG, Insall JN, Kelly MA. The total condylar prosthesis. 10 to 12 year results of a cemented knee replacement. *J Bone Joint Surg* 1989;71B:93–797.

12 Ritter MA, Faris PM, Keating EM, Meding JB. Post-operative alignment of total knee replacement. Its effect on survival. *Clin Orthop* 1994;299:153–6.

13 Picard F, Leitner F, Saragaglia D, Cinquin P. Mise en place d'une prothèse totale du genou assistée par ordinateur. A propos de 7 implantations sur cadavre. *Rev Chir Orthop* 1997;83(Suppl. II):31.

14 Insall JN, Ranawat CS, Aglietti P, Shine J. A comparison of four models of total knee replacement prostheses. *J Bone Joint Surg* 1976;58A:754–65.

15 Laskin RS, Turtel A. The use of an intramedullary tibial alignment guide in total knee replacement arthroplasty. *Am J Knee Surg* 1989;2:123.

16 Hungerford DS, Kenna RV. Preliminary experience with a total knee prosthesis with porous coating used without cement. *Clin Orthop* 1990;255:215–27.

3.2 Conventional surgical approaches for the knee reconstruction

Sorin Blendea, Anthony M. DiGioia III, and Branislav Jaramaz

In the past 10 years, the surgical approaches to knee reconstruction have been continually modified with increasing focus on improving recovery, less trauma to the soft tissues, and better ligament balancing.

3.2.1 Total knee replacement

Total knee replacement is usually performed through a midline incision. It offers a good access to either side of the joint, without affecting the skin flaps. Generally, it is recommended to keep these skin flaps as minimal as possible, to avoid skin necrosis. The skin incision is most important for the integrity of the skin flaps. Some authors suggest that making the incision with the knee in flexion allows the subcutaneous tissue to fall medially and laterally, improving the exposure. If required, the incision can be extended proximally or distally, as far as necessary. The approach to the knee joint itself is determined more by the arthrotomy incision. It can be done on the medial or lateral side of the patella. Generally, the incision is made over the midline, using a median parapatellar approach. The approach is carried on through the quadriceps in its tendinous portion, around the medial border of the patella and continued down, along the patellar tendon. A small rim of tendon is left attached to the vastus medialis for the closure. The synovium is then opened and patella is everted, if sufficiently released proximally (see Fig. 3.1).

The major drawback of the parapatellar approach is that once the quadriceps tendon is incised there will be possibly a certain degree of weakening of the extensor mechanism.

To avoid interfering with the extensor mechanism, Engh described the technique of midvastus arthrotomy.[1] In this approach, the dissection separates the vastus medialis muscle in the direction of it's fibers, beginning at the superior pole of the patella. In a retrospective study[2] there were compared the medial

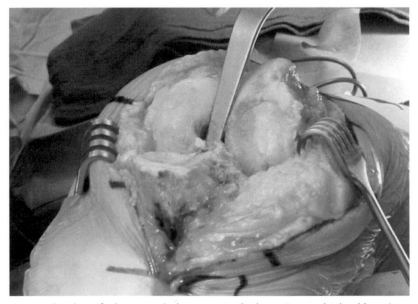

Fig. 3.1 Intra-operative view of a large surgical eposure to the knee. It was obtained by using a classic medial parapatellar approach.

parapatellar arthrotomy and the midvastus splitting arthrotomy. Lateral retinacular release of the patella was done in 50% of the parapatellar approaches and in just 3% of the midvastus. Another report[1] showed a quicker return of quadriceps muscle control and a more stable patello-femoral articulation.

Another technique, which tries to avoid damaging the quadriceps tendon, is the subvastus medialis approach. It is generally done on patients who are thin and have fairly loose tissues.[3] The inferior incision along the patellar tendon is the same as for the parapatellar approach, but when reaching the inferior border of the vastus medialis the incision is moved medially and superiorly parallel to the border of the fibers.

Other less used approaches for special indications include lateral parapatellar arthritomy for genu valgum, quadriceps snip,[4] V–Y turndown quadriceps-plasty or extended tibial tubercle osteotomy.

3.2.2 Partial knee replacement

Early failures of unicompartmental implants have been secondary to less accurate technical technique and poor design of the prosthetic components. Recent progress in both surgical approaches and design led to promising results in well-selected patients. For the unicondylar implants a longitudinal is performed, just medial to the midline of the patella. The arthrotomy is medial parapatellar, without damaging the vastus medialis, allowing the eversion of the patella. The coronary ligament is incised on the affected side, but leaving it intact on the other side. Alternatively, some surgeons recommended a lateral parapatellar incision for a valgus deformity and lateral compartment arthritis.[5] After carefully removing the osteophytes, the affected compartment (medial or lateral) is resurfaced. Implant positioning is vital for the postoperative outcomes and wear rates. It was shown that many failures of unicompartmental replacement are caused by *components malpositioning, **attributable to poor instrumentation**.*[6]

Isolated patello-femoral arthritis occurs in approximately 10% of cases. In some of these cases associated with severe pain and limitation of daily activities, isolated patello-femoral arthroplasty can be considered.[7] This arthroplasty is the resurfacing of the patella and the femoral groove. The approach generally used is a medial parapatellar with lateral eversion of the patella. Lateral release it is also performed during surgery. A major technical pitfall is again, **the lack of instrument guidance**, especially while performing the femoral groove plasty, this being done in a 'free-hand' manner.

Conventional surgical techniques for knee reconstruction require large surgical exposures and extensive soft tissue dissection to visualize, access, and prepare the bone surfaces. Despite important advances, surgeons and researchers still lack accurate measurement tools, to assess the actual orientation of the implants, both intra- and postoperatively. Less and minimally invasive surgery (L/MIS) for knee reconstruction is an important development that promises significant changes in partial and total knee replacement.

References

1 Engh GA, Parks NL. Surgical technique of midvastus arthrotomy. *Clin Orthop* 1998;351:270–4.

2 Engh GA, Parks NL, Ammeen DJ. Influence of surgical approach on the lateral retinacular release in total knee arthroplasty. *Clin Orthop* 1996;331:56–63.

3 Jordan C, Mirzabeigi E (eds.). The knee; anterior approach. In: *Atlas of orthopedic surgical exposures.* New York: Thieme; 2000:137–9.

4 Garvin KL, Scuderi G, Insall JN. Evolution of the quadriceps snip. *Clin Orthop* 1995;321:131–7.

5 Keblish PA. Valgus deformity in total knee replacement: the lateral retinacular approach. *Orthop Trans* 1985;9:28.

6 Laskin RS. Unicompartmental knee replacement; some unanswered questions. *Clin Orthop* 2001;392:267–71.

7 Argenson JN, Guillaume JM, Aubaniac JM. Is there a place for patellofemoral Arthroplasty. *Clin Orthop* 1995;321:162–7.

3.3 **Less invasive surgical approaches for the knee reconstruction**

Sorin Blendea, Branislav Jaramaz, and Anthony M. DiGioia III

3.3.1 **Introduction**

Joint reconstructive surgery is experiencing new and important developments. Less and minimally invasive techniques for knee replacement have been recently described. Eventually, this would lead to the improvement of patient outcomes and possible long-term cost reduction of the treatment. However, there are also drawbacks that have emerged with the introduction of these new techniques such as the prolonged learning curve, increased cost of equipment and disposable instruments, and longer operating times. There is a special concern about the accuracy of implant positioning and the possible additional complications when using smaller approaches. Performing total knee replacement through 8–10 cm incisions is a more challenging task than wide conventional approaches (see Fig. 3.2).

3.3.2 **Partial knee reconstruction**

The development of less invasive surgical approaches took first place in the field of unicompartmental knee replacement. Repicci described a minimally invasive technique for unicondylar replacement, in selected individuals.[1] The surgical technique involves a limited medial parapatellar incision that was reported to reduce peri-operative morbidity and bone preparation techniques that emphasize preservation of bone for future arthroplasty procedures. A 3-inch incision is required for bone preparation and implant insertion and the patella is not dislocated, avoiding the suprapatellar pouch which reduces morbidity.[2] The major advantages reported were avoiding normal tissue sacrifice (opposite compartment, patellar bone, and cruciate ligaments), and decreasing morbidity (no patellofemoral disruption). It was done as an outpatient procedure in 80% of cases; since postoperative physical therapy is minimal or unnecessary, recovery time was shorter (90% independent function at 2 weeks after operation). With this type of surgical approach there was reported a 7% failure rate, at 8-year follow-up.[3] Similar to other minimally invasive procedures, the authors mention the improved results through learning and the need for adapted instrumentation. In a recent symposium,[2] the future role of computer guidance was outlined as a future option for minimally invasive unicompartmental arthroplasty.

(a)

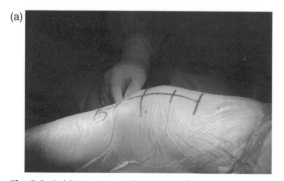

(b)

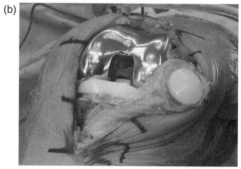

Fig. 3.2 (a,b) Intra-operative views of a wide classic exposure for total knee replacement. Using this common type of implant by much smaller incisions can be challenging.

3.3.3 **Total knee replacement**

Less invasive techniques for total knee replacement were developed recently by a number of authors, but only a few preliminary reports are available. The technique developed by Bonutti uses a 6–10 cm anterior incision, two times the patellar length.[4] It's driving force is reported to be the limited soft tissue damage, and reduced quadriceps exposure. A vastus medialis snip is done and the patella is retracted laterally, but not everted. The author shows that the increase in quadriceps stress, with retraction of patella is 8.7% compared to 16.7% length stress, with a classic patellar eversion. To enhance knee distraction, the leg is hanging over the edge of the table, in an arthroscopic knee holder. In a 2-year follow-up of 210 mini-incision total knee arthroplasties (TKA), the author mentioned no revision, loosening, or catastrophic failures. However, this was an early report and no detailed information about results and complications was available.

Tria[5] uses a similar technique to the unicondylar minimally invasive approach. The arthrotomy is performed in line with the skin incision. The author outlined that the true MIS surgery for the knee does not violate the quadriceps mechanism in any way. The patellar surface is removed first, to allow more space in the knee joint. An intramedullary guide is used for the femur and an extramedullary guide for the tibia. The trial reduction and final cementing of the components is done in the order: tibia first, patella second, and the femur at the end. Patients are discharged on the first or second postoperative day. Preliminary data on 60 minimally invasive total knee replacements show a 9 months longest follow-up. The range of motion was 20 degrees greater than a matched cohort and the blood loss was one half of the standard procedure. There were reported, however, one peroneal nerve neuropraxia, but no infections or wound compromise.

Although promising these data represent very early results. Further prospective, controlled studies are required to validate the techniques. Performing precise bone cuts and correctly aligning implants within a smaller workspace, is not an easy task, even for experienced surgeons. The proof is represented by difficult learning curves, reported by authors and in some cases, extended operative times.

References

1 Repicci JA, Eberle RW. Minimally invasive surgical technique for unicondylar knee arthroplasty. *J South Orthop Assoc* 1999;8(1):20–7.

2 Repicci JA. Mini-incision unicompartmental arthroplasty. Evolution to less invasive approach. *AAOS 70th Annual Meeting Proceedings*, New Orleans; 2003;4:35.

3 Romanowski MR, Repicci JA. Minimally invasive unicondylar arthroplasty. Eight-year follow-up. *J Knee Surg* 2002;15:17–22.

4 Bonutti PM. Total knee arthroplasty minimally invasive approach. 70th Annual *Meeting Proceedings*. New Orleans: AAOS; 2003:127.

5 Tria AJ. MIS TKR: Is it feasible? *70th Annual Meeting Proceedings* 2003:36. New Orleans: AAOS: 2.

3.4 **Biological issues of cartilage repair and new challenges for knee regenerative surgery**

Sorin Blendea, Branislav Jaramaz, and Anthony M. DiGioia III

3.4.1 **Introduction**

As mentioned earlier in the book (Section 2.4), a great deal of basic science research is oriented towards the biological mechanisms of prosthetic wear and implant fixation. Hence, this section will focus mostly on issues regarding knee cartilage regeneration. The knee joint is the center of interest for clinical applications of cartilage regeneration, mainly because of the relatively easy access and the advances in arthroscopic knee surgery. The articular cartilage is a unique biological structure and although a number of substitutes have been developed for the treatment of cartilage defects, none has integrally replaced normal chondral tissue. Articular cartilage defects that are symptomatic and refractory to nonoperative treatment represent a clinical challenge. The surgical goal is to replace these defects with cartilage-like substitutes, to provide pain relief, reduce inflammation, restore function, and postpone the need for prosthetic replacement.

3.4.2 **Natural cartilage repair**

The cartilage injury outcome is affected by the extent, depth and location of the damaged area. Generally, injury only to the matrix components, not to the chondrocytes, has the potential of a new matrix synthesis and to restore normal proprieties. Articular cartilage is isolated from the marrow cells by a dense subchondral bone and has no access to its vascular supply. Therefore, lesions of chondrocytes and matrix but without penetrating the subchondral bone have very little capacity to heal.[1] Larger osteochondral defects are often filled with fibrocartilage, formed mainly by collagen I, sometimes collagen II. Mechanically, the new reparative tissue is structurally different and less durable than cartilage. Growth factors like transforming growth factors (TGFs) or bone morphogenic proteins (BMPs) influence articular cartilage regeneration by regulating cell migration, proliferation and matrix synthesis. Sellers[2] investigated the effect of rhBMP-2 on the healing of full thickness osteochondral defects in rabbits. At 24 weeks, the thickness of the healing cartilage was 70% of the normal adjacent cartilage.

3.4.3 **Surgical options**

Articular lavage and arthroscopic debridement are considered palliative options, providing temporary relief of the symptoms. This is believed to be due to the removal of cartilage debris, proteolytic enzymes, inflammatory mediators.[3]

Repair stimulation, by drilling, abrasion arthroplasty or microfracture,[4] could potentially induce migration of high concentration repair cells into the defects. The usual result of these techniques is partial filling of the defect with fibrocartilage, that contains mostly type I collagen with poor biomechanical characteristics.

Cell and tissue transplantation techniques require living cells or tissues containing living cells. These biological structures may be implanted in the defect and need to remain viable and replicate and also synthesize the matrix. It was shown that both autologous chondrocytes and undifferentiated mesenchymal cells placed in articular cartilage defects survive and are capable of producing a new matrix.[5] The autologous chondrocyte implantation technique preserves the subchondral bone plate. In a retrospective study[6] there were evaluated clinical, arthroscopic and histological results in 101 patients who underwent autologous cultured chondrocyte transplantation. There were observed good or excellent results in 92% of isolated lesions, 65% of patellar lesions, and 67% of multiple lesions.

Osteochondral plugs can be used to treat large, untreated lesions, created in weight-bearing surfaces of the medial femoral condyles. Osteochondral allografts are another surgical option big articular cartilage defects, underlying bone. Best results were observed in single, well-demarcated, full-thickness osteochondral defects that are 2–5 cm in diameter.[7]

3.4.4 Integrating modern imaging and navigation tools

There are justified hopes that more reliable cartilage repair techniques will soon be available. The biologics advances and existing microsurgical techniques would eventually be combined with modern guiding technologies, to add more accuracy to present techniques. Better understanding of knee MRI with precise mapping of cartilage defects could lead to development of new minimally invasive, image-guided techniques for cartilage repair. Biologic resurfacing of the knee joint is probably today's goal of many research labs. Computer-assisted technologies could play an important role in making this technically possible.

References

1 Goldberg VM, Caplan AI. Biologic restoration of articular surfaces. *Instr Course Lect* 1999;48:623–7.

2 Sellers LS, Peluso D, Morris EA. The effect of recombinant human bone morphogenetic protein-2 (rhBMP-2) on the healing of full-thickness defects of articular cartilage. *J Bone Joint Surg Am* 1997;79:1452–63.

3 Hubbard MJ. Articular debridement versus washout for degeneration of the medial femoral condyle. *J Bone Joint Surg Br* 1996;78:217–9.

4 Steadman JR, Rodkey WG, Singleton SB, Briggs KK. Microfracture technique for full-thickness chondral defects: technique and clinical results. *Oper Tech Orthop* 1997;7:300–4.

5 Buckwalter JA, Lohmander S. Operative treatment of osteoarthrosis: current practice and future development. *J Bone Joint Surg Am* 1994;76:1405–18.

6 Peterson L, Minas T, Brittberg M, Nilsson A, Sjogren-Jansson E, Lindhal A. Two to nine-year outcome after autologous chondrocyte transplantation of the knee. *Clin Orthop* 2000;374:212–34.

7 Garret JC. Osteochondral allografts for reconstruction of articular defects of the knee. *Instr Course Lect* 1998;47:517–22.

Chapter 4

Clinical classification of CAOS systems

F. Picard, James E. Moody, Anthony M. DiGioia III, and
Branislav Jaramaz

Emerging CAS systems for the hip and for the knee already include multiple applications in adult
reconstruction and trauma surgery. Following an extensive survey of the literature regarding the classifications of computer-assisted systems, we have set out a general scheme to classify computer-assisted
hip and knee systems currently in use or under development. In order to explain the computer-assisted
surgery concepts in simple terms, we chose a classification scheme that relies upon clinical, instead of
solely technical (localizer properties, computer specifics, . . .) criteria. We believe that new concepts in
computer-assisted hip and knee surgery will easily fit into this classification framework.

Several classifications for computer-assisted orthopaedic systems have been tentatively established in
the literature depending on the state of the art at the time. Below is an overview of the main classification
schemes from the recent past:

4.1 Stulberg's classification (1995)

David Stulberg[1] classified computer-assisted orthopaedic systems according to (1) surgeon/patient
interaction and (2) the type of function the system is able to perform. In the first approach, and
depending on the degree of robot involvement in the surgical action with respect to surgeon's role, two
types were defined:

(1a) Active or 'surgeon-replacing' systems are those in which the robot itself performs the final action,
such as machining the bone to accept an implant or drilling screw holes.

(1b) Passive or 'surgeon-assisting' systems utilize the robot as a measuring device or an aid in accurately
directing the surgeon. The surgeon is the final performer of the surgical action. This differentiation
between active and passive systems was important with respect to safety considerations.

The second classification involves positioning versus machining systems:

In a positioning system, the robot might be used to identify the exact location of a resection or
a drill hole or to indicate the placement of implants.

In a machining system, the robot might shape a cavity or make multiple resections of the bone. The
distinction entails an important technical difference between higher accuracy and geometric complexity
of machining devices in comparison with positioning systems. This classification of computer-assisted
orthopaedic systems did not differentiate between robotic and navigation systems. But back in 1995,
computer-assisted ACL reconstruction systems and most of the computer-assisted orthopaedic systems
in use or under development were robotics assistive based.[2,3]

4.2 Cinquin's classification (1995)

Taking into account new developments in robotics and computer-assisted surgery, Cinquin[4] introduced an additional category between passive and active computer-assisted systems called semi-active

computer-assisted systems. However, navigation and robotic systems were still not differentiated. Three categories were defined:

1) *Active systems* are capable of performing individual tasks autonomously.

2) *Semi-active systems* physically constrain the surgical action to follow a predefined strategy.

3) *Passive systems* perform no action independently, but provide the surgeon with additional information before and during a procedure.

Semi-active systems, for example, directly control a saw during a resection, but may limit the depth of cut. Most systems in this category restrict a task within a predetermined envelope. In other words, they enforce constraints specified in the preoperative plan.

This classification was very practical and easy to use, but it did not differentiate robotic assistive technology from navigation technology, the two being really quite different from each other in terms of usability.

In 1998, DiGioia[5] extended Cinquin's classification with additional subclasses of passive systems: navigators and aiming devices. Navigators are image guided systems which address the missing link between image information, accessible anatomy, and the action of surgical instruments by combining imaging with position sensing techniques. Aiming devices provide the surgeon with not only a map but also a set of directions to follow to arrive at the desired destination.

4.3 **Taylor's classification (1998)**

Taylor *et al.*[6,7] clearly differentiated navigation technology from robotics assistive technology in their classification:

1) *Intern replacement.* systems primarily focused on assistive tasks such as instrument holding, limb positioning.

2) *Navigational aids.* 'many of the most promising applications of "robotic technology" to surgery do not involve the use of a moving robot. The goal is simply to provide the surgeon with accurate positional feedback about location of surgical instruments relative to the patient's anatomy'.

3) *Precise positioning systems.* passive devices may be used with (or without) navigational aids to achieve precise alignment of surgical instruments with a desired target position on the patient's anatomy; active robot devices have some obvious advantages for these purposes.

4) *Precise path systems.* the use of robots in applications that require bone to be machined accurately to a desired shape.

This classification defines the different computer-assisted systems with respect to functionality. However, certain concepts developed since then could fit into several categories.

4.4 **Delp's classification (1998)**

Scott Delp[8] divided computer-assisted knee technology into three categories:

1) *Computer integrated instruments.* Integrating mechanical instruments with highly accurate measurement equipment can significantly enhance their capabilities.

2) *Image guided replacement.* Based on a preoperative plan, three-dimensional computer models of the patient's femur and tibia are constructed from computed tomography (CT) data.

3) *Robot assisted knee replacement.* Utilization of robots for performing surgical tasks.

This classification took into account functional considerations, in particular with respect to surgeon/patient interaction and to system function. However, some new concepts include both image guidance as well as computer integrated instruments.

4.5 **Troccaz's classification (1999)**

Somewhat later, Troccaz[9] extended the concept of passive systems for applications other than those used in orthopaedic surgery. She defined passive systems as systems allowing comparisons between the planned and executed strategy. With the navigator, the surgeon sees the location of the tip of a tool on a pre-operative image (computer-aided bronchoscopy was given as an example). Aiming systems require a predefined strategy to be followed. To guide the surgeon intra-operatively, three crosses are displayed on a screen.

4.6 **Bainville's classification (1999)**

According to the technological improvements, navigation technology generated multiple types of registration processes. Bainville *et al.*[10] made a classification based on technical (registration) considerations:

1) Point registration using a 3D localizer (paired points)

2) Surface registration using a 3D localizer

3) Surface registration using a range imaging sensor

4) Surface registration using 2.5D ultrasound images

5) 2D/3D registration using calibrated X-ray images acquired with a C-arm

6) 2D/3D registration using video images

7) Registration using individual templates

This classification was very clear but limited to the registration aspect and too technical for explaining different systems from a functional point of view.

4.7 **Nolte's classification (1999)**

Nolte[11] differentiates navigation from robotic technology in orthopaedic surgery, and introduced the notion of preoperative and intraoperative models:

1) Navigation systems based on preoperatively acquired three-dimensional tomographic data sets.

2) Navigation systems based on intra-operative images (fluoroscopy, ultrasound, and endoscopy).

3) Navigation systems based on 'surgeon-defined anatomy'.

4.8 **Vannier's classification (1999)**

Vannier recognizes three major categories of surgical robots:

1) *Autonomous*, which perform fixed functions that involve precise movements and planning, like drilling through a bone.

2) *Telemanipulators*, that mimic and refine a surgeon's hand movements, whether the physician is in the OR or at a remote location.

3) *Microbots*, tiny experimental devices that perform tasks like delivering drugs within the body.

Table 4.1 CAOS systems classification

	Preop. image	Intra-op. image	Image free
Active robotic	*	–	–
Semi-active robotic	*	–	–
Passive (SNS)	*	*	*

* systems in use – systems in not use

This classification was theoretically applicable for all different computer-assisted systems and not only orthopaedic systems. There is currently no system in CAOS in the second and the third categories.

In 2000, we proposed a classification for computer-assisted knee systems that we extended to all CAOS systems.[12] Several reasons motivated us to modify the current classifications: (1) there is a number of CAOS systems available based on different principles; (2) insufficient understanding of CAOS systems by most orthopaedic surgeons; and (3) the necessity to explain in simple and practical terms the differences between the systems.

Recognizing that the surgical navigation systems incorporate many of the same technical components included in the robotics systems, we adopted Cinquin's classification that distinguishes the systems based on how active is the robotic component, and added the other dimension that classifies the systems based on the type of medical images used. The resulting classification is a matrix presented in Table 4.1.

1. Active robotic systems perform some surgical task, such as drilling or milling, without the direct intervention of the surgeon.[13–23] This group in CAOS includes active robots like RoboDoc, CASPAR (described in this book), etc.

2. Semi-active robotic systems are not autonomous and they increase the surgeon's control of the tool. Such a system may, for example, not directly control a saw during a resection, but may limit the depth of cut. The systems in this category can act to enforce constraints by restricting a task within a predetermined envelope[24–26] or they can mimic the surgeon's hand motion, scaling and filtering it in the process (telesurgery). The important characteristic is that the control is shared between the robotic tool and the surgeon, increasing both the flexibility and adaptability of the tool and the accuracy and precision of surgical action.

3. Passive the surgical procedures support the procedure, but no part of surgery is overtaken by a machine, and the surgeon is in full control of the surgical action at all times. The most frequent examples of these systems are surgical navigation systems. The 'individual templates' introduced by Radermacher[27] also fall into this category. Although the template needs to be in contact with the patient, this is a mechanical instrumentation in addition to the traditional instrumentation and the surgeon uses it in the same way as traditional mechanical guides.

With respect to how the information is acquired and used in planning and when the reference system and surgical plan is defined, we divide the systems into the following three groups:

1. *Preoperative image systems* rely on models generated preoperatively, usually from large 3D data sets (CT or MRI). They can provide a wealth of detailed information, and typically include a preoperative planning system.[6,28–30]

2. *Intra-operative image systems* rely on intra-operative data collection to develop anatomical reference models. For example, a set of coordinated fluoroscopic images generated during the surgical procedure can be used to construct a frame of reference and define the surgical plan.[31,32]

3. *Image-free systems* derive all model information required for the task from direct measurements of the bone surface (using, for instance, a tracked probe), or from direct measurement of limb kinematics (e.g., computing rotational centers from relative bone movement).[2,12,33–36]

4.9 Discussion

Not all the possibilities in this categorization matrix are currently realized, but they should not be ruled out. Future computer-assisted systems will certainly cross the categorization boundaries by combining different features of navigation systems and robotic technology, or by mixing and combining preoperative and intra-operative images.

References

1 Stulberg SD, Picard F, Saragaglia D. Computer assisted total knee arthroplasty. Operative techniques. *Orthopaedics* 2000;10(1):25–39.

2 Dessenne V, Lavallee S, Julliard R, *et al*. Computer assisted knee anterior cruciate ligament reconstruction: first clinical tests. *J Image Guided Surg* 1995;1:59–64.

3 Stulberg SD, Kienzle TC. In: Taylor, Lavallee, Burdea, Mosges, eds. *Computer integrated surgery, technology and clinical applications*. Cambridge: MIT Press Publishers, 1995;374–8.

4 Cinquin P. Gestes médico-chirurgicaux assistés par ordinateur. *Société d'Edition de l'Association d'Enseignement Médical des Hôpitaux de Paris* 1993;63:386–405.

5 DiGioia A, Jaramaz B, Blackwell M, *et al*. Image guided navigation system to measure intraoperatively acetabular implant alignment. *Clin Orthop Relat Res* 1998;355:8–22.

6 Taylor RH. Robotics in orthopedic surgery. In: Nolte LP and Ganz R, eds. *Computer assisted orthopaedic surgery (CAOS)* 1998;35–41. Hogrefe and Huber Publishers.

7 Troccaz J. Man-machine interfaces in computer augmented surgery. In: Nolte LP, Ganz R, eds. *Computer assisted orthopaedic surgery*. Hogrefe and Huber Publishers, 1999;53–68.

8 Delp SL, Stulberg SD, Davies B, Picard F, Leitner F. Computer assisted knee replacement. *Clin Orthop Relat Res* 1998;354:49–56.

9 Tso CY, Ellis RE, Rudan J, *et al*. A surgical planning and guidance system for high tibial osteotomies. In: *Proceedings Medical Image Computing and Computer–Assisted Intervention-* MICCAI 1998;39–50.

10 Bainville E, Bricault I, Cinquin P, Lavallee S. Concepts and methods of registration for computer integrated surgery. In: *Computer Assisted Orthopedic Surgery (CAOS)*, Part I. Nolte LP, Ganz R, eds. Bern: Hogrefe and Huber Publishers, 1999;15–34.

11 Paul HA. Surgical robot for total hip replacement surgery. *Proceedings IEEE International Conference on Robotics and Automation* 1992;Nice, France, 606–11.

12 Picard F, Moody J, Jaramaz B, DiGioia A, Nikou C, LaBarca S. A classification proposal for computer assisted knee systems. Medical Image Computing and computer assisted intervention. MICCAI 2000, 3rd International conference. Pittsburgh, PA, USA: *Springer Publishers,* 2000;1145–51.

13 Bargar W, Bauer A, Borner M. Primary and revision total hip replacement using the Robodoc system. *Clin Orthop* 1998;354:82–91.

14 Bauer A. Robot assisted total hip replacement in primary and revision cases. Techniques. *Orthopaedics,* 2000;10(1):9–13.

15 Fadda M, Bertelli D, Martelli S, Marcacci M, *et al*. Computer assisted planning for total knee arthroplasty. In: *First Joint Conference of CVRMed and MRCAS*. Grenoble, France: Springer, 1997: 619–28.

16 Glozman D, Shoham M, Fischer A. Efficient registration of 3-D objects in robotic-assisted surgery. In: DiGioia, ed. *Proceedings CAOS/USA*, UPMC Shadyside Medical Center, 1999: 248–52.

17 Gotte H, Roth M, Brack CH, *et al.* A new less-invasive approach to knee surgery using a vision-guided manipulator. *IARP Workshop on Medical Robotics*, 1996; Oct, 99–106. Vienna (Austria).

18 Kober R, Meister D. Total knee replacement using the Caspar-system. Computer assisted total knee arthroplasty. In: *International Symposium on CAOS*. 2000 February, 17–19. Davos.

19 Martelli S, Beltrame F, Dario P, Fadda M. A system for computer and robot assisted knee implantation. *Proceedings of the 14th IEEE Medicine and Biology Conference*, 1992. Paris.

20 Peterman J, Kober R, Heinze, *et al.* Computer assisted planning and robot assisted surgery in the reconstruction of the anterior cruciate ligament. Operative techniques. *Orthopaedics* 2000;10(1):50–5.

21 Picard F, Leitner F, Raoult O, Saragaglia D. Computer assisted knee replacement. Location of a rotational center of the knee. Total knee arthroplasty. In: *International Symposium on CAOS* 2000;February 17–19, Davos.

22 Sati M, Staubli H, Bourquin Y, Kunz M, Kasermann S, Nolte LP. Clinical integration of computer-assisted technology for arthroscopic anterior cruciate ligament reconstruction. *Oper Tech Orthop* 2000;10:40–9.

23 Van Ham G, Denis K, Vander Sloten J, Van Audekerche R, Van Der Perre G, De Schutter J, Aertbelien E, Demey S, Bellemans J. Machining and accuracy studies for a tibial knee implant using a force controlled robot. *Comput Aided Surg* 1998;3:123–33.

24 Cinquin P, Bainville E. Computer assisted medical intervention: passive and semi-active aids. *IEEE Eng Med Biol Mag* 1995;14:254–63.

25 Davies BL, Harriss J, Lin WJ, *et al.* Active compliance in robotic surgery—the use of force control as a dynamic constraint. *J Eng Med* 1997; *Proc H Institut Mech Eng*, UK, 211:H 4.

26 Kienzle TC, Stulberg SD, Peshkin M, *et al.* A computer-assisted total knee replacement surgical system using a calibrated robot. Orthopaedics. In: Taylor RH, *et al.* eds. *Computer integrated surgery*. 409–416. Cambridge, MA: MIT Press, 1996:409–16.

27 Radermacher K, Portheine F, *et al.* Computer assisted orthopaedic surgery with image based individual templates. *Clin Orthop Rel Res* 1998;354:28–38.

28 Amiot LP, Labelle H, DeGuise JA, Sati M, *et al.* Computer-assisted pedicle screw fixation: a feasibility study. *Spine* 1995;10:1208–12.

29 Jaramaz B, DiGioia A, Blackwell M, Nikou C. Computer assisted measurement of cup placement in total hip replacement. *Clin Orthop Rel Res* 1998;354:70–81.

30 Tucker Anthony. Analysis of the Orthopedic Industry Equity Research 11.

31 Hofstetter R, Slomczykowski M, Sati M, Nolte LP. Fluoroscopy as an imaging means for computer-assisted surgical navigation. *Comput Aided Surg* 1999;4:65–76.

32 Klos TVS, Banks AZ, Banks SA, *et al.* Computer and radiographic assisted anterior cruciate ligament reconstruction of the knee. In: Nolte LP, Ganz R, eds. *Computer Assisted Orthopaedic Surgery*, Hogrefe and Huber Publishers, 184–9;1999; 84–89.

33 Krackow K, Serpe L, Phillips MJ, *et al.* A new technique for determining proper mechanical axis alignment during total knee arthroplasty. *Orthopedics* 1999;22(7):698–701.

34 Kuntz M, Sati M, Nolte LP, *et al.* Computer assisted total knee arthroplasty. In: *International Symposium on CAOS*, February, 17–19, Davos.

35 Leitner F, Picard F, Minfelde R, *et al.* Computer-assisted knee surgical total replacement. In: *First Joint Conference of CVRMed and MRCAS*. Grenoble, France: Springer, 1997:629–38.

36 Taylor RH, Brendt D, Mittelstadt BD, Paul H, Hanson W, Kazandides P, Williamson B, Musits B, Glassman E, Bargar W. An image directed robotic system for precise orthopaedic surgery. In: Taylor, Lavallee, Burdea and Mosges, eds. *Computer integrated surgery, technology and clinical applications*. Cambridge: MIT Press Publishers, 1995;379–91.

Chapter 5

Hardware components

5.1 Imaging devices, computers, peripherals, interfaces

Branislav Jaramaz

In this chapter we discuss the hardware components typically encountered in computer assisted and robotic surgery systems. Most of the components are shared across different types of CAOS systems and clinical applications. The key components of all navigation systems are the computer and the tracking device. Robotics systems also include a robot and in many cases substitute tracking with rigid fixation. Figure 5.1 illustrates typical configurations, without exhausting all the possibilities. For example, the planning station is frequently the same as the navigation station, i.e. the planning is performed on the navigation cart. Furthermore, robotic devices can be used in combination with trackers, with the trackers being used to detect bone motion or in a more advanced setting, to compensate for it. Most systems rely on medical images, obtained either pre- or intra-operatively, as a basis for planning and navigation.

5.1.1 Imaging devices

Computed tomography (CT), magnetic resonance imaging (MRI), and fluoroscopy are the most commonly used imaging modalities in computer assisted orthopaedic surgery. In computed tomography, a three-dimensional image is created by mathematical reconstruction of X-ray images acquired from a source–detector assembly that rotates around the body. Its relatively high accuracy and capability to clearly distinguish bones from other structures make CT imaging suitable for many CAS applications in orthopaedics.

Magnetic resonance imaging is also suitable for applications in orthopaedics. MRI constructs images from the magnetic resonance signal produced by the hydrogen atoms primarily from water and fat. MRI is especially suitable for imaging of soft tissues, such as ligaments and tumors. Defining the surfaces of bones is more difficult with MRI than with CT, and consequently the construction of 3D bone models from MRI can be more labor intensive (in most cases it can be entirely automated with CT).

Fluoroscopy is two-dimensional imaging modality that is being used with increasing frequency in CAS applications. It is basically a digital X-ray, obtained with a machine that has the X-ray source and detector on the opposite sides of the rigid C-shaped arm. Fluoroscopes were not originally developed for CAS

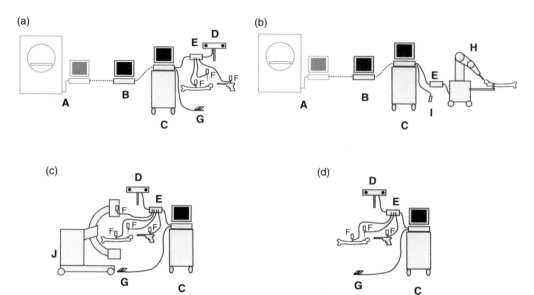

Fig. 5.1 Typical hardware configurations in computer assisted and robotic surgery: (a) preoperative image based—navigation; (b) preoperative image based—robotic; (c) intra-operative image based navigation; (d) image free navigation. A—imaging station; B—planning station; C—computer (navigation) cart; D—tracking device; E—controller; F—tracking markers; G—foot pedal; H—robot; I—safety switch; J—fluoroscope.

applications, and the images frequently include significant distortions. However, it is possible to correct image distortions and use the corrected images as a basis for surgical navigation. State of the art fluoroscopes have significantly reduced image distortion. The imaging field (typically 9–12 in) is at the lower limit of typical adult reconstructive surgery needs, but positional tracking of the image acquisition enables the creation of a bigger virtual navigation space that may incorporate all the areas and volumes of interest. New hybrid devices have been recently introduced[1] that allow CT-like volumetric reconstruction using C-arms. Given their capability to provide intra-operative 3D visualization while avoiding the need for registration, these applications could play a significant role in some CAOS applications.

5.1.2 **Computers, peripherals, interfaces**

Computers are the brains of CAOS systems—information from medical images, implant data, tracking information, and surgical plans are combined with the surgeon's input into meaningful instructions using the computer's information processing power. The speed of computing, memory, storage capacity and communication speed have reached a point where even a mid-range personal computer can satisfy the needs of most current CAOS applications. The emphasis is now being shifted to the 3D rendering speed, stability of performance, and the portability of computers, but even in these categories computing hardware can deliver satisfactory performance.

In terms of operating systems, current CAOS applications run under a range of platforms: mostly under different flavors of Unix or the Windows operating system. In most cases contemporary commercial CAOS systems are packaged in transportable carts on wheels that include the computer with the monitor, keyboard, and a mouse, power transformer and isolation unit, and the tracker controller unit with the ports to plug in the tracker and the tracking markers. In some cases, the tracker is attached to the cart with a flexible arm and in some cases it is placed on a separate stand.

During surgery, trackers provide a continuous stream of positional measurements of relevant anatomy and surgical tools. These data are placed in the context of the surgical plan and are processed in concurrence with the surgical flow. To achieve this, CAOS systems have to enable the communication of the surgeon with the computer throughout the procedure, without slowing down the surgery. Typically, the surgeon is presented with a monitor showing a graphical user interface that supports the current step and provides options to proceed from that step. There are several different ways the surgeons can communicate back to the computer: single and double foot pedals, keypads, touch screens, pointer integrated controls, voice-activated controls.

The single foot pedal allows the surgeon to step through an already determined sequence of events. A double foot pedal allows the sequence of events to be organized as a binary tree, in which at every step of the procedure the surgeon can choose between two options how to proceed. A similar effect can be achieved if a distinction is introduced between say long and short pedal presses on a single foot pedal. Of course, combining the double foot pedal with variable pedal press outcome allows for more complex decision flow, but also requires more difficult 'dancing' with the foot pedal.

The foot pedals are still a simple and effective choice that leaves the surgeon's hands free for other work, which is especially important when data are collected during surgical action (point collection for registration, recording tool positions).

Sterile touch screens are becoming more popular because they bring more complex interfaces directly under the surgeon's control. Similar results can be inexpensively achieved with the sterile keypad, although this requires some customization of interfaces, and requires some additional eye/hand coordination. Voice-activated controls are being introduced in computer assisted surgery[2] but haven't yet achieved high acceptance, probably because of the limitations it imposes to other OR communication and the state of voice recognition software.

5.2 Localizers and trackers for computer assisted freehand navigation

Frank Langlotz

Ever since surgery entered the human body and surgeons tried to operate on deep structures onto which they did not have direct visual access, there was a great demand for aids to improve orientation. Surgeons had to trust in their experience and their knowledge of anatomy when working in the dark. However, already articles published at the end of the nineteenth and the beginning of the twentieth century report on targeting devices that attempted to intra-operatively apply a surgical plan, which had been prepared preoperatively on an image of the anatomy. Clarke and Horsley[3] presented an example of such a 'stereotactic apparatus' in 1906. It consisted of a rigid frame into which a patient's head was supposed to be mounted. A tumor—the target of a biopsy or similar intervention—was marked on a brain image taken from an anatomical atlas, and its location within the head was calculated. The apparatus then facilitated guiding a biopsy needle towards the computed target position.

With the advent of modern imaging technology, especially the invention of computed tomography (CT), precise and three-dimensional representations of an individual patient's anatomy became available and allowed for accurate preoperative planning of interventions. Combining the digital CT data with technological improvements that were made in the area of position measurement enabled the development of the first computer aided surgical navigation systems. Such a CAS navigation system is an aiming device that enables real-time visualization of surgical action within an image of the operated structures.

For successful surgical navigation it is essential to determine the position and orientation of an instrument to be visualized with respect to the anatomical structures it acts on. Technically there are several ways this task can be achieved, and although the usage of such a device in a clinical environment sets up a considerable number of constraints (e.g., reliability, accuracy, sterilizability), various concepts have been implemented in surgical navigation systems.

The easiest way to follow an instrument in the hand of a surgeon is by direct contact. If the tool is mounted onto the end of a multilinkage arm, encoders at each joint of the arm can measure the angle between two adjacent links, which enables the calculation of the instrument's position and orientation in space relative to the pedestal of the arm. Obviously such a construct can easily become bulky, and its theoretical accuracy depends on the number and quality of joints as well as on the stiffness of each link. A second arm to measure eventual movements of the patient on the operating table is normally not feasible. Consequently, the usage of multilinkage arms as localizing devices requires rigid fixation of the operated structures and has therefore been limited to neurosurgery.[4]

The variety and flexibility, which are required from a localizing system for orthopaedic surgery, demand for contactless tracking. Associated navigation systems based on ultrasound, magnetic fields, or infrared light have been proposed and introduced into clinical usage. All of them allow observing several objects simultaneously, which is important for measuring an instrument's movements relative to possible motions of the anatomy. Local coordinate systems (COS) are defined on each object of interest, and their positions may be expressed mathematically as coordinate transformations into a global COS.

One research group presented an ultrasound based navigation system for femoral osteotomies.[5] A frame holding microphones is placed in the operating theater and calibrated. Arrays of three ultrasound emitters are attached to the surgical chisel to be tracked and—using a bone screw—to the femur distally to the planned osteotomy. Measuring the duration that each sound pulse needs to travel between emitter and microphone and knowing the speed of sound in air allows calculating the position of each tracked object. The authors report an accuracy of less than 0.5°. However, no commercially available ultrasound based navigation system is available to date, since there are a number of systematic drawbacks that have to be mentioned: The system requires a delicate calibration procedure, and its precision depends upon the speed of sound, which may vary depending on temperature differences. Last but not least, sterilization of the equipment is difficult.

Alternatively, magnetic fields can be used to measure position and orientation of an object in space. A generator coil is used to erect a homogenous magnetic field. 'Receiver' coils that are attached to the objects of interest then measure the field characteristics. One company has presented a navigation system for orthopaedic surgery based on magnetic tracking.[6] At first sight, several advantages let magnetic tracking appear superior over the other technologies: The equipment to be attached to surgical tools and the operated anatomy is rather small and compact. The achievable accuracy is sufficient, and objects such as the surgeon's arm located between the two coils hardly affect the measurement. However, the presence of ferromagnetic items such as implants, instruments, or other OR equipment made from steel, can disturb precise measurement dramatically and in an unpredictable way. Consequently, the aforementioned navigation system now features an optical localizer in its latest version.

Optical localization using infrared light (Fig. 5.2) is nowadays used in each commercially available navigation system for orthopaedic surgery. Two conceptually different approaches have to be distinguished: active and passive tracking. For active tracking, light emitting diodes send out light pulses that are registered by camera arrays. Three or (for redundancy reasons) more of these LEDs are

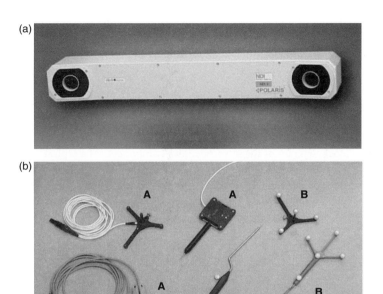

Fig. 5.2 (a) Optical localizer (Hybrid Polaris, Northern Digital, Ontario, Canada) and (b) various active (A) and passive (B) tracking markers.

attached to the objects of interest and are flashing sequentially. The camera systems consist of three linear or two planar charge coupled devices (CCDs) that are rigidly mounted into a solid housing allowing these systems to be delivered in a precalibrated state.

Passive systems use reflecting spheres that are fixed onto the objects which are to be tracked. Infrared flashes sent out by LED arrays on the camera housing illuminate the spheres. As for active tracking, CCD pairs or triplets observe the reflections and interpolate the spatial location of each light source. Reliability, flexibility, high accuracy, and good OR-compatibility are the main advantages of optical localization systems. A major obstacle is the necessity to guarantee free line-of-sight between the LEDs/spheres and the CCD array. In addition, active tracking to date requires cables to the instruments in order to power and synchronize the LEDs, which may be cumbersome especially when several surgical tools or bony structures are traced simultaneously. On the other hand, automatic tool identification is more difficult for passive systems, because all spheres in view reflect the light flashes equally, and no unique identification is possible as for the sequentially pulsed LEDs. Moreover, reflecting spheres are considered disposables and add considerable per-case costs.

In summary infrared light based tracking systems currently are the technologies of choice. Neither magnetic nor acoustic systems have proven to be superior over the optical ones. In the future, localizing devices can be expected which combine the advantages of passive and active navigation. Using battery-powered LED shields and remotely triggered diodes the construction of cableless, active instruments will be possible. Since the line-of-sight issue remains, magnetic tracking would be an alternative provided that the negative influence of metal objects on the measurement accuracy could be eliminated.

5.3 **Medical robots**

Russell H. Taylor

As we will discuss in Chapter 7, medical robot systems are, first and foremost, computer-integrated surgery (CIS) systems that share many properties with nonrobotic CIS systems. We will defer most discussion of broader systems and applications issues to that chapter. In this section, we will discuss some of the design and implementation issues associated with the specifically 'robotic' components intra-operative components of these systems.

Figure 5.3 gives a block diagram of the intra-operative components of a typical surgical robot similar to the ISS ROBODOC system for hip and knee surgery. Medical robot systems have the same basic components as any other robot system: manipulators, end-effectors, controllers, communications interfaces, etc.). Many of the design challenges are familiar to anyone who has developed an industrial system. However, the unique demands of the surgical environment, together with the emphasis on cooperative execution of surgical tasks, rather than unattended automation, do create some unusual challenges.

5.1.3 **Manipulator**

The most obvious part of a surgical robot system is the robot manipulator itself. This is the part that moves surgical instruments. There are many different robot manipulator designs, but all designs have some common elements.

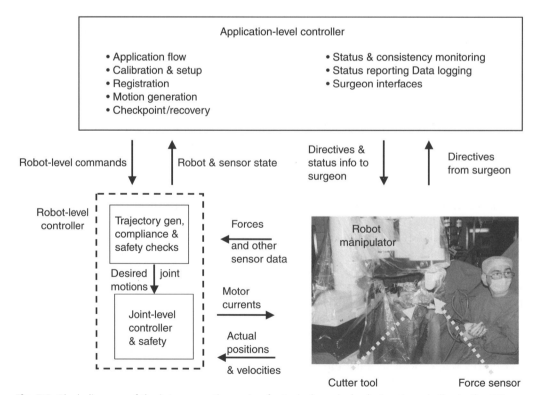

Fig. 5.3 Block diagram of the intra-operative parts of a typical surgical robot system similar to the ISS ROBODOC. (Photo credit BGU Frankfurt.)

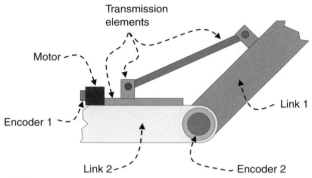

Fig. 5.4 Surgical robot joint.

Robot manipulators usually comprise multiple joints, each of which can be moved under computer control. Figure 5.4 illustrates the components a typical medical robot joint between two structural elements, here labeled 'link 1' and 'link 2'. There are many different joint designs providing various ways in which link 1 can move relative to link 2. The most common motions are revolute (shown here) and rectilinear or sliding. The joint is moved by a drive mechanism consisting of a motor and some transmission elements, here shown schematically as a lead-screw and connecting rod arrangement. Unlike most unmodified industrial robots, surgical robots for orthopaedic applications usually do not have to move rapidly, and it is usually good practice to choose very high gear reductions in joint transmission elements. This tends to make the robot stiff, precise, and incapable of very high speed or acceleration. These speed and acceleration limitations can be a significant safety advantage since both the computer and the surgeon can then have more time to detect an unsafe situation and take appropriate action (usually, to stop all motion). There are usually at least two encoders giving position feedback for each joint. Again, this is an important safety consideration. An arrangement similar to that shown in the figure, in which one position encoder is mounted on the motor output shaft and the other is mounted directly on the joint, is common, although other arrangements are also found.

The way that the joints and links of the robot are connected together to cause motion of a tool held by some distal part of the robot relative to its base is often referred to as the *kinematic design* of the robot. The computer controlling the robot can combine information about the kinematic design with positional feedback from the joint encoders to determine the position and orientation of the tool relative to the robot's base. This computation is often called the *forward kinematic solution* for the robot. Given a desired tool position and orientation, the computer can also find the *inverse kinematic solution* to determine the corresponding set of joint positions.

The most common kinematic designs resemble the *serial linkage* structures found in most industrial robots. The ROBODOC manipulator shown in Fig. 5.3 is a typical example. One important design feature that has become increasingly popular in medical robots is incorporation of a *remote-center-of-motion* (RCM) mechanism (e.g.,[7–9]). The advantage of such a mechanism is that it permits one to change the orientation of a surgical tool without moving one point such as the tool tip or the point at which the tool enters a patients's body. The IBM/JHU LARS robot shown in Fig. 5.5 is one frequently cited example. It is also possible to construct *parallel linkage* structures for orthopaedic surgery (e.g.,[10–12]). One typical example is shown in Fig. 5.6.

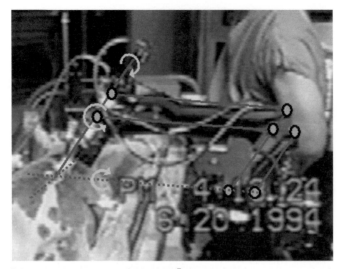

Fig. 5.5 Close-up of the IBM/JHU LARS surgical robot,[7] showing the remote-center-of-motion (RCM) linkage.

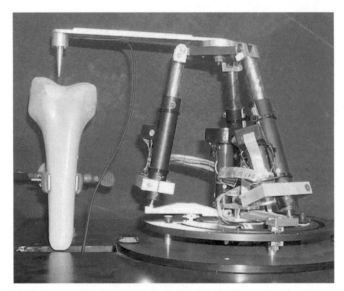

Fig. 5.6 Typical parallel linkage robot for medical applications.[11,12]

5.1.4 **End effectors**

The term 'end effector' is used somewhat loosely to refer both to the surgical tool being manipulated by the surgical robot and the device or interface used to attach tools to the robot, although the former use is more common. For orthopaedic applications, common end effectors include rotary surgical cutters, saws, drills, saw guides, drill guides, biopsy devices, and tissue ablation devices.

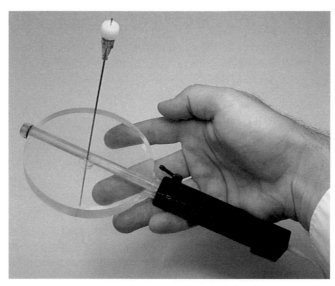

Fig. 5.7 PAKY radiolucent end-effector (Photo credit: Dan Stoianovici).[13]

Sterility is a crucial concern both for end effectors and the robot manipulator. Usually, covering most of the robot with a sterile bag or drape and then separately sterilizing the instruments or end-effectors provide sterility. Autoclaving, which is the most universal and popular sterilization method, can unfortunately be very destructive for electromechanical components, force sensors, and other components. Other common methods include gas (slow, but usually kindest to equipment) and soaking.

Because medical robots are often used together with imaging, materials are an important concern in surgical manipulator and end-effector design (e.g.,[14]) shows one example of a simple 1-degree-of-freedom radiolucent mechanism that can be used to drive needles into soft tissue (Fig. 5.7). This device is designed for use with fluoroscopic X-rays or CT scanners, and it can be employed either with a simple support clamp or as the end effector of an active robot. Fiducial geometry can be added easily to the robot or end-effectors to assist in registration of the robot to the images (e.g.,[15–21]). Further discussion may be found in Chapter 7.

5.1.5 **Controller**

The different levels of a typical medical robot control hierarchy are illustrated in Fig. 5.3. These elements are usually packaged into at least two or three computers, although there is no hard and fast rule. Generally, it is good practice to have a separate computer or computational process whose only job is safety and consistency checking, although *all* levels of the control hierarchy should perform at least some measure of safety checking and should have the ability to halt or pause the surgical procedure if something does not seem to be right.

At the bottom-most level one finds electrical interfaces connecting the robot manipulator to the controller. These are generally similar to those one might find in an industrial robot, although the amount of power that must be delivered to the joint motors is often relatively low and there are multiple encoder interfaces for each joint. Generally, extremely rigid electrical safety, electrical isolation and electrical noise standards must be followed, and it is not unreasonable for a controller design to include a dedicated microprocessor to check such things as power supply and interlock status.

At the next higher level one finds software or a mixture of software and dedicated electronic circuitry responsible for positional control of the robot joints. Above this, one finds software that is responsible for kinematic control of the robot and coordination of multiple joints. This level usually receives commands specifying trajectories giving desired positions and orientations of surgical tools relative to the robot's base. The trajectory control software calls the inverse kinematic solution software described above to produce desired joint trajectories or to repeatedly produce position set points for each joint. Usually, there is some sort of *application programming interface* (API) defined within the robot controller software for specifying commands to the trajectory control software. This interface is not commonly exposed to outside parties by the medical robot vendor, but is used internally to provide a modular interface to higher-level application-specific software.

References

1 Rock C, Linsenmaier U, Brandl R, Kotsianos D, Wirth S, Kaltschmidt R, Euler E, Mutschler W, Pfeifer KJ. Introduction of a new mobile C-arm/CT combination equipment (ISO-C-3D). Initial results of 3-D sectional imaging. Unfallchirurg; 2001;104(9):827–33. [German.]

2 Allaf ME, Jackman SV, Schulam PG, Cadeddu JA, Lee BR, Moore RG, Kavoussi LR. Laparoscopic visual field. Voice vs foot pedal interfaces for control of the AESOP robot. *Surg Endosc* 1998;12(12):1415–18.

3 Clarke RH, Horsley V. On a method of investigating the deep ganglia and tracts of the central nervous system (cerebellum). *Br Med J* 1906;2:1799–1800.

4 Zamorano L, Jiang Z, Kadi AM. Computer-assisted neurosurgery system: Wayne State University hardware and software configuration. *Comp Med Imaging Graph* 1994;18(4):257–71.

5 Wallny T, Klose J, Steffny G, Schulze Bertelsbeck D, Perlick L, Schumpe G. Dreidimensionaler ultraschall und intraoperative navigation: Ein neuer Einsatz des Ultraschalltopometers bei Umstellungsosteotomie des proximalen Femurs. *Ultraschall Med* 1999;20(4):158–60.

6 Amiot LP, Labelle H, DeGuise JA, Sati M, Brodeur P, Rivard CH. Computer-assisted pedicle screw fixation. A feasibility study. *Spine* 1995;20(10):1208–12.

7 Eldridge B, Gruben K, LaRose D, Funda J, Gomory S, Karidis J, McVicker G, Taylor R, Anderson J. A remote center of motion robotic arm for computer assisted surgery. *Robotica* 1996;14(1):103–9.

8 Stoianovici D, Whitcomb LL, Anderson JH, Taylor RH, Kavoussi LR. A modular surgical robotic system for image guided percutaneous procedures. *International Conference on Medical Image Computing and Computer-Assisted Intervention.* Cambridge, MA, USA, 1998.

9 Taylor RH, Funda J, Eldridge B, Gruben K, LaRose D, Gomory S, Talamini MD, Mark A. Telerobotic assistant for laparoscopic surgery. In: Taylor R, *et al.*, eds. *Computer-integrated surgery.* MIT Press; 1996:581–92.

10 Brandt G, Radermacher K, Lavallee S, Staudte H-W, Rau G. A compact robot for image-guided orthopaedic surgery: concept and preliminary results. *Proceedings of the First Joint Conference of CVRMed and MRCAS.* Grenoble, France: Springer, 1997, March 19–22:767.

11 Simaan N, Glozman D, Shoham M. Design considerations of new types of six-degrees-of-freedom parallel manipulators. *IEEE International Conference on Robotics and Automation.* Belgium; 1998:1327–33.

12 Shoham M, Roffman M, Goldberger S, Simaan N. Robot structures for surgery. In *First ISRACAS, Israeli Symposium on Computer Assisted Surgery, Medical Robotics and Medical Imaging.* Haifa, Israel, 1998.

13 Stoianovici D, Cadeddu JA, Demaree RD, Basile SA, Taylor RH, Whitcomb LL, Sharpe WN, Kavoussi LR. A novel mechanical transmission applied to percutaneous renal access. *1997 ASME Winter Annual Meeting,* 1997.

14 Stoianovici D, Cadeddu JA, Demaree RD, Basile SA, Taylor RH, Whitcomb L, L, Sharpe WN, Kavoussi LR. An efficient needle injection technique and radiological guidance method for percutaneous procedures. *First Joint Conference: CRVMed II & MRCAS III, March.* Grenoble, France: Springer, 1997;295–8.

15 Gueziec A, Kazanzides P, Williamson B, Taylor R. Anatomy-based registration of CT-scan and intraoperative X-ray images for guiding a surgical robot. *IEEE Trans Med Imag* 1998;17(5):715–28.

16 Gueziec AP, Kazanzides P, Williamson B, Taylor RH. *Registration of computed tomography data to a surgical robot using fluoroscopy: a feasibility study*. 1996. IBM Research: New York.

17 Joskowicz L, Taylor RH, Williamson B, Kane R, Kalvin A, Gueziec A, Taubin G, Funda J, Gomory S, Brown L, McCarthy J. Computer-integrated revision total hip replacement surgery: preliminary results. *Proceedings of the Second International Symposium on Medical Robotics and Computer Assisted Surgery*. Baltimore, MD: MRCAS1995 International Symposium, C/O Center for Orthop Res, Shadyside Hospital, Pittsburgh, PA. Nov 4–7;1995:193–202.

18 Masamune K, GF, Patriciu A, Susil R, Taylor R, Kavoussi L, Anderson J, Sakuma I, Dohi T, Stoianovici D. Guidance system for robotically assisted percutaneous procedures with computed tomography. *Comp Assisted Surg* 2001;6:370–83.

19 Solomon S, Patriciu A, Masamune K, Whitcomb L, Taylor RH, Karoussi L, Stoianovici D. CT guided robotic needle biopsy: a precise sampling method minimizing radiation exposure. *Radiology* 2002;225:277–82.

20 Taylor RH, Joskowicz L, Williamson B, Gueziec A, Kalvin A, Kazanzides P, Vorhis RV, Yao J, Kumar R, Bzostek A, Sahay A, Borner M, Lahmer A. Computer-integrated revision total hip replacement surgery: concept and preliminary results. *Med Image Anal*, 1999;3(3):301–19.

21 Yao J, Taylor RH, Goldberg RP, Kumar R, Bzostek A, Vorhis RV, Kazanzides P, Gueziec A. A C-arm fluoroscopy-guided progressive cut refinement strategy using a surgical robot. *Comp Aided Surg* 2000;5(6):373–90.

Chapter 6

Software infrastructure for computer-assisted orthopaedic surgery

Branislav Jaramaz and Scott L. Delp

6.1 Introduction

Computer assisted surgery (CAS) systems are used in a variety of surgical specialities, including neurosurgery, craniofacial surgery, and orthopaedics. Although the clinical applications span several surgical disciplines, many of the software components are common. These common software components can facilitate the development of new systems and enable deployment into novel clinical applications if a robust software platform can be defined and developed.

Computer assisted surgery systems are created from a software infrastructure that integrates medical images and mathematical algorithms with surgical tools and clinical methods. Although a diverse array of computer assisted surgical systems have been developed, a relatively small number of software components underlie virtually all of these systems. The purpose of this chapter is to provide an overview of these basic software components. Our goal is to provide an introduction to the elements of the software infrastructure required to create CAS systems for orthopaedics, so that the common elements among the systems described in later chapters can be more easily recognized; it is not our intention to provide a comprehensive review.

Computer assisted surgical systems provide a wide range of capabilities. Some CAS systems allow the development of sophisticated preoperative plans on the basis of three-dimensional models constructed from medical images. Others simply enhance intra-operative measurements. Only the most comprehensive systems use all of the components described here; most systems include only a subset. The basic software components used for preoperative planning are medical image segmentation and analysis, surgical planning, and outcome simulation. The software components used in the operating room provide registration, navigation, procedure guidance, safety, and—in the case of robotic surgery—robot control. All of these intra-operative features are accessed through a graphical user interface, an important software component for all CAS systems.

6.2 Image segmentation, preoperative planning, and simulation

Surgical planning is typically based a computer model of the patient's anatomy. This model can be created from three-dimensional medical images, such as CT or MRI (Fig. 6.1), from co-registered two-dimensional images (fluoroscopy), or without images—using intra-operative kinematic measurements. If the model is based on three-dimensional images, the first step in preoperative planning is the creation of a three-dimensional model. This may involve segmentation of the medical images into distinct anatomical structures. Segmentation of medical images is an area of intensive research.[1]

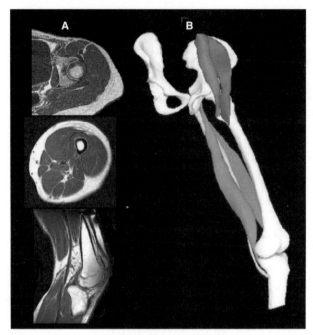

Fig. 6.1 Three-dimensional surface reconstruction of the pelvis, femur, and several muscles from MR images. Surface models of the bones and muscles were generated from two-dimensional outlines that were defined in each image (A). Surfaces from overlapping series were registered to obtain a representation of the subject's anatomy (B).[2]

Three-dimensional medical images are typically presented in two ways, often simultaneously: (1) as cross-sections through the image volume and (2) as 3D perspective renderings. Less used, but also helpful, are pseudo-X-ray views, synthesized from CT scans. The first mode allows insight inside the bone volume, which is helpful in understanding the interaction between the tools, implants and the bones. The cross-sections usually move based on the position and orientation of tools, or are selected by the user. The perspective rendering is helpful in global orientation within the bone of interest and in identifying bony landmarks. This mode requires that the bone of interest is separated or segmented from other bones and tissues, so that it can be displayed without being obscured by other objects. This segmentation is also useful in some other components of CAOS surgery, such as implant placement and range of motion simulation and image registration. Because the bone shows as the highest intensity tissue in a CT scan (in absence of any metallic objects) it is easy to segment from other tissues, such as muscle, ligaments, etc. However, the separation between bones can be difficult, especially in arthritic joints, and may require sophisticated software or manual interaction. Once the bone is segmented, it can be displayed directly, using volume rendering techniques, or a surface model of the bone can be constructed using connected triangles or surface patches. The user can usually preset the views or interactively select the point of view.

The best user interaction is typically achieved when a combination of cross-sectional and perspective views is used. Pseudo-X-rays can be used when cumulative understanding of the image is required, for instance when the user needs to select a subvolume of interest; or when this form is helpful because it relates to postoperative X-rays, as the most often used form of postoperative imaging.

Construction of a three-dimensional model allows for detailed surgical planning. For example, the optimal size of prosthetic components and their positions and orientations relative to the bones can be determined based on a three-dimensional model.[3] Some CAS applications have introduced planners enhanced with simulators, which provide analytical capability that can aid the surgeon in making the critical preoperative planning decisions. For example, the planning software of one system for total hip replacement has a range of motion simulator that can aid the surgeon in selecting the position and orientation of implant components.[4] Other systems have incorporated patient-specific finite element models to predict the load transfer after a pelvic osteotomy,[5] or examined the effects of tilting the tibial component on knee range of motion.[6]

Once a surgical plan is developed, it becomes the blueprint for surgical intervention. The performance of the plan is typically dependent on several steps, the first of which is registration.

6.3 Registration

Registration is the process of determining the geometrical transformation between two sets of data. Tracking devices provide a continuous stream of positional measurements of tracking markers rigidly attached to tools and bones. In order to perform the surgery as it was planned, the geometrical transformation between the computer model of the patient's anatomy and the patient's actual anatomy must be determined through a registration process. Rigid registration algorithms assume that the anatomical structures have not deformed between imaging and surgery, whereas nonrigid registration algorithms allow for deformation of anatomical structures. Since the deformation of bones is generally negligible, most computer assisted orthopaedic systems use rigid registration algorithms.

Fiducial-based registration is a simple rigid registration algorithm. It involves the insertion of physical markers (i.e., 'fiducials') into the bone before the images are obtained. The coordinates of these physical markers are determined in the image data and during the surgical procedure. Fiducial registration requires that at least three markers be implanted into each bone to determine the bone's position and orientation. Although fiducial-based registration is conceptually and computationally simple, it requires that screws be placed into each bone, typically several days before surgery. To avoid this additional procedure alternative methods have been developed.

Shape-based registration is an alternative to fiducial-based registration. In this procedure, the shape of part of the bone surface is measured intra-operatively and matched to the surface model created from the medical images (Fig. 6.2). Intra-operative measurement of the shape of the bone surface can be done using a pointing probe, an ultrasonic probe, or any other technology that acquires the three-dimensional shape of the bone surface. If a pointing probe is used, the coordinates of a set of points are acquired. Given this set of sampled points (S_i), an iterative closest point algorithm[7] finds the rotation (R) and the translation (T) that minimizes the mean squared distance between the sampled points and the set of closest points on the computer model of the bone surface (M_i). That is, R and T are determined that minimize the function:

$$f(R, T) = \frac{1}{N_s} \sum_{i=1}^{n} ||M_i - (RS_i + T)||^2$$

where N_s is the number of sampled points.

Ultrasonic registration is a promising new method based on measuring bone surface profiles with an ultrasonic probe.[8] This technology is especially attractive for minimally invasive applications, in which the bone surface exposure is not sufficient to acquire a widely distributed cloud of points.

Some CAS applications use intra-operative imaging (such as fluoroscopy) for navigation and therefore obviate the need for registration to preoperative image data.

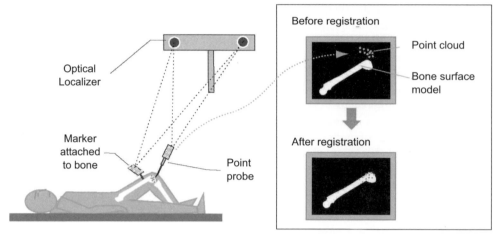

Fig. 6.2 Example of shape-based registration used in TKR surgery. Bone surface coordinates are measured using a point probe. The resulting point cloud is matched with the surface model created from the medical image data.

6.4 **Operating room interface**

The software used in the operating room manages procedural flow and allows access to various algorithms and visualization techniques throughout the surgical procedure. The specific algorithms and visualization techniques depend on the clinical application, but the overall function of the system software is application independent. The system software takes input from the user, reads data from the various hardware components, provides visual feedback on the state of the system, and may guide the surgeon through the steps of the procedure. While there is a wide variety of user interfaces, surgeons frequently interact with this software through foot switches or a sterilizable 'virtual keyboard'.[9]

Navigation is one of the key functions generally provided. Once registration is performed, the surgeon can identify the position of tracked surgical tools relative to the target bones. The enables the surgeon to reposition the tools to match the planned positions and trajectories and provides assistance navigating the patient's anatomy. Typical interfaces show the current positions of the tools in the cross-sections through the patient's image, or as a three-dimensional view from the chosen point of view. Simple interfaces similar to those used by airplane pilots guide the surgeon to the desired tool alignment.

The system software frequently provides additional capabilities as well. CAS systems frequently provide enhanced visualization, which can be accessed during the case. Systems that include active robotic elements require specialized control software. In addition, this software is also responsible for the overall safety of the system.

References

1 Pham DL, Xu C, Prince JL. Current methods in medical image segmentation. *Ann Rev Biomed Eng* 2000;2:315–37.
2 Arnold AS, Salinas S, Schmidt DJ, Delp, SL. Accuracy of muscle moment arms estimated form MRI-based musculoskeletal models of the lower extremity. *Comput Aided Surg* 2000;5:108–19.

3 Delp SL, Stulberg SD, Davies B, Picard F, Leitner F. Computer assisted knee replacement. *Clin Orthop Rel Res* 1998;354:49–56.

4 DiGioia AM III, Jaramaz B, Nikou C, LaBarca RS, Moody JE, Colgan B. Surgical navigation for total hip replacement with the use of HipNav. *Oper Tech Orthop* 2000;10(1):3–8.

5 Hipp JA, Sugano N, Millis MB, Murphy SB. Planning acetabular redirection osteotomies based on joint contact pressures. *Clin Orthop Rel Res* 1999;64:134–143.

6 Piazza SJ, Delp SL, Stulberg SD, Stern SH. Posterior tilting of the tibial component decreases femoral rollback in posterior-substituting knee replacement. *J Orthop Res* 1998;16:264–70.

7 Besl PJ, McKay ND. A method for registration of 3D shapes. *IEEE Trans Pat Anal Mach Intell* 1992;14:239–56.

8 Amin DV, Kanade T, DiGioia AM III, Jaramaz B, Nikou C, LaBarca RS. Ultrasound based registration of the pelvic bone surface for surgical navigation. *1st Annual Meeting, International Society for Computer Assisted Orthopaedic Surgery* (CAOS-International), 2001. Davos, Switzerland.

9 Visarius H, Gong J, Scheer C, Haralamb S, Nolte LP. Man-machine interfaces for computer assisted surgery. *Proceedings of the Second International Symposium on Medical Robotics and Computer Assisted Surgery* 1995:181–5.

Chapter 7

Robotic systems for orthopaedic surgery

R.H. Taylor

7.1 Systems paradigms: surgical CAD/CAM and surgical assistants

Robotic systems for orthopaedic surgery are Computer-Integrated Surgery (CIS) systems first, and 'medical robots' second. In other words, the robotic manipulator itself is just one element of a larger system that typically includes preoperative planning based on medical images, intra-operative registration to presurgical plans, a combination of robotic assist and manually controlled tools for carrying out the plan, and patient verification and follow-up.

The basic information flow of CIS systems is illustrated in Fig. 7.1. Typically, one starts with information about the patient in the form of 3D medical images. These images are combined with anatomical atlas information to produce a computer model of the individual patient, which is then used in surgical planning. All this information (images, model, and plan) is brought into the operating room, and registered to the actual patient. This registration step usually involves additional sensing, either through the use of a 3D localization device (see Chapters 5 and 8), X-ray or ultrasound images, or the use of the robot itself. If necessary, the surgical plan can be updated. Then a variety of means can be used to help the surgeon carry out the surgical plan. In this chapter, we will mostly be concerned with the use of robots, but it is important to note that surgical navigation systems are otherwise very similar. Additional

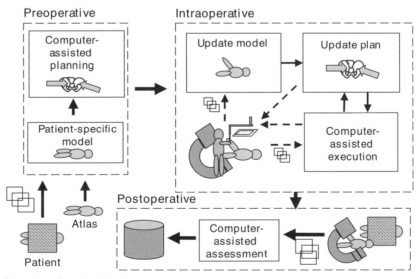

Fig. 7.1 Information flow in CIS systems.

Table 7.1 Comparative strengths and limitations of humans and robots in surgical applications

	Strengths	Limitations
Humans	Excellent judgment	Prone to fatigue and inattention
	Excellent hand-eye coordination	Tremor limits fine motion
	Excellent dexterity (at natural 'human' scale)	Limited manipulation ability and dexterity outside natural scale
	Able to integrate and act on multiple information sources	Bulky end-effectors (hands)
	Easily trained	Limited geometric accuracy
	Versatile and able to improvise	Hard to keep sterile
		Affected by radiation, infection
Robots	Excellent geometric accuracy	Poor judgment
	Untiring and stable	Hard to adapt to new situations
	Immune to ionizing radiation	Limited dexterity
	Can be designed to operate at many different scales of motion and payload	Limited hand-eye coordination
	Able to integrate multiple sources of numerical and sensor data	Limited ability to integrate and interpret complex information

images or sensing can be used to verify that the surgical plan is successfully executed and to assist in post-surgical follow-up.

We refer to this process of building a model of the patient, planning, registration, execution, and follow-up as 'surgical CAD/CAM', emphasizing the analogy to the processes in computer-integrated manufacturing. Of course, the analogy is not perfect. Surgery is a highly interactive process and many surgical decisions are made on the spot. As the late Hap Paul frequently remarked, '. . . the robot is not the surgeon; the robot is a surgical tool to improve the efficacy of [a] procedure'. Thus, we also speak of these systems as 'surgical assistants' intended to work cooperatively with the surgeon to improve or simplify specific tasks. The paradigms of surgical CAD/CAM and surgical assistants are not mutually exclusive. Many, if not most, robotic systems used in orthopaedics have aspects of both, although the surgical CAD/CAM paradigm tends to predominate.

In considering what sort of robotic system to select for a particular application (or, indeed, whether to use a robot at all) it is important to consider the specific advantages that will be gained from the use of the robot. Here, it is helpful to consider the relative strengths and limitations of robots and humans in performing surgical tasks, as illustrated in Table 7.1.

7.2 General engineering considerations for medical robot systems

Medical robots are both robots and medical devices. Like industrial robots, they are intended to be reasonably versatile without being 'universal' machines. In other words, medical robots are often designed for particular classes of surgical procedure (e.g., bone machining, placing needles into targeted positions) that are broad enough to cover an important market but also narrow enough to permit economic design and simplicity of use. There is no one obvious design point, and medical robot manufacturers have taken different approaches to striking the right balance. Nevertheless, medical robots, like surgical navigation systems, are more complicated than most equipment in current operating rooms. Consequently, system designers, prospective users, and regulators need to pay careful attention to issues such as safety, usability and maintainability, and interoperability.

Safety is a primary consideration in any medical system. Medical robot systems both must be safe, in the sense that system failures will not cause harm to the patient or operating room staff and must be perceived to be safe. Just as in any other medical system, designers must conduct careful analyses of potential failures and of the consequences of such failures. Care must be taken to ensure that system component failures will not go undetected and that the system will remain under control at all times. Wherever possible, redundancy in both hardware and software should be provided and the system design should include intensive real time consistency checking. Rigorous adherence to good software engineering practice is crucial. Further discussion of safety issues for medical robots may be found in Section 5.3 and references.[1–5]

Many discussions of safety in medical robotics tend to focus on a concern that the robot might 'run away', i.e., begin to move in an uncontrolled manner. This is a valid concern, and generally robots should be designed not to move faster than they need to. If this is done, and if good engineering practice is otherwise followed, the chance of an out-of-control situation is remote.

The more important challenge is to assure that the system will not do exactly what it told to do, but in the wrong place. This problem is the same in both robotic and navigation assistance systems that rely on the accuracy of registration. A human surgeon acting on incorrect information can place a screw into the spinal cord just as easily as a robot can. This means that registration software and sensing must be analyzed just as carefully as motion control. Surgeons must be fully aware of the limitations as well as the capabilities of their systems and system design should include appropriate means for surgeon 'sanity checking' of surgical actions.

System usability and maintainability are also important design considerations. Good ergonomic design of the system from the surgeon's perspective is important (e.g.,[6,7]). One must also provide easy-to-use interfaces for the operating room staff who must set up, maintain, and help operate the systems.

At another level, medical robots should include interfaces to assist field engineers trouble-shoot and service equipment. The ability of computer-based systems to log data during use can be especially useful in post-failure analysis and in scheduling preventative maintenance, as well as in providing data for improvement in surgical outcomes and techniques. Although most systems make some use of such facilities, they are probably under-used in present-day commercial systems.

System interoperability is currently a major challenge that will become increasingly important, especially when one considers the close potential synergy between medical robots, surgical navigation, and other forms of CIS. Commonly accepted open standards permitting different equipment to work together in a variety of settings are badly needed. Although several companies have proposed proprietary standards and there have been some academic and government-supported efforts to provide common software tool kits, standardization efforts are still very fragmented. As with image data formats, a strong 'demand pull' from customers will probably be needed to promote such standards. But their development will ultimately be essential in promoting broad and rapid dissemination of this new technology.

7.3 Robotic systems for precise machining of bone

Because bone is rigid and relatively easy to image in CT, and because geometric precision is often an important consideration in preparing bones for joint replacement surgery, robotic systems for machining bone were among the first medical robots introduced for clinical use. For example, the ROBODOC® system discussed in Chapter 10 has been used clinically since 1992. ROBODOC combines CT-based preoperative planning with robotic machining of bone for primary and revision total hip surgery.[8–13] Both ROBODOC and a very similar subsequently introduced system called CASPAR®[14] have also been applied to knee surgery.[15–20] Other robotic systems that have been proposed or (in a few cases) applied for hip or knee surgery include.[21–30]

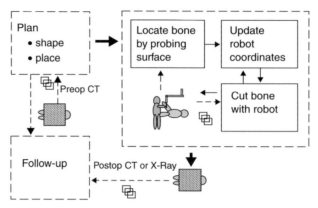

Fig. 7.2 ROBODOC information flow (example of surgical CAD/CAM).

These applications fit naturally within the context of surgical CAD/CAM systems, as illustrated by the ROBODOC information flow diagram in Fig. 7.2. CT images are read into a planning workstation and a simple segmentation method is used to produce an accurate surface model of the patient's bones. The surgeon makes some key anatomical measurements from the images and selects an implant design from a library. The surgeon determines its desired placement in the patient's femur by manipulating a CAD model of the implant with respect to selected mutually orthogonal cross-sections through the CT data volume. The planning workstation computes a cutter trajectory relative to CT coordinates and all of the planning information is written to a magnetic tape along with the patient images and model.

In the operating room, robotic hip replacement surgery proceeds much as manual surgery until after the head of the femur (for the case of primary hip surgery) or failing implant (for revision surgery) is removed. Then the femur is fixed to the base of the robot and a redundant position sensor is attached to the bone to detect any slipping of the bone relative to the fixation device. A 3D digitizer is used to locate points on the bone surface, and these points are used to compute the coordinate transformation between the robot and CT images used for planning and (thus) to the patient's bone. The surgeon hand-guides the robot to an approximate initial position using a force sensor mounted between the robot's tool holder and the surgical cutter. The robot cuts the implant shape while monitoring cutting forces, bone motion, and other safety sensors. The surgeon also monitors progress and can interrupt the robot at any time. If the procedure is paused for any reason, the system instructs the surgeon on what appropriate corrective actions to take and provides menus permitting the procedure to be resumed or restarted at one of several defined checkpoints. Once the desired shape has been cut, surgery proceeds manually in the normal manner.

An alternative approach to the use of robots in accurate shaping of bone is discussed in Section 7.5. Again, the particular method used to control a cutting tool is only one element of the overall system. Whatever method is chosen, planning, registration, and the other elements of a complete surgical CAD/CAM system must be supported.

7.4 Robotically assisted percutaneous therapy systems

One of the first uses of robots in surgery was positioning of needle guides in stereotactic neuro-surgery.[31–33] This is a natural application, since the skull provides a rigid frame-of-reference. However, the potential application of localized therapy is much broader, and there is now a fairly broad research community exploring the use of robots for percutaneous procedures (e.g.,[34–46] including applications in the spine (e.g.,[47]).

Surprisingly, there has been relatively little focus on the use of such robot systems for tool path guidance in hip and knee applications. A few examples include the ORTHOSISTA™ system for hip pinning,[48] the use of a CASPAR robot for ligament replacement surgery, and work at Johns Hopkins University on percutaneous access to osteolytic lesions.[49] Because of the widespread use of X-ray imaging modalities (C-arm fluoroscopy, CT) in orthopaedics, robots offer several potential advantages beyond simple geometric accuracy. In particular, the robot can tolerate large cumulative doses of radiation that a surgeon cannot. Although care must still be taken to avoid excessive radiation to the patient, the use of a robot to place biopsy needles, drills, or other under real time X-ray fluoroscopic guidance[40,43,46,50,51] or CT guidance (e.g.,[42,52–54]) can potentially improve both the accuracy and efficiency of many orthopaedic procedures.

Figure 7.3 shows an experimental setup in our laboratory at Johns Hopkins University using a robot to assist the surgeon in treatment of osteolytic lesions in the periacetabular portion of the pelvis.[49] In this case, the access path is planned from preoperative CT images. In the operating room, multiple X-ray images are registered to the robot and to the preoperative CT scan. The robot then positions a cannula to provide the correct tool path for access to the lesion. Such a system can be made to track motions of the pelvis to maintain the correct tool-to-anatomy relationship. Registration of multiple X-ray images to the robot and to each other can be facilitated by the use of appropriate X-ray fiducial objects mounted on the robot and/or the patient. Figure 7.4 shows an X-ray 'corkscrew' fiducial pattern originally developed as part on an IBM/Integrated Surgical Systems/Johns Hopkins collaboration for use with the ROBODOC system.[40,42,52–54] If the X-ray source-to-detector relationship and image distortion are known, there is

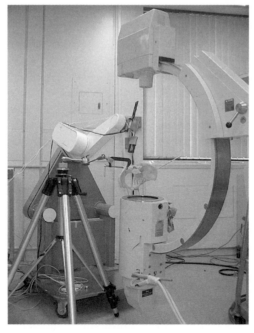

Fig. 7.3 Experimental setup at Johns Hopkins University showing a feasibility study of the use of a robot to access osteolytic lesions in the periacetabular region of the hip.

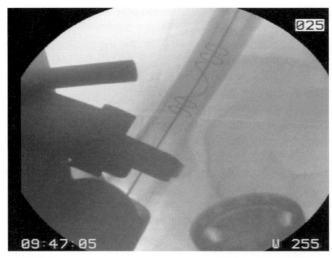

Fig. 7.4 'Corkscrew' fiducial object used for X-ray image pose recovery.[50,51,68–70]

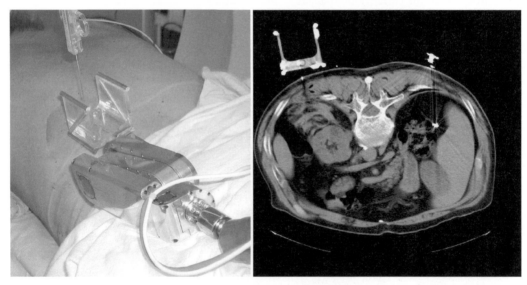

Fig. 7.5 In-scanner percutaneous therapy. The photo on the left shows a clinical application at Johns Hopkins University of a novel in-scanner percutaneous therapy robot, combining a modular robotic manipulator[71] with a specialized needle driver permitting the pose of the robot relative to the patient to be determined from a single CT image, as shown on the right.[42,52] Although the application shown is kidney biopsy,[53] the approach has significant promise for spine, long bone, and other orthopaedic procedures. Photos courtesy S. Solomon.

sufficient information in a single image to recover the relative pose of the X-ray system and the fiducial, which may be mounted on the robot, on a surgical instrument, or on the patient's bone.

Figure 7.5 shows a clinical example of the use of a robot with intra-operative CT image guidance in a percutaneous biopsy. A fiducial pattern on the robot's end-effector provides a direct registration between the robot and the CT images without an extensive calibration process.[40,42,52–54] This system could be used with relatively little modification in other CT-guided orthopaedic procedures.

7.5 **Robotic systems for human augmentation**

There have been a number of efforts to use robotic systems to extend a surgeon's sensory-motor capabilities or to simplify the manipulation of instruments in minimally invasive surgery. Many of these systems (e.g.,[56–63]) have involved master–slave robotic systems in which the surgeon manipulates handles at a control console and the robot manipulates surgical instruments touching the patient. Such systems have so far found little (if any) application in hip and knee surgery, although they might possibly be useful in some arthroscopic applications.

Several groups have, however, explored schemes to improve the ability of a surgeon to make very precise surgical motions (e.g., in preparing a bone for a surgical implant) while preserving much of the immediacy of hands-on surgery. Many of these efforts (e.g.,[24,64,65]) have involved one form or another of cooperative manipulation, in which a surgeon holds a handle located on the robot or on the surgical instrument. The robot's controller senses forces exerted on the handle by the surgeon and moves the robot in the direction pushed, so long as the robot's tool obeys prescribed constraints. This produces very smooth, precise, and tremor-free motions of the surgical instrument, and the scheme can be modified to enable the surgeon to control tool-to-tissue forces as well as positions.[65] Perhaps the earliest use of this mode of operation was the hand guiding used in ROBODOC for approximate positioning of the robot (Fig. 7.6, left). An example of the use of this mode in actual bone preparation is the ACROBOT system of Davies *et al.* (Fig. 7.6, right).[23,24,64,66,67]

Several other groups have explored an alternative approach that provides some of the benefits of cooperative manipulation but without an actively powered robot.[64] In these approaches, the computer is able to control a robotic steering device or controllable brake that constrains the motion of the 'robot' tool, but that require all motive power to be provided by the surgeon. The advantage of such an approach for bone shaping is not clear, but it may possibly have some advantages in certain instrument positioning tasks.

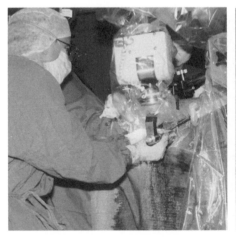 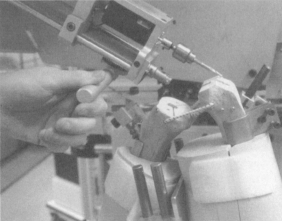

Fig. 7.6 Two examples of cooperative hand guiding of a surgical robot. (left) ROBODOC;[8,9] (right) ARTHROBOT.[23,24,64] Photo credits: BGH, Brian Davies.

7.6 **Acknowledgments**

Any survey or critical summary must necessarily draw upon the work of many people. I would like especially to acknowledge the contributions of many colleagues over the past decade who have helped develop an evolving shared understanding of medical robotics and computer-integrated surgery. I am especially grateful to those individuals who generously provided photographs and other information about the specific systems that we have used as examples. In some cases, these colleagues have also contributed to the development of some of these systems.

I also gratefully acknowledge the many agencies and organizations that have contributed financial and other support to the development of much of the work that we have reported. The National Science Foundation's support of the Engineering Research Center for Computer-Integrated Surgical Systems and Technology under cooperative agreement number EEC9731478 is especially appreciated. Other US Government funding came from NSF grants #IIS9801684 and #ST32HL07712 (with Whitaker Foundation), and NIST cooperative agreement #94-01-228. Other support from IBM Corporation and Johns Hopkins University is also gratefully acknowledged.

References

1 Taylor RH. Safety. In: Taylor RH *et al.*, eds. *Computer-integrated surgery*. Cambridge, MA: MIT Press, 1996:283–6.

2 Taylor R, Kazanzides P, Mittelstadt B, Paul H. Redundant consistency checking in a precise surgical robot. *12th Annual Conference on Engineering in Medicine and Biology*, 1990. Philadelphia: IEEE Press.

3 Taylor R, Paul H, Kazanzides P. *et al.* Taming the bull: safety in a precise surgical robot. *International Conference on Advanced Robotics (ICAR)*, 1991. Pisa, Italy.

4 Davies B. A discussion of safety issues for medical robots. In: Taylor R, *et al.*, eds. *Computer-integrated surgery*. Cambridge, MA: MIT Press, 1996:287–96.

5 Varley P. Techniques of development of safety-related software in surgical robots. *IEEE Trans. Inform Technol Biomed*, 1999;3(4):261–7.

6 Rau G, Radermacher K, Thul B, Pichler CV. Aspects of ergonomic system design applied to medical work stations. In: Taylor RH, *et al.*, eds. *Computer-integrated surgery*. Cambridge, MA: MIT Press, 1996:203–22.

7 Sheridan T. Human factors in telesurgery. In: Taylor RH, *et al.*, eds. *Computer-integrated surgery*. Cambridge, MA: MIT Press, 1996:223–30.

8 Taylor RH, Paul HA, Kazandzides P, Mittelstadt BD, Hanson W, Zuhars JF, Williamson B, Musits BL, Glassman E, Bargar WL. An image-directed robotic system for precise orthopaedic surgery. *IEEE Trans Robot and Automation* 1994;10(3):261–75.

9 Mittelstadt B, Kazanzides P, Zuhars J, Williamson B, Cain P, Smith F, Bargar W. The evolution of a surgical robot from prototype to human clinical use. In: Taylor RH, *et al.*, eds. *Computer-integrated surgery*. Cambridge, MA: MIT Press, 1996:397–407.

10 Taylor RH, Joskowicz L, Williamson B, Gueziec A, Kalvin A, Kazanzides P, Vorhis RV, Yao J, Kumar R, Bzostek A, Sahay A, Borner M, Lahmer A. Computer-integrated revision total hip replacement surgery: concept and preliminary results. *Medi Image Anal* 1999;3(3):301–19.

11 Bargar W, DiGioia A, Turner R, Taylor J, McCarthy J, Mears D. Robodoc multi-center trial: an interim report. *Proceedings of the 2nd International Symposium on Medical Robotics and Computer Assisted Surgery*, 1995: Nov 4–7, 208–14. Baltimore, MD: MRCAS'95 Symposium, C/O Center for Orthop Res, Shadyside Hospital, Pittsburgh, PA.

12 Boerner M, Wiesel U. European experience with an operative robot for primary and revision total hip—a summary of more than 3800 cases at BGU Frankfurt. *Proceedings of CAOS USA*, 2001, July 6–8, 95–8. Pittsburgh: CAOS International.

13 Krismer M, Nogler M, Kaufmann C, Ogon M. Cement removal by robot vs manual procedure. *Proceedings of CAOS USA*, 2001, July 6–8, 99–102. Pittsburgh: CAOS International.

14 Peterman J, Kober R, Heinze P, Heekt P, Gotzen L. Implementation of the CASPAR system in the reconstruction of the ACL. *CAOS/USA*, 2000, 86–7. Pittsburgh: Shadyside Hospital.

15 Wiesel U, Lahmer A, Tenbusch M, Borner M. Total knee replacement using the robodoc system; *Proceedings of the 1st Annual Meeting of CAOS International*, 2001, 88. Davos.

16 Tenbusch M, Lahmer A, Wiesel U, Borner M. First results using the robodoc system for total knee replacement. *1st Annual Meeting of CAOS International*, 2001, 133. Davos.

17 Mai S, Lorke C, Siebert W. Motivation, realization, and first results of robot assisted total knee arthroplasty. *Proceedings of the 1st Annual Meeting of CAOS International*, 2001, 90. Davos.

18 Mai S, Siebert W. Planning and technique using the robot-system 'CASPAR' for TKR. *Proceedings of CAOS. USA*, 2001, July 6–8, 278–88. Pittsburgh: CAOS International.

19 Siebert W, Mai S. One year clinical experience using the robot system 'CASPAR' for TKR. *Proceedings of CAOS USA*, 2001, July 6–8, 141–2. Pittsburgh: CAOS International.

20 Wiesel U, Boerner M. First experiences using a surgical robot for total knee replacement. *Proceedings of CAOS USA*, 2001, July 6–8, 143–6. Pittsburgh: CAOS International.

21 Garbini JL, Kaiura RG, Sidles JA, Larson RV, Matson FA. Robotic instrumentation in total knee arthroplasty. *Proceedings of 33rd Annual Meeting, Orthopaedic Research Society*, 1987, 413. San Francisco.

22 Fadda M, Wang T, Marcacci M, Martelli S, Dario P. *et al.* Computer-assisted knee arthroplasty at Rizzoli institutes. *Proceedings of 1st International Symposium on Medical Robotics and Computer Assisted Surgery*, 1994, 26–31. Pittsburgh.

23 Harris SJ, Lin WJ, Fan KL, Hibberd RD, Cobb J, Middleton R, Davies BL. Experiences with robotic systems for knee surgery; *Proceedings of 1st Joint Conference of CVRMed and MRCAS*, 1997, March 19–22, 757–66. Grenoble, France: Springer.

24 Ho SC, Hibberd RD, Davies BL. Robot Assisted Knee Surgery. *IEEE EMBS Mag Spl Issue on Robot Surg*, 1995;(April–May):292–300.

25 Kienzle TC, Stulberg SD, Peshkin A, Quaid A, Wu CH. An integrated CAD-robotics system for total knee replacement surgery. *Proceedings on IEEE International Conference on Robotics and Automation*, 1993, 889–94. Atlanta.

26 Leitner F, Picard F, Minfelde R, Schulz H-J, Cinquin P, Saragaglia D. Computer-assisted knee surgical total replacement. *Proceedings of 1st Joint Conference of CVRMed and MRCAS*, 1997, March 19–22, 629–38. Grenoble, France: Springer.

27 Kienzle TC, Stulberg SD, Peshkin A, Quaid A, lea J, Goswami A, Wu CH. Total knee replacement. *IEEE EMBS Mag Spl Issue Robot in Surg* 1995;(April–May):301–6.

28 Marcacci S, Dario P, Fadda M, Marcenaro G, Martelli S. Computer-assisted knee arthroplasty. In: Taylor RH *et al.*, eds. *Computer-integrated surgery*. Cambridge, MA: MIT Press, 1996:417–23.

29 Brandt G, Radermacher K, Lavallee S, Staudte H-W., Rau G. A compact robot for image-guided orthopaedic surgery: concept and preliminary results; *Proceding of 1st Joint Conference of CVRMed and MRCAS*, 1997, March 19–22, 767. Grenoble, France: Springer.

30 Yoon YS, Shin HC, Park YB, Kwon DS, Lee JJ, and Won CH. Robot assisted THA surgery using gauge based registration; *Proceedings of CAOS USA*, 2001. July 6–8, 117–20. Pittsburgh: CAOS International.

31 Kwoh YS, Hou. J, Jonckheere EA, *et al.* A robot with improved absolute positioning accuracy for CT guided stereotactic brain surgery. *IEEE Trans Biomed Eng* 1988;35(2):153–61.

32 Cinquin P, Troccaz J, Demongeot J, Lavallee S, Champleboux G, Brunie L, Leitner F, Sautot P, Mazier B, Perez A, Djaid M, Fortin T, Chenic M, Chapel A. IGOR: image guided operating robot. *Innovation et Technonogie en Biologie et Medicine* 1992;374–94.

33 Lavallee S, Troccaz J, Gaborit L, Cinquin P, Benabid AL, Hoffman D. Image-guided operating robot: a clinical application in stereotactic neurosurgery, In: Taylor RH *et al.* eds. *Computer-integrated Surgery*. Cambridge, MA: MIT Press, 343–52.

34 Bzostek A, Barnes AC, Kumar R, Anderson JH, Taylor RH. A testbed system for robotically assisted percutaneous pattern therapy. In: *Medical Image Computing and Computer-Assisted Surgery*. Cambridge, England: Springer, 1999:1098–107.

35 Schreiner S, Anderson J, Taylor R, Funda J, Bzostek A, Barnes A. A system for percutaneous delivery of treatment with a fluoroscopically-guided robot. *Joint Conference of Computer Vision, Virtual Reality, and Robotics in Medicine and Medical Robotics and Computer Surgery*, 1997. Grenoble, France.

36 Bzostek A, Schreiner S, Barnes AC, Caddedu JA, Roberts W, Anderson JH, Taylor RH, Kavoussi LR. An automated system for precise percutaneous access of the renal collecting system. *Proceedings of 1st Joint Conference of CVRMed and MRCAS*, 1997, March 19–22 Grenoble, France: Springer.

37 Bishoff JT, Stoianovici D, Lee BR, Bauer J, Taylor RH, Whitcomb LL, Cadeddu JA, Chan D, Kavoussi LR. RCM-PAKY: clinical application of a new robotics system for precise needle placement. *J Endourol*, 1998;12:S82.

38 Cadeddu J, Stoianovici D, Taylor R, Whitcomb L, Jackman S, Lee B, Bishoff JT, Fabrizio MD, Jarrett TW, LR Kavoussi, A robotic system for percutaneous renal access incorporating a remote center of motion design. *J Endourol* 1998;12:S237.

39 Fichtinger G, Stoianovici D, Taylor RH. Surgical CAD/CAM and its application for robotically assisted percutaneous procedures. *IEEE 30th Applied Imagery Pattern Recognition Workshop (AIPR)*, 2001, October 10–12, 3–8. Washington, DC.

40 Fichtinger G, Masamune K, Patriciu A, Tanacs A, Anderson JH, DeWeese TL, Taylor RH, Stoianovici. Robotically assisted percutaneous local therapy and biopsy. *IEEE 10th International Conference of Advance Robotics*, 2001;133–51. ISBN 963-7154-043.

41 Fichtinger G, DeWeese TL, Patriciu A, Tanacs A, Mazilu D, Anderson JH, Masamune K, Taylor RH, Stoianovici D. System for robotically assisted prostate biopsy and therapy with intra-operative CT guidance. *J Acad Radiol* 2002;9:60–74.

42 Masamune K, GF, Patriciu A, Susil R, Taylor R, Kavoussi L, Anderson J, Sakuma I, Dohi T, Stoianovici D. Guidance system for robotically assisted percutaneous procedures with computed tomography. *Comput Assisted Surg* 2001;6:370–83.

43 Patriciu A, Stoianovici D, Whitcomb L, Jarrett T, Mazilu D, Stanimir A, Iordachita I, Anderson J, Taylor R, Kavoussi L. Motion-based robotic instrument targeting under c-arm fluoroscopy. In: *Medical Image Computing and Computer-Assisted Interventions*, 2000, October 11–14, 988–98. Pittsburgh: Springer.

44 Stoianovici D, Whitcomb L, Anderson J, Taylor R, Kavoussi L. A modular surgical robotic system for image-guided percutaneous procedures. In: *Medical Image Computing and Computer-Assisted Interventions (MICCAI-98)*, 1998, October 11–13, 404–10. Cambridge, MA: Springer.

45 Kaiser WA, Fischer H, Vagner J, Selig M. Robotic system for biopsy and therapy of breast lesions in a high-field whole-body magnetic resonance tomography unit. *J Invest Radiol* 2000;35(8):513–19.

46 Loser M, Navab N, Bascle B, Taylor R. Visual servoing for automatic and uncalibrated percutaneous procedures. *Proceedings of SPIE Medical Imaging*, 2000:270–81.

47 Cleary K. ed. *Workshop Report: Technical Requirements for Image-Guided Spine Procedures (April 17–20, 1999)*. Washington, DC: Georgetown University Medical Center, 1999:113.

48 Finlay P. *et al.* Orthosista: an active surgical localiser for assisting orthopaedic fracture fixation. In: *Medical Robotics and Computer-Assisted Surgery*, 1995.

49 Prasad S, Li M, Ramey N, Frassica F, Taylor R. A minimally invasive approach to pelvic osteolysis. *Proceedings of Computer-Assisted Orthopaedic Surgery*, 2002:349–50.

50 Joskowicz L, Taylor RH, Williamson B, Kane R, Kalvin A, Gueziec A, Taubin G, Funda J, Gomory S, Brown L, McCarthy J. Computer-integrated revision total hip replacement surgery: preliminary results. *Proceedings of 2nd International Symposium on Medical Robotics and Computer Assisted Surgery*, 1995, November 4–7, 193–202. Baltimore, MD: MRCAS '95 Symposium, C/O Center for Orthop Res, Shadyside Hospital, Pittsburgh, PA.

51 Taylor RH, Joskowicz L, Williamson B, Gueziec A, Kalvin A, Kazanzides P, VanVorhis R, Yao JH, Kumar R, Bzostek A, Sahay A, Borner M, Lahmer A. Computer-integrated revision total hip replacement surgery: concept and preliminary results. *Med Image Anal* 1999;3(3):301–19.

52 Susil RC, Anderson JH, Taylor RH. A single image registration method for CT guided interventions. *Second International Symposium on Medical Image Computing and Computer-Assisted Interventions (MICCAI99)*, 1999, 798–808. Cambridge, England: Springer.

53 Solomon S, Patriciu A, Taylor RH, Kavovssi L, Stoianovici D. CT guided robotic needle biopsy: a precise sampling method minimizing radiation exposure. *Radiology* 2002;225:277–82.

54 Masamune K, Patriciu A, Stoianovici D, Susil R, Fichtinger G, Kavoussi L, Anderson J, Taylor R, Sakuma I, Dohi T. Development of CT-PAKY frame system—CT image guided needle puncturing manipulator and a single slice registration for urological surgery. *Proceedings of 8th Annual Meeting of JSCAS*, 1999, 89–90. Kyotop.

55 Masamune K, Patriciu A, Stoianovici D, Susil R, Taylor R, Fichtinger G, Kavoussi LR, Anderson J, Sakuma I, Dohi T. CT image guided needle puncturing manipulator and a single slice registration for needle placement therapy. *J Comput Aided Surg* 2001;6:370–83.

56 Green P. Telepresence surgery. *NSF Workshop on Computer Assisted Surgery*, 1993. Washington, DC.

57 Green P, Jensen J, Hill J, Shah A. Mobile telepresence surgery. *Proceedings of 2nd International Symposium on Medical Robotics and Computer Assisted Surgery*, 1995, Nov 4–7, 97–103. Baltimore, Md.: MRCAS '95 Symposium, C/O Center for Orthop Res, Shadyside Hospital, Pittsburgh, PA.

58 Guthart GS, Salisbury JK. The intuitive telesurgery system: overview and application. *Proceedings of the IEEE International Conference on Robotics and Automation (ICRA2000)*, 2000, April. San Francisco.

59 Reichenspurner H, Demaino R, Mack M, Boehm D, Gulbins H, Detter C, Meiser B, Ellgass R, Reichart B. Use of the voice controlled and computer-assisted surgical system zeus for endoscopic coronary artery surgery bypass grafting. *J Thoracic Cardiovas Surg* 1999;118(1).

60 Charles S, Williams RE, Hamel B. Design of a surgeon-machine interface for teleoperated microsurgery. *Proceedings of the Annual International Conference of the IEEE Engineering in Medicine and Biology Society* 1989;11:883–4.

61 Mitsuishi M, Watanabe T, Nakanishi H, Hori T, Watanabe H, Kramer B. A telemicrosurgery system with colocated view and operation points and rotational-force-feedback-free master manipulator. *Proceedings 2nd International Symposium on Medical Robotics and Computer Assisted Surgery*, 1995, November 4–7, 111–18. Baltimore, MD: MRCAS '95 Symposium, C/O Center for Orthop Res, Shadyside Hospital, Pittsburgh, PA.

62 Salcudean SE, Ku S, Bell G. Performance measurement in scaled teleoperation for microsurgery. *First Joint Conference Computer Vision, Virtual Realtiy and Robotics in Medicine and Medical Robotics and Computer-Assisted Surgery*, 1997, 789–98. Grenoble, France: Springer.

63 Ku S Salcudean SE. Dexterity enhancement in microsurgery using a motion-scaling system and microgripper. *IEEE International Conference on Systems, Man and Cybernetics*, 1995, October 22–25. Vancouver, BC, Canada: IEEE.

64 Troccaz J, Peshkin M, Davies BL. The use of localizers, robots, and synergistic devices in CAS. *Proceedings of First Joint Conference of CVRMed and MRCAS*, 1997, March 19–22, 727–9. Grenoble, France: Springer.

65 Taylor R, Jensen P, Whitcomb L, Barnes A, Kumar R, Stoianovici D, Gupta P, Wang Z, deJuan E, Kavoussi L. A steady-hand robotic system for microsurgical augmentation. *Int J Robotics Res* 1999;18(12).

66 Davies B, Harris S, Jakopec M, Fan K, Cobb J. Intra-operative application of a robotic knee surgery system. In: *Medical Image Computing and Computer-Integrated Medical Interventions (MICCAI)*, 1999. Cambridge: Springer.

67 Davies B, Harris S, Jakopec M, Cobb J. A novel hands-on robot for knee replacement surgery. In: *Computer Assisted Orthopaedic Surgery USA (CAOS USA)*, 1999, 70–4, Pittsburgh: UPMC Medical Center.

68 Yao J, Taylor RH, Goldberg RP, Kumar R, Bzostek A, Vorhis RV, Kazanzides P, Gueziec A, Funda J. A progressive cut refinement scheme for revision total hip replacement surgery using C-arm fluoroscopy.

In: *Medical Image Computing and Computer-Assisted Interventions (MICCAI-99)*, 1999, October 11–13, 1010–19, Cambridge, England: Springer.

69 Yao J, Taylor RH, Goldberg RP, Kumar R, Bzostek A, Vorhis RV, Kazanzides P, Gueziec A, A C-arm fluoroscopy-guided progressive cut refinement strategy using a surgical robot. *Comput Aided Surg* 2000;5(6):373–90.

70 Joskowicz L, Taylor RH, Williamson B, Kane R, Kalvin A, Gueziec A, Taubin G, Funda J. Computer integrated revision total hip replacement surgery: preliminary report. *Second Annual International Symposium on Medical Robotics and Computer Assisted Surgery*, 1995, 193–202. Baltimore, MD.

71 Stoianovici D, Whitcomb LL, Anderson JH, Taylor RH, Kavoussi LR. A modular surgical robotic system for image guided percutaneous procedures. *International Conference on Medical Image Computing and Computer-Assisted Intervention*, 1998. Cambridge, MA, USA.

Chapter 8

Surgical navigation systems

Branislav Jaramaz

8.1 **Preoperative-model systems**

Preoperative-model systems rely on three-dimensional preoperative images (CT or MR) for surgical planning and navigation. In most cases images are processed so that the 3D models of bones can be viewed in a perspective view from an arbitrary viewpoint, in addition to cross-sectional views through the scan volume. During the preoperative planning phase the elements of surgical intervention are specified relative to the preoperative medical image, and the derived 3D bone models. In most cases, it is necessary to define the anatomic landmarks and bone reference systems first, and use them as a basis of the preoperative plan. For example, to plan the placement of the acetabular cup in THR, the anatomic reference system of the pelvis is defined first, based on the anterior pelvic plane. The implant model is then selected from a database and its position and orientation within the bone model is specified. In some cases, a simulation of postoperative performance, such as the range of motion, is a part of the planner. Once the preoperative plan is developed, it serves as a blueprint for surgical intervention. Its execution during surgery requires several technical steps: tracking, tool calibration, registration, and navigation interfacing. The tracking is achieved by attaching tracking markers to bones of interest and to the surgical tools, and by tracking those markers using a positional tracking device. However, while the tracking device can measure the positions of tracking markers in space, the system does not initially know where the associated tools or bones are relative to those markers. To resolve that issue, the tools need to be calibrated, i.e. the key geometric features of the tool (axis of a drill, cutting plane of a saw, etc.) are specified relative to the tool's tracking marker. Similarly, the surgical plan and the reference bone model needs to be mapped to the position of the target bone in the operating room through the registration process described in the previous chapter.

The orientation of tools relative to the bone of interest can then be calculated and compared to the planned one and presented to the user in a visual form. In addition, the positions of the tools relative to the preoperative plan can be displayed in real time, both numerically and visually, enabling surgical navigation. Figure 8.1 illustrates a typical preoperative model system: (1) A tomographic scan of the patient is obtained and (2a) transferred to the planning station. (2b) The bone model is segmented from the scan, and (2c) the anatomic reference system is defined. (2d) The surgical plan is specified and (2e) tested in a virtual simulation. (3) Intra-operatively, the tools and bones are tracked using a position measurement system. Tools are calibrated and the preoperative plan is registered to the target bones. (4) The tools are then navigated in the planned position. Because these systems rely on preoperative images, instead of ones taken during surgery, they are sometimes called 'canned reality' systems.

8.2 **Intra-operative-model systems**

In intra-operative model systems, the anatomic reference system is established and the surgical plan is specified during surgery. The key information is obtained after the tracking markers are rigidly attached

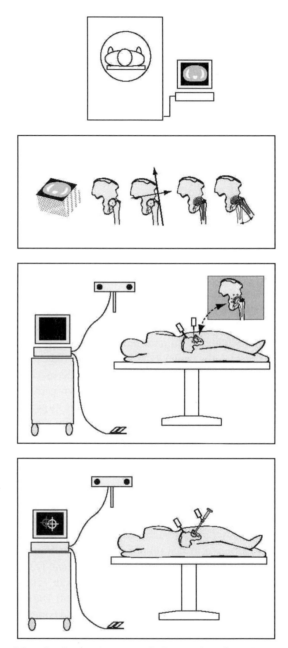

Fig. 8.1 Preoperative-model navigation system—a typical procedure flow. A tomographic scan of the patient is obtained and transferred to the planning station. The bone model is segmented from the scan, and the anatomic reference system is defined. The surgical plan is then specified and tested in a virtual simulation. Intra-operatively, the tools and bones are tracked using a position measurement system. The plan model is registered to the target bones. The tools are guided in the planned position.

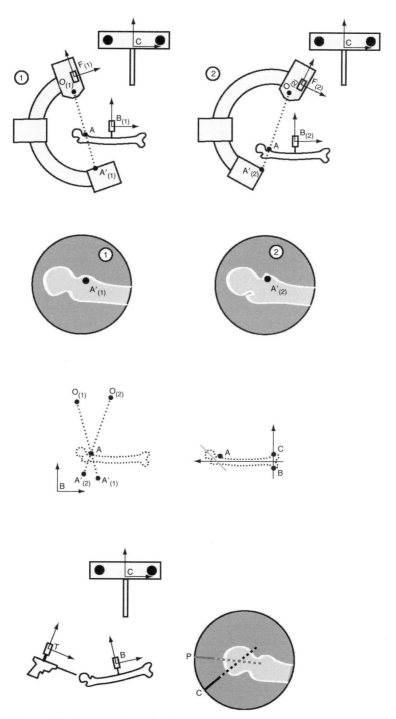

Fig. 8.2 Typical steps of the fluoroscopic navigation procedure.

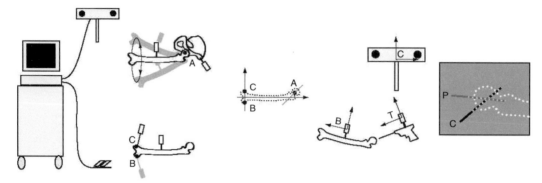

Fig. 8.3 Image-free navigation procedure.

to the target bones, hence eliminating the need for registration. The image based systems rely on intra-operative images, while the image-free systems obtain the key information and establish references without the use of imaging devices. The intra-operative imaging devices used in surgical navigation to date include CT and MR scanners and fluoroscopes. Obtaining images intra-operatively is particularly beneficial in trauma surgery, where the geometric configuration of the target bones may change from the time of imaging, and additional transporting and scanning of the patient may not be desirable. Due to their size and cost, intra-operative MR and CT scanners are not widely used in orthopaedic surgery, while fluoroscopy-based navigation is gaining in popularity. In order to avoid the need for registration, the position of the imaging device in the frame of the localizer needs to be known and the imaging device needs to be calibrated, so that the position of the image can be reconstructed in the localizer space. Figure 8.2 shows the typical flow of the fluoroscopic navigation procedure. Using a tracked and calibrated fluoroscopy imager, pairs of two nearly orthogonal images are obtained of the target area and of all bony landmarks of interest and used to define the anatomic reference system. In the example shown, an anatomic landmark A is imaged using the positions 1 and 2. The user identifies the landmark position A' in the views 1 and 2, and the corresponding rays connecting the X-ray source and the imaging plane (OA') can be identified for both positions and transformed into the reference system of the bone. The landmark point is then defined at the intersection of these rays. Building on this basic procedure, reference systems and surgical plans can be specified. Finally, the actual positions of the tracked tools can be displayed in real time and correctly overlaid on the original fluoroscopic views (C), together with the surgical plan (P), enabling surgical navigation.

Image-free navigation does not use any medical imaging. Instead, the bone landmarks are either specified directly, by using a tracked pointer, or found as centers of relative rotation of two tracked limbs. Figure 8.3 shows a typical system (1); the landmark point A (hip center) is determined as a center of rotation of the femur relative to the pelvis, after the femur is manipulated in a spherical motion and the tracking data are collected for both the pelvis and the femur. The landmark points B and C are collected directly using the tracked pointing probe (2). The bone reference system is derived from the landmark points, and used to specify the surgical plan (3). The navigation step then compares the position of the tracked tools to the surgical plan and to the bone reference system, only without using patient-specific images.

More sophisticated approaches to image-free navigation are currently being introduced, that use statistical atlases of bone shapes and create a synthetic bone shape that fits the information collected in the operating room. While these applications cannot guarantee that the bone shape will be correct outside the areas where the shape is measured, they can in most cases create the bone models that approximate the specific case with sufficient accuracy, and provide better visual models for the user.

Chapter 9

Total hip replacement—robotic-assisted technique

André Bauer

9.1 Clinical challenges

Historically, total hip replacement was the first procedure performed in humans to remove destroyed joints and restore function through implanting an artificial joint surface. After a short period of partial replacement only of the femoral head's surface, THR in the way we still perform it today was introduced: the acetabulum is replaced by a polyaethylen or metal cup with a plastic inlay, and the proximal femur with neck and head is replaced by a component, which is placed into the proximal part of the bone, after head and neck were cut of above the trochanteric level. Early attempts of cementless fixation were less successful, and only after Charnley's invention of bone cement, THR proved to be a safe and reliable method that soon would be performed by thousands of surgeons. The use of bone cement showed a lot of advantages: 1. The cancellous bone in the proximal femur, supposedly to soft to give enough support to the implant, was fortified by the cement. 2. The cavity could be prepared without high accuracy, as the cement would fill any gaps between bone and implant. 3. The use of cement allowed for immediate weight bearing, as fixation was perfectly tight after hardening of the cement. Yet the use of bone cement was not without side effects: during polymerization toxic reactions were encountered, with a common, sometimes fatal cardiovascular depression in that period. In addition, the cement itself created problems: one more interface was added, and the elasticity module of cement neither matched the ones of bone or implant. The cement therefore always was prone to wear. Positioning of the implant was more difficult, because the implant was 'swimming' in the cement mantle. And finally, in the event of loosening and revision, all the cement had to be removed, this itself being in many cases a major undertaking. Although alterations in cement preparation, cement placement and implant design improved the cemented technique a lot, many surgeons regard cementless fixation and primary healing between bone and implant as the ideal solution in THR, specifically in younger patients.

In the development of cementless techniques, numerous variations in design of the implant and surface modeling were performed. This lead to an overwhelming variety of implants, with almost every orthopedic celebrity boasting his own implant. As the overall performance only can be judged after a period of 10 to 15 years, a lot of confusion was created with only view reliable and proven results. Even the invention of the so-called custom-made implants, created individually after CT data, could not solve the main problems cementless techniques were facing:[1]

1. Preparation of the femoral cavity with hand held reamers and broaches was inaccurate regarding the form of the implant (Fig. 9.1). Hard bone could deflect the reamer without the surgeon even noticing it. Although reaming techniques were constantly improved, studies showed the poor performance and the lack of tight contact between bone and implant.

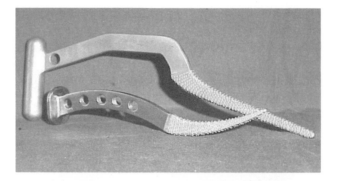

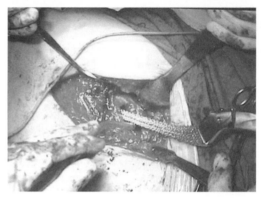

Fig. 9.1 Traditional instruments for preparation of femoral cavity during THR.

2. Planning was performed with acetate templates, laid over X-rays of the femur. The surgeon had to apply this two-dimensional plan to the real world at the patient. During surgery, the surgeon had to rely on certain anatomic landmarks in order to orient the implant and try to transform the preop plan. This orientation was impeded by the fact that only small parts of the bone were actually visible and the most of it hidden under soft tissue.

3. Many studies showed that the attempt of tight fixation of the implant in the femur led to a significant number of femur fractures, this fact in itself presenting a major factor for early failure of the implant.[2]

4. Finally modern reaming techniques, i.e. high-speed cutters, cannot be precisely applied by hand but need machine guidance.

Despite various changes in techniques and designs, certain principals in cementless THR were finally established: 1. To achieve primarily healing between implant and bone, close initial contact between prosthesis and bone is crucial. Thus any micro-motion can be excluded, and there is no room for rotational instability, which is seen as one of the major factors in aseptic loosening. 2. As important is the correct placement of the implant. Varus or valgus orientation have to be strictly avoided, and the proper antetorsion of the implant has to be considered. 3. Femur fractures must not occur. Obviously it is hard to meet these principals using the traditional techniques. Therefore, the rationale for the use of a robotic system was given.

9.2 **System description**

The Robodoc system consists of the actual robot, a computer cabinet, which is guiding the robot, and the Orthodoc workstation, which is the planning part of the system.

Orthodoc is a Linux based workstation, which transforms CT based data into images that will serve planning purposes. On the screen the image of the proximal femur of the patient is displayed in an a.p., a lateral and a cross-sectional view, and the level of the cross-section can be chosen freely (Fig. 9.2). Also displayed is a 3D reconstruction of the proximal femur. The system allows marking the center of rotation, measuring antetorsion, offset, leg length, as well as the marking of the site of the acetabular component. An implant library incorporated in the system currently consists of nine implant families, with all available sizes or modular combinations. The software allows the virtual placement of any selected implant into the bone and the control of all relevant parameters.

Data from Orthodoc to the robot are transferred by a tape or intranet. The robot is a modified industrial robot, specifically adapted for the use in surgery. On a five-degree-of-freedom arm the tools (either a probe or a high-speed cutter) are installed. The motion of the robot arm is reduced drastically, and a force sensor introduced between the tool and the robot arm prevents any application of exceedingly strong forces. The surgeon communicates with the robot by screen prompts and a remote control. Once the process of registration (see below) is finalized, the robot performs autonomously according to the preoperative established plan. Only application of strong forces, or detection of bone motion, will stop

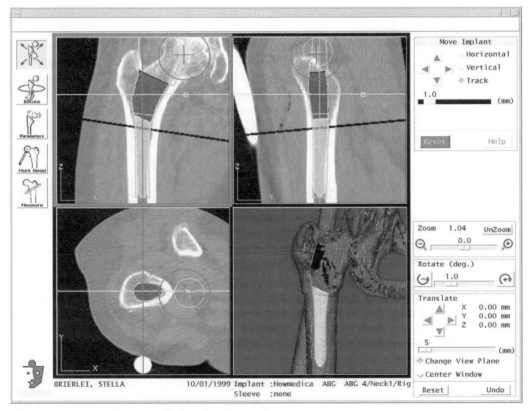

Fig. 9.2 Planning surface on Orthodoc planning workstation.

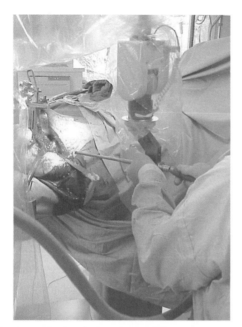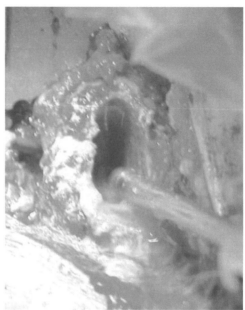

Fig. 9.3 Robodoc during surgery: the surgeon guides the reamer to the bone (left) and the high-speed cutter reams the cavity under constant irrigation (right).

the reaming process. The tool applied to the robot is an air driven high-speed cutter (70,000 r.p.m) with one-time use disposable cutters introduced into the motor. The system itself is not fit for sterilization, as the overall size is two meters and the weight more than 250 kg. Yet the system can be covered with sterile drape, through which the sterile motor assembly can be attached to the covered robot arm (Fig. 9.3). Also attached to the robot base are the bone motion monitors, checking any relevant motion of the bone, and a digitizer arm, which is used during surface finding in pinless registration.[3,4]

9.2.1 Indications

In principle, the robot procedure is indicated in every patient where a cementless total hip replacement is possible. As cementless stems require certain strength of the bone to support the implant, therefore elderly patients with clearly visible osteoporotic bone should be excluded from the procedure and provided with a cemented implant. The cutoff-age is somewhere between 65 and 70, but the selection is made individually for every patient according to the finding on the standard X-rays. Another critical point in relation to the indication is the weight of the patient. As will be pointed out later, the access for the robot to the bone, especially in the use of straight stems, is sometimes critical and extended soft tissue might either prevent the robot from reaching the bone or requires extensive skin and soft tissue release. Therefore, in some cases patients with extensive soft tissue layers at the proximal femur and over the hip joint should be excluded from the procedure.

9.3 Preparation

Planning on the Orthodoc workstation is the crucial part in the Robodoc procedure. As in any computer-assisted surgery, digital data are required from the patient in order to perform the procedure. In general, these data are retrieved from images. These can be ultrasound data, fluoroscopy data, MRI data, or the data from plain X-rays. In the Robodoc procedure, CT data are required to establish a plan and guide the robot. CT data have been selected, because currently they allow for higher precision than ultrasound, fluoroscope, or MRI data. Before the CT is performed, the surgeon has to decide on the mode of registration. The term registration describes the intra-operative matching between the virtual world in the computer and the real world, which the robot encounters during surgery. In the original Robodoc procedure, three pins, inserted before the CT scan in both femoral condyles and the greater trochanter, served these purposes. In an attempt to simplify this pin-based method, the two distal pins were later exchanged for one long pin, inserted into either the medial or lateral condyle. Today the standard is a pinless method of registration (DiGi Match Technology), which was developed and tested three years ago and is currently available to all users.

9.4 **Pin procedure**

The pin procedure itself is a simple procedure that can either be performed in local or regional anesthesia. The small titanium pins are canulated and can be inserted over a K-wire through stab wounds. In the proposed area at the condyles and the greater trochanter the exact position can be chosen freely, as this procedure is performed before the CT scan. Yet, a few precautions should be monitored: at the condyles an opening of the joint should be avoided. During insertion of the pin the position of the leg during pin finding (usually the ballet position) should be somewhat simulated, to ensure easy access to the pin during surgery. At the greater trochanter the rotation of the femur during surgery should be kept in mind to avoid burying the pin in soft tissue. Both pins (in the two-pin procedure) have to be touched by the robot in the center and on the plane, therefore an unlimited access to the pin during surgery and the pinfinding is mandatory. The DiGi Match Technology allows the performance of the CT without prior insertion of pins.

9.5 **CT scan**

During CT scan of the femur slices have to be taken from the top of the femoral head down to the knee. The CT has to follow exactly the scan protocol supplied by Integrated Surgical Systems (ISS). Slices through the knee are necessary both in pinless and pin-based referencing, as the orientation of the knee provides information on the femoral axis and the antetorsion. To avoid motion of the patient during the scan, the leg of the patient is comfortably, but securely fixed to the CT table. Also an aluminum rod is placed next to the patient. A specifically designed routine loaded into the CT allows the fast calculation of the data of this rod and thus detection of any motion of the patient. Patient motion was a major issue in the beginning of the Robodoc procedure, when the scan took between 30 and 45 minutes. Modern spiral CTs perform the necessary scan in less than 2 minutes, therefore scan motion is hardly detected anymore.

CT data (images are not required) are loaded on a MOD (multiple optical disc) or transferred to Robodoc via a network.

9.6 **Planning**

Planning starts with the importation of the CT data. Again, scan motion is checked. In the pin-based procedure, the two pins are identified by the system; this identification has to be acknowledged by the surgeon. Problems can be caused by metal artifacts in the femur, i.e. K-wires or screws. These are detected by the system; the surgeon has to use a special routine to exclude them and tell the system which metal pieces are the inserted pins and that the calculation should only be based on these two parts. During importation of the data, the surgeon also has the possibility to create a 3D model of the proximal femur and the joint. Once imported, the surgeon starts the actual planning procedure by opening Ortho 500, the planning software. On the screen he sees the images of the proximal femur in an AP, a lateral and a cross-sectional view. By moving the current axis in any image, views of the femur and the level of the cross-section can be easily adjusted.

9.7 Planning in the pin-based procedure

Once the images of the proximal femur are adjusted, the surgeon identifies the center of rotation by choosing this function and placing a red circle as a marker. He also can measure the current antetorsion by comparing the axis of the femoral neck and the condyles. The surgeon selects an implant from the implant library that currently contains the implant of eight different manufacturers. In anatomic implants the surgeon has to select the proper side. He tries to place the implant into a correct position on the screen. By watching all three images, he can correct the axis, the height, the distance to cortical bone, the offset, the leg length, and the centering of the distal tip. For every chosen implant he can select different sizes of heads and different neck length. By rotating the implant he can correct antertorsion. A separate function shows the outline of the reaming for every selected implant according to the recommendations of the implant manufacturer. This outline of the cutting path also gives information on the situation at the greater trochanter during surgery. This planning procedure normally takes between 10 and 15 minutes. If the surgeon is satisfied with the selection and the position of the implant in the bone, he saves the files and creates a transfer tape. He also has to check whether the proximal pin interferes with the cutting path or the implant. The finally created tape is then transported into the OR.

9.8 Pinless planning (Digimatch Technology)

The selection of the implant and positioning of the implant is identical to the pin-based procedure. In addition to the pin-based procedure, the surgeon also has to select a certain area at the femoral neck, which will during surgery serve the purpose of surface point identification. In this process the surgeon has to cut virtual slices through the femoral neck and outline the boundaries of solid bone. Very important for the surface identification is the differentiation between the solid bone and ostheophytes, which might be removed during luxation of the hip and capsular resection (Fig. 9.4). This surface identification is currently a rather cumbersome process, which will be automated in the near future.

9.9 Preparation of the robot

Before the surgery starts, the robot has to perform a routine of nonsterile and then, after draping, sterile calibration. Normally these calibration processes are done parallel to the usual preparations for the surgery. The sterile draping of the robot has to be done by the nurse, who also attaches the sterile motor unit and the probes.

9.10 Surgery

The surgical approach is at the discretion of the surgeon. Robodoc can be utilized with all standard approaches. The initial standard approach in the US trial was the dorsal approach with the patient in lateral decubitus, while in Germany and Austria the majority of surgeons use Robodoc with a standard antero-lateral approach.

Skin incision is similar to the hand surgery. Yet it is advisable, that the access of the robot to the bone is kept in mind when performing the skin incision. In the antero-lateral approach, a skin incision slightly more proximal and dorsal is recommended to facilitate the access. The joint is then exposed in the usual manner.

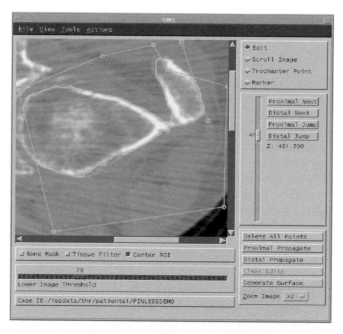

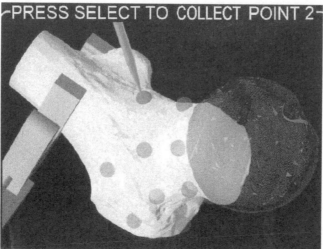

Fig. 9.4 Pinless registration: the screen for pinless planning (top); the screen guiding surface point matching during surgery (bottom).

9.11 **Pin-based surgery**

In pin-based surgery, the neck resection is performed in a level related to the preoperative plan. When a collared implant is used, the robot is preparing the neck file during the reaming. In collarless implants the neck is not further prepared by the robot, but at the end of the reaming the robot indicates the correct height of the neck resection. After neck resection the acetabular component is placed by hand in the usual technique. The leg is then brought carefully into the so-called ballet position. The lower leg of the patient is carefully placed on a leg holder and fixed there with sterile drapes. At the proximal femur the leg fixator is cautiously slid under the muscles a few centimeters below the lesser trochanter. It is there tightened with the screw. Fixation has to be tight enough to secure the clamp to the bone without any motion, yet a bending or fracturing of the bone strictly has to be avoided. The robot is brought to the table and the leg fixator is connected to the robot. All connections have to be tightened. The surgeon can verify manually whether the bone is fixed without any relative motion to the robot. A Homann retractor has to be placed under the greater trochanter to protect the medial gluteus muscle. An incision of the medial gluteus should be avoided. The surgeon inserts the probe of the bone motion monitor into the proximal femur with a minimum distance to the leg-fixator of 2 cm. He also has to make sure that the proximal pin is accessible. All these steps completed, the actual robot procedure starts. The surgeon is guided through the next steps by screen prompts on the computer mounted next to the robot. He has to expose the pins and guide the tip of the probe to the pin centers. After this process of pin finding the robot calculates the distances and angles of these two pins and compares the data to the data that he calculated from the CT slices. Only if these data match precisely, will the computer allow the continuation of the procedure. The probe is removed and a high-speed drum cutter is attached to the motor assembly. The surgeon has to connect compressed air and irrigation to the motor. He has to guide the cutter in front of the bone, from where the robot takes over. The robot moves to the top of the bone and starts cutting under constant irrigation. The surgeon can monitor the progress of the work on the screen holding in his hand a remote control. With this he can interrupt the reaming process instantly at any time of the procedure.

Difficult and critical in this phase is the access of the cutter to the bone. Especially in straight stems the robot chooses a straight approach to the bone, which is, correctly though, a very lateral approach. In patients with a very small or medially bowed greater trochanter the robot's cutting path might interfere with this structure and this could compromise the insertion site of the medial gluteus. As already mentioned, the surgeon should select in these cases an anatomic implant. The cutting path of the anatomic implants is more medially located and also allows for a different angle of the cutter. The orientation of the cutter in relation to the greater trochanter in these implants is between 0.5 and 1 cm more medially.

At the end of the reaming the robot is removed from the table, the proximal fixator is removed and the implant placed into the bone. Reduction is then performed with the preoperatively chosen neck length of the modular head.

9.12 Pinless surgery (DiGimatch Technology)

The pinless procedure differs significantly from the pin-based. The approach is the same. Yet, as a proximal femur and the femoral neck serve as registration surface, the hip should be either dislocated completely or only a very high neck resection can be performed. In pinless surgery it is advisable to do the femoral preparation before the acetabular preparation. The leg is positioned and fixated according to the pin-based procedure. The bone motion monitor is attached. The surgeon is then prompted by the computer to guide a separate digitizer arm, which is attached to the robot base, to certain points at the femoral neck. With a slim percutaneous probe also few point at the distal femur have to be digitized. This process of surface point registration is guided by prompts on the screen and is easily performed within 5 minutes. At the end of registration the surgeon places two small pins into the bone, one at the proximal femur and another one percutaneously at the distal femur. These pins serve as recovery markers in case a bone motion occurs during surgery. Simply by touching the tip of these pins with the digitizer any bone motion can be corrected. Thus with the Digimatch technology restart of the procedure after a bone motion is much faster. Once registration is completed, the surgery with the robot is performed in the same way as with the pin-based system. After finalizing the reaming of the femoral canal, first the acetabular component is placed and then finally the femoral stem is inserted.[5]

9.13 Animal experiment

The author performed an animal experiment in the years 1996/97 in cooperation with Dr. Ron Montgomery at the Auburn University in Auburn, Ala. Hand-broached hemiarthroplasty was evaluated vs. robot-assisted hemiarthroplasty in 20 greyhounds. Histology was performed at 35 days, 84 days, and 365 days. OR time was an average of 30 minutes longer in the robot group, and blood loss slightly higher. Two fractures occurred in the hand-broached group vs. none in the robot group. Positioning and reconstruction of the center of rotation was better in the robot group. Force plating 6 weeks after surgery showed a significant higher load transfer through the operated leg in the robot group. Finally histological examination showed a smoother and more accurate preparation of the interface, leaving strong unhurt trabeculae to support the implant and transfer load in the robot group, while destruction of trabeculae at the interface with consecutive remodeling impaired load transfer and led to large atrophy zones in the periphery.[6]

9.14 Clinical trials (United States)

In the context of a feasibility study for the FDA Dr. William Bargar performed the first Robodoc surgery on a human patient in the year 1992. This feasibility study with ten patients was followed by a randomized clinical trial, which was performed in three orthopedic centers in the United States. Follow-up for two years was documented in these cases. Significant differences were found in OR time and blood loss, with clear disadvantages in the robot group. Yet this higher blood loss and longer OR times were not reflected in the postoperative course, which, at least in the monitored follow-up, showed no significant differences in the group. The evaluation of the postoperative X-rays by a neutral observer showed better positioning, better selection of implant size, and less reaming artifacts in the robot group.[7,8]

9.15 Clinical trials (Germany)

The largest group of patients in a single arm study was operated at the BG-Unfallklinik in Frankfurt, Germany from 1994 on. The author was involved in this study until 1998 and reported early results in 1996 and in 1998. Boerner reported on the evaluation of 3800 primary and revision cases, operated in a period ending March 2001. Main results in this series are the development from three-pin-based over two-pin-based to pinless registration without sacrificing accuracy. A few pinless cases that showed a postoperative lateral shift of the implant finally could be identified as user errors. OR time in this series showed a constant improvement and is now steady at an average time of 90 minutes. No robot-specific complications were reported, but earlier weight bearing and faster rehabilitation were attributed to the accurate positioning of the implant and the precise preparation of the interface. The midterm results of the group operated in 1994 show no fractures and no loosening of implants. The overall results are favorable, yet the long term results are pending.[7,9–11]

9.16 Pitfalls

Main pitfalls are seen in the area of planning, men-machine interaction, and soft tissue management. Planning is the most important process in the whole procedure, yet the planning possibilities are more

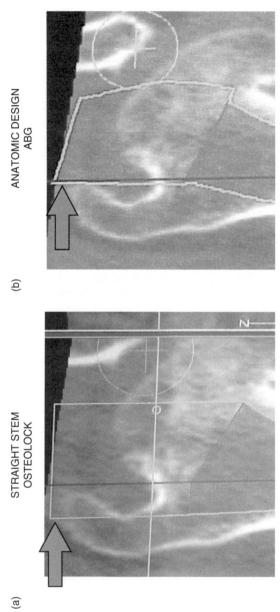

Fig. 9.5 Outline of cutting path (green line) in relation to the greater trochanter (arrow) in straight stem design vs. anatomic stem design. (See Plate 1.)

developed than the criteria established by surgeons. The possibility to plan for up to one tenth of a millimeter or 0.5 degrees ask for clear criteria in preoperative planning. These criteria still have to be established by the surgeons and validated in the further process.

Men-machine interaction or ergonomy is a crucial part of robot-assisted surgery. OR space is limited, and the current systems are rather bulky and cumbersome to use. Further research and development is necessary to enhance the integration of the system into daily routine and to promote men-machine interaction with the goal to make this type of surgery as smooth and fast as traditional surgery.

Finally soft tissue management in surgery involving robots reaches a new dimension. The robot is functioning to a preoperative established plan, but the surgeon has to guarantee free access to the bone. Already during the planning process possible interference between the cutting tool and soft tissue, for example the insertion site of the medial gluteus, has to be checked by the surgeon and precautionary steps have to be taken. These for example can be a selection of a different implant with a more medially oriented cutting path, as it is common in anatomic implants (Fig. 9.5). During surgery the surgeon has to control the access of the robot to the bone, and make sure that no soft tissue is compromised by any means. Insufficient soft tissue management might cause transitory or permanent damage, which would compromise the benefits of robot-assisted surgery.

9.17 **Discussion**

Cementless total hip replacement requires a thorough preoperative planning, exact preparation of the interface and positioning of the implant, with high degree of initial stability to facilitate healing between implant and bone. Clearly these goals are not easy to achieve with the traditional hand-broached method. Therefore a system offering computer based planning and robot assisted execution of the plan was developed. The system is based on images derived from CT scans. Based on these images a preoperative plan is established on a workstation, and this plan is executed by the robot within a tight tolerance frame.

Although the system comprises advanced technology and the success of the surgery relies on an intense man-machine interaction, animal experiment and clinical study have demonstrated that the technology is feasible and can be applied safely in routine surgery. Training of the surgical team, as routinely provided by the industry, is obviously sufficient and successful in preventing malfunction. The dramatic longer OR times in the US clinical trial can be explained by two facts:

1. The system itself was still a rather crude prototype, which proved to be cumbersome especially in the process of fixation and registration.

2. Because of the study set-up, intervals between surgeries were rather long and prevented formation of routine in the surgical team. The longer OR times shown in the animal experiment, with an average of 30 minutes, reflect the necessary time for fixation, registration, and reaming. The learning curve from the German study shows the same effect, with an average OR time of 90 minutes robot assisted surgery remained 20 to 30 minutes longer than hand-broached surgery. No clinical sequels like higher infection rates or higher incidence of thrombosis were monitored.

The animal experiment showed that fractures could securely be avoided. It also showed that despite a seemingly equal postoperative course, force plating revealed significant difference between the groups: unaware of the significance of their performance, the dogs in the robot group allowed significantly higher load transfer on the operated leg than the dogs in the hand-broached group. A possible reason for this might be the better fit of the implant and the undestroyed interface with continuous load transfer through the bone. The German study also showed the feasibility of robot assisted surgery in daily routine. No fractures were monitored, and no robot specific complications were reported. The learning curve not only led to shorter OR times but also helped to improve the planning process and selection of the implant, specifically regarding their situation at the greater trochanter.

Robot-assisted surgery now has to compare to navigator assistance during THR. A striking difference between robot-assisted and navigated surgery is the preparation of the cavity: in navigational systems this is done with traditional handheld broaches, that are guided by the navigational system. The system gives information to the surgeon about the orientation and location of the broach, thus enhancing the surgeon's abilities to guide the instruments. Yet he is still confined to the traditional instruments, while robot assisted surgery allows the use of a high-speed cutter, which performs a sparing preparation of the interface. On the other hand one has to see clearly that navigational systems are cheaper, easier to apply, and more flexible regarding applications.

In the nine years after the first surgery on a human patient in more than 7000 surgeries worldwide robot assisted surgery has demonstrated its feasibility and safeness. A striking advantage is the unavoidable necessity to establish a valid preoperative plan. Planning the computer based 3D planning is undoubtedly superior to the traditional templating over X-rays. The established plan is executed by the robot with highest precision, and this has been demonstrated in many surgical series. Fractures can securely be avoided; the position of the implant reflects precisely the preoperative plan. The interface is prepared without reaming artifacts and cancellous bone is cut precisely without causing any destruction. Whether this good performance in the 'surrogate variables (Bargar) will be reflected in better long term clinical outcome, will be answered within the next years. 2002 ten year results from the first series in Sacramento will be available and the ten-year follow-up after the randomized clinical trial will be finalized in the year 2004. By this time also ten year results from Unfallklinik in Frankfurt will be available.

9.18 Summary

Total hip replacement was the first application of robot-assisted surgery in orthopedics. The application of Robodoc was the first use of a robot within surgery worldwide. Since 1992, more than 7000 surgeries using Robodoc have been performed, and the system was also tested in animal experiment. The system underwent refinements, which helped to reduce OR time and facilitated the use of the system. The application of the system in routine surgery is safe and reliable. Robot specific complications were not reported. The clinical outcome is favorable, yet long term results are not available.

References

1 Freeman MAR, Railton GT. Die zementlose Verankerungin der Endoprothetik Orthopäde 1987;16:206–19.

2 Schutzer SF, Grady-Benson J, Hasty M, O'Connor DO, Bragdon C, Harris W. Influence of intra-operative femoral fractures and cerclage wiring on bone ingrowth into canine porous-coated femoral components. *J Arthroplasty* 1995;10(6):823–9.

3 Mittelstadt BD, Kazanzides P, Zuhars JF, *et al.* The evolution of a surgical robot from prototype to human clinical use. In Taylor RH, Lavalle S, Burdea GC, Mosges R eds. *Computer-integrated surgery.* pp. 397–407, Cambridge, MA: The MIT Press; 1996:397–407.

4 Paul HA, Bargar WL, Mittelstadt BD, Musits B, *et al.* Development of a surgical robot for cementless total hip arthroplasty. *Clin Orthop Rel Res* 1992;285:57–66.

5 Bauer A. Robot-assisted total hip replacement in primary and revision cases. *Oper Techniq Orthop* 2000; 10(1):9–13.

6 Bauer A, Boerner M, Montgomery R. Tierexperimentelle Untersuchungen zur Gestaltung des Interfaces bei roboterunterstuetzter Hemiarthroplastik. *Orthopaedische Praxis* 2000;36(12):762–6.

7 Bargar WL, Bauer A, Boerner M. Primary and revision total hip replacement using the Robodoc® system. *Clin Orthop Rel Res* 1998;354:82–91.

8 Bargar WL, Bauer A, DiGioia A, *et al.* Robodoc clinical results: domestic multicenter trial, European trial. AAOS Meeting, 1996. San Francisco, California.

9 Bauer A, Lahmer A, Boerner M. Robot-assisted surgery in total hip replacement-concept and clinical experience. *Comput Aided Surg* 1996;3(1):13–17.

10 Boerner M, Bauer A, Lahmer A. Computer assisted robotics in hip endoprosthesis. Unfallchirurg 1997; 100:640–5.

11 Boerner M, Wiesel U. European experience with an operative robot for primary and revision total hip replacement. *Proceedings of 5th Annual North American Program on Computer Assisted Orthopedic Surgery*, 2001. Pittsburgh.

Chapter 10

Total hip replacement—navigation technique

Branislav Jaramaz and Anthony M. Digioia III

10.1 Clinical challenges

10.1.1 State of the art in standard THR surgery

Consistently achieving correct alignment of implant components in Total Hip Replacement (THR) is still one of the main challenges orthopaedic surgeons face today. Clinical problems that stem from the lack of correct component alignment include reduced safe range of motion, implant impingement, dislocation, and accelerated wear.

Despite clinicians' and researchers' attempts to understand and prevent dislocation after total hip replacement, it remains the most common early post-operative complication. The incidence of dislocation is reported in the range from 1 to 5% following primary total hip replacement.[1–4] The causes of dislocation are multifactorial and include component malposition, patient related positional factors, soft tissue or bone impingement, soft tissue laxity, and implant design parameters such as the head to neck ratio of the femoral implant and acetabular liner design.[1,5–7] Of all the factors associated with dislocation, component malposition has been reported to be the leading cause. It is also the most easily correctable factor, and when corrected, yields a good post-operative result.[1,8–12] Prevention of malalignment has also been shown to be important because nearly all patients with recurrent dislocation associated with component malposition require revision surgery.[9,13] Although improvements continue to be made in the design of implants, methods of fixation and development of materials that better resist wear, little effort has been made to provide surgeons with more accurate tool guides or strategies to improve implant alignment.

One important factor affecting acetabular implant alignment is the orientation of the pelvis on the operating room table. McCollum and Gray[14] reported that the pelvis may not be reproducibly or correctly aligned with the patient in the lateral decubitus position and that the pelvic malalignment could lead to improper cup alignment. In the lateral position the pelvis may be flexed, and increased implant flexion would be necessary to achieve the desired anatomic anteversion of the acetabular component.

The position of the pelvis during activities of daily living may also influence dislocation rates by changing the 'functional' cup alignment. There are significant changes in the orientation of the pelvis especially in the direction of flexion and extension during sitting, standing, and lying supine.[14,15] These functional positions of the pelvis may play an important role in a patients' positional instability after total hip replacement.

All of these factors need to be taken into account by the surgeon in planning for and performing a total hip replacement.

Reducing the invasiveness of the surgical procedure is becoming an important aspect of hip replacement surgery, both for surgeons and patients. This should be achieved while maintaining or increasing the accuracy of component placement. In the current attempts, the surgeons lack preoperative and intra-operative tools which would permit surgeons to plan, test and validate functional implant alignment strategies on a patient-specific basis. Furthermore, there is a lack of proper intra-operative orientation landmarks to guarantee the correct placement of implant components. This is especially pronounced on the acetabular side of the joint. During surgery, bony anatomic landmarks of the pelvis are relatively obscured. Despite many techniques of stabilizing and positioning the patient's pelvis on the operating room table, most surgeons will admit that it is very difficult to precisely know how the patient's pelvis is oriented during surgery. The current mechanical guides provided by implant manufacturers are designed to align the acetabular component with respect to the coronal (abduction) and sagittal (flexion) planes of the patient. However, these devices assume that the patient's trunk and pelvis are aligned in a known orientation on the operating room table, and do not take into account the actual position of the pelvis or consider the individual variations in patients' anatomy.

The post-operative outcome is typically related to implant placement variables by correlating the outcome measurements to the implant alignment parameters measured from post-operative X-rays. However, in most cases the links between clinical outcome and implant related variables are not based on solid technical grounds. The measurements of implant alignment are based on post-operative X-rays and suffer from all inherent inaccuracies, the effects of one component are evaluated without considering the other implant component, etc. Although it is intuitive to surgeons that component alignment is an important factor, several large clinical series have concluded that component orientation is not associated with the risk of dislocation.[13,16–20] Other studies have shown a more direct relationship between malalignment and the risk of dislocation.[1,10,21–24] These studies, however, and nearly all prior clinical series, have been limited to using radiographic measures of acetabular alignment as opposed to true anatomic alignment.[10,13,16,19,20,25,26] Radiographic measures of cup alignment are dependent on the position of the patient's pelvis on the X-ray table and the angle of the X-ray beam with respect to the pelvis. These errors can lead to potentially significant variations in measured component alignment.[25–32] Radiographic measurements of version are especially sensitive to the position of the patient on the X-ray table.[27,28,31,32] Of numerous studies that tried to relate the radiographic measurements of cup orientation to the incidence of dislocation, only Lewinnek and coworkers[25] attempted to standardize the position of the patient with respect to the X-ray table and beam by leveling the anterior pelvic plane (defined by the anterior superior iliac spines and the pubic tubercles) to maintain a standardized pelvic alignment. The inability to measure accurately true acetabular alignment from the radiographic measures of alignment may be one of the reasons that the influence of component position on dislocation was not detected in some of these large clinical series. In addition, researchers have shown that there is significant motion of the human pelvis during activities of daily living such as sitting, standing, and lying supine.[14,15] These functional positions of the pelvis also may play an important role in instability following total hip replacement.

Therefore, clinicians and researchers need to know the true alignment of the acetabular component and account for functional changes of pelvic position during normal activities in order to relate implant alignment to patient outcomes.

10.1.2 Computer assisted orthopaedic THR surgery applications

Several surgical navigation systems for THR surgery have been developed over the last decade. The HipNav system is the first computer assisted and image guided clinical system used to assist in precise

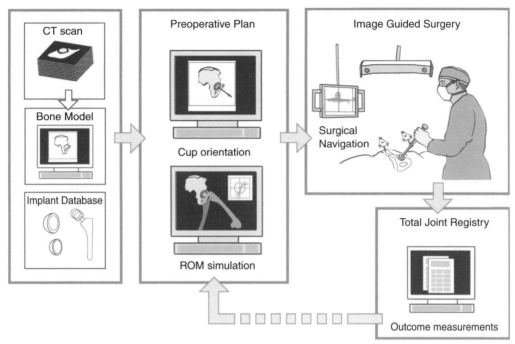

Fig. 10.1 Schematic drawing of the HipNav system (B. Jaramaz).

planning and placement of implant components in total hip replacement surgery.[33] Using position track-ing devices, HipNav provides surgeons with the tools to place the implants precisely within the bone and to measure its relative orientation. As a measurement tool, it also provides the insight into current practice, measuring the position of the patient's pelvis on the operating room table, the performance of traditional mechanical cup positioners, or the validity of radiographic measurements of cup alignment (Fig. 10.1).

10.2 System description

10.2.1 Classification

Currently available surgical navigation (passive robotic) systems for THR can be classified as either preoperative model, CT-based; intra-operative model, fluoroscopy-based; or image-free systems. HipNav is a CT-based system, using patient-specific preoperative-model and image based navigation.

10.2.2 Important concepts

10.2.2.1 Definitions and reference systems

All THR systems share some basic concepts regarding the anatomic references and definitions of implant alignment. Orientation of prosthetic components in THR is measured with respect to anatom-ically based reference systems. For the acetabular cup, the system is based on the anterior pelvic plane (APP). The plane is defined by the left and right anterior iliac spines and the middle point between the two pubis symphysys points. The transverse axis connects the anterior iliac spine points, and the other two axes are perpendicular to it and either laying in the APP or perpendicular to it (Fig. 10.2).

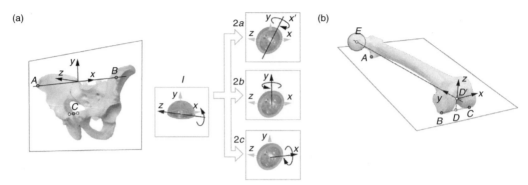

Fig. 10.2 Reference systems used in THR: (a) Pelvic reference system and the common definitions of cup orientation: (1, 2a) radiographic; (1, 2b) anatomic; and (1,2c) operative. (b) Femoral reference system.

There are three different definitions of cup orientation in common use, stemming from different practical approaches to the measurement of cup orientation:[35] anatomic, operative and radiographic. Like any rigid body, cup orientation can be defined in terms of three rotation angles. Given the axial symmetry of the cup and ignoring the rotation about the symmetry axis, the cup orientation can be simplified and specified in terms of only two anatomic angles. In all three definitions, the first angle is the cup abduction, followed by version (anatomic definition), flexion (operative definition) or rotation around the abducted axis (radiographic definition), as shown in Fig. 10.2.

For the femur, the coordinate system is based on the mechanical axis of the femur defined by the line connecting the femoral head center and the knee center. The transverse plane is defined by the lesser trochanter and the medial and lateral posterior condyle points. The knee center is defined as the midcondyle point translated with the transverse plane, as the plane is translated perpendicularly to pass trough the center of the femoral head.

The stem orientation is defined in terms of two angles of the stem axis and the version of the stem defined as the angle between the stem neck axis and the transverse plane of the femur. It is commonly assumed that the anterior pelvic plane coincides with the transverse plane of the body. However, since the flexion of the pelvis can vary individually and functionally, it should be treated in planning and simulation as a separate variable.

The HipNav system relies on three-dimensional CT images to create a patient-specific surgical plan. The system has two components: (1) a preoperative planner with range of motion (ROM) simulator and (2) intra-operative surgical navigation. The preoperative planner allows the surgeon to select the implant components and test the performance of the artificial joint and optimize the outcomes before the surgery. The navigation technology has been incorporated into a regular surgical routine and does not add significantly to the total time of surgery, since there are only few additional steps for the image guided procedure, and most of them are performed in parallel with the regular surgical flow.

10.2.2.2 Preoperative planning and simulation

Conventional planning for THR surgery with planar x-ray images and acetate implant templates only permits the surgeon to get an approximate implant size, and no orientation. The orientation of the components is left to be decided intra-operatively, based on the limited exposure to bony landmarks, surgical positioning guides, and the surgeon's ability to understand the spatial relationship between the patient's bones and implants. In the HipNav patient-specific preoperative plan, the implant size,

(a) (b)

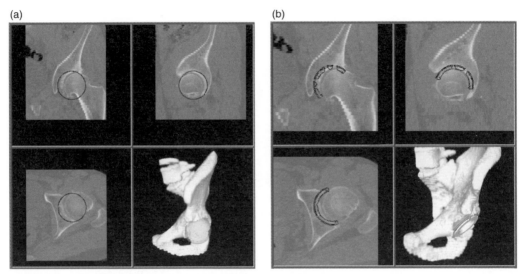

Fig. 10.3 Cup planning: (a) reamer position; (b) cup orientation.

position (Fig. 10.3a) and orientation (Fig. 10.3b) is determined using the CT scan and three-dimensional models of the pelvis and femur. The range of motion is then simulated for a given set of implant components using traditional ROM tests for anterior and posterior instability.[36] The procedure is fully interactive and allows the surgeon to search for an optimal size and orientation of both the femoral and acetabular components, by varying all the relevant parameters and immediately observing the effects on ROM, offset and leg length.

The patient's CT scan is electronically transferred to the planning site and processed during the planning procedure to extract the bone surfaces. Separate surface models of the pelvis and the femur are generated and used subsequently for visualization, simulation of ROM and intra-operative registration. The CT scan, surface models and implant database are used for preoperative planning. The planner comprises the following main steps:

(1) acetabular plan;

(2) femoral plan; and

(3) combined range of motion simulation and final implant adjustments.

In the acetabular part of the planner, anatomic landmarks are identified and used as reference points for the definition of the pelvic coordinate system. The orientation of the acetabular component is expressed in terms of the previously described anatomic APP reference system. The landmark points are identified automatically and verified by the surgeon. The position of the reamed acetabular cavity is planned by fitting a sphere into the acetabulum in three orthogonal CT cross-sections. This position is then used for placement of the acetabular component. The acetabular cup is then oriented in the full 3D pelvic model. The exact model and size of the acetabular component and liner is selected from the implant database.

The femoral planner follows parallel steps, with the identification of bony landmarks followed by the placement of the femoral stem. The femoral coordinate system is defined by the plane tangent to the lesser trochanter center and the posterior femoral condyles and by the axis parallel to that plane passing through the center of the femoral head and mid condyles. To define a femoral head center,

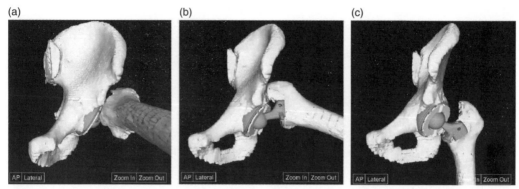

Fig. 10.4 ROM simulation: (a) internal rotation after 90° flexion (bone impingement); (b) max. abduction; (c) max. external rotation. The red dot indicates the impingement point. (See Plate 2.)

a sphere is fitted to the native femoral head using the orthogonal CT views and the three-dimensional femoral model. The other landmark points and the axis of the femoral canal are identified automatically and verified by the surgeon. After the make and size of femoral stem is selected and placed in its initial position, the planner permits the surgeon to interactively reposition and reorient both components, as well as adjust neck lengths. The information about the change in the leg length and the hip offsets relative to the preoperative position is displayed and continuously updated.

In the final step of the planner, the full 3D virtual anatomic model of the pelvis and femur with the artificial joint implanted is taken through the test of ROM. The range of motion simulation is interactively performed for a number of preselected leg motion paths that test for the anterior and posterior instability (Fig. 10.4). The surgeon can optimize the orientation of components with respect to both implant and bone impingement. Any desired leg motion path can be constructed as an ordered sequence of basic leg motions: flexion/extension, abduction/adduction, internal/external rotation and rotation in flexion. Leg motion is defined relative to the body and independent of pelvic position because there can be significant differences in pelvic orientation for various functional positions (e.g., sitting vs. standing positions). Pelvic flexion and extension is treated as an independent variable and controlled separately. All defined leg motion paths with the impingement limits are displayed on a single two-dimensional plot as well as on the three-dimensional model of the pelvis and the femur, and interactively updated for any change in surgical variables (i.e. implant size and design, neck length, femoral head size, implant orientation, acetabular hooded liners.) The interactive simulation permits for the fast and intuitive search for an optimal placement of all components. All leg motion paths are animated and the entire ROM path until impingement is displayed, with the impingement point marked on the three-dimensional patient model. Once the surgeon has finalized the plan and placement of implant components, all relevant parameters are stored for the image guided surgical procedure.

10.2.3 Surgical technique

The HipNav intra-operative guidance system has been designed to minimize the impact on the surgeon's normal routine. By attaching the tracking devices, the tools currently used in traditional THR are converted from 'passive' mechanical devices into 'smart' tools.

While any surgical approach can be utilized with HipNav, a posterolateral approach to the hip was used in our ongoing clinical tests. Over 250 cases have been performed to date. The patient is placed on the operating room table according to the surgeon's typical routine. Prior to dislocation of the hip,

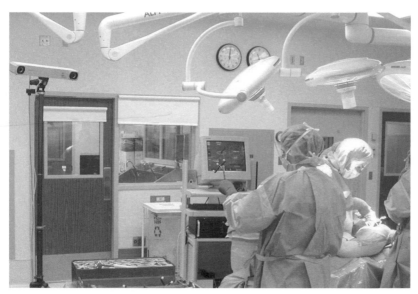

Fig. 10.5 HipNav setup. Probe calibration step.

a small counter incision is made near the wing of the ilium on the operative side. A small fixator and tracking marker are attached to the pelvis to permit real time tracking of the pelvic position during surgery. In general, a 2-millimeter pressfit technique was used to initially fix the cup and screws were used as supplemental fixation as needed. An optical tracking system and camera (Polaris, Northern Digital, Ontario, Canada) is used to monitor any bone or tool position (Fig. 10.5). The camera can determine the spatial location of markers with light emitting diodes (LEDs) with a submillimeter accuracy. The LEDs are attached to rigid frames (markers) and sequentially activated, providing the 3D spatial position and orientation of every marker. Any object can then be continuously tracked in space as long as an LED marker is rigidly attached. Alternatively, wireless 'passive' markers with reflective spheres are used for tracking.

A surface based registration technique is used[37,38] to relate the position of the patient's pelvis to the CT scan and preoperative plan. Surface points on the pelvis are acquired by touching the bone surface around the acetabulum using the pointing probe. In HipNav, 46 points are collected within three to five minutes in three zones on the pelvis: the superior acetabular rim, sciatic notch and percutaneously on the iliac crest. Surface based registration matches the cloud of measured points with the bone surface to establish the proper transformation between the position of the pelvis in the operating room and the CT based surface model in which the planned cup orientation was defined (Fig. 10.6).

After registration is completed, the pelvis can be continuously tracked in the operating room, and the relative position and orientation of any other tracked object (tools, instruments, bones) can be calculated and continually updated. To verify the registration process, the pointing probe can be used to point to known anatomic landmarks. The tip of the probe is displayed within the orthogonal planes of the CT and on the 3D surface model. This visual check permits for a quick test of the registration accuracy. This 'wand' capability also brings the three-dimensional medical images directly into the operating room as an on-line visualization aid for surgeons and gives the surgeon the ability to have direct access to a CT scan of the patient on the OR table.

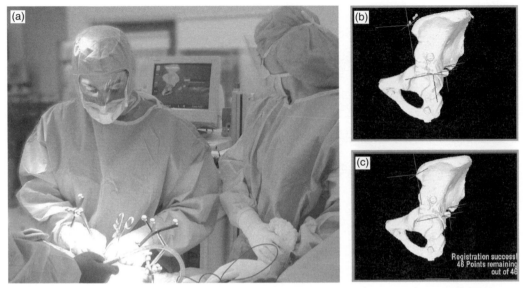

Fig. 10.6 Registration process: (a) collection of points; (b) before registration; (c) after registration.

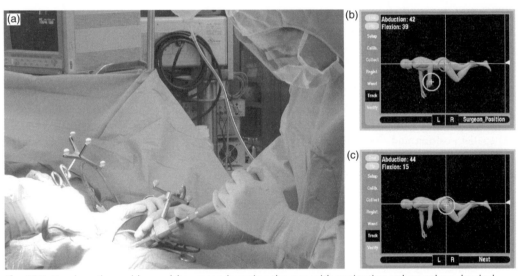

Fig. 10.7 Cup insertion guidance: (a) surgeon inserting the cup with navigation enhanced mechanical tool; (b) and (c) navigation interface.

The conventional mechanical alignment handle used to implant the acetabular cup is also instrumented with LED markers to allow its tracking in space. This permits continuous measurement of the orientation of the guide relative to the pelvis, and hence allows for active tool guidance (Fig. 10.7). HipNav permits the precise measurements and placement of the acetabular component in the preoperatively planned orientation. Alternatively, cup orientation can be adjusted during surgery based on any unexpected intra-operative findings.

By introducing femoral tracking and navigation using the same principles, the system extends its usability to intraperative control of stem placement. In addition to control of the femoral neck resection depth and version of the femoral component, the system can provide updated information on combined effects of both components to ROM, offset and leg length change.

10.2.4 Validation and accuracy

A series of experiments are being performed to validate the basic software component and to establish the accuracy bounds of both the individual system components and the system as a whole. The experiments include:

(1) validation of a range of motion simulator using a physical model covered with conductive paint, so that the low voltage electrical current is closed at the point of impingement;

(2) test of a surface reconstruction procedure;

(3) tests of tracking accuracy: testing the accuracy of point collection an a grid of known points;

(4) test of accuracy of registration: repeatability, sensitivity to the point selection process and distribution of points;

(5) factors affecting implant placement—final implant position vs. planned position;

(6) end-to-end accuracy of the system: the implant position in the sawbones model is measured using a coordinate measurement machine;

(7) post-operative measurement of implant alignment: preoperative CT scan and implant 3D geometric models are registered to post-operative X-rays in order to get precise three-dimensional measurements of implant position in an anatomic reference frame.

Probably the most important quantity to the practicing surgeon is the end-to-end accuracy measurement, which indicates how far off the final measured orientation of the implant may be from its actual location. For the HipNav system, we measured the end-to-end accuracy of the cup alignment using the navigation system, in the laboratory environment and by using plastic bone models and standard HipNav tools and procedures. We found that the end-to-end square root of the mean square error was 0.82° in abduction and 0.76° in version.[39]

10.3 Comparison with traditional techniques

Part of the protocol for the first 80 HipNav cases was the additional measurements of cup alignment using the traditional mechanical guide. The true orientation of the guide was measured when it was placed in accordance with the manufacturer's specification. (The intended cup orientation with the mechanical guide is 45° of abduction and 20° of flexion,* with the orientation frame aligned with respect to the patient's long axis and the operating room table.)

The acetabular implant is then placed in the planned position with the aid of a simple interface. In order to align the cup in the preoperatively planned orientation, the surgeon only needs to align the two sets of cross-hairs on the monitor screen. The actual measurements of version and abduction angles are also displayed. HipNav guides the surgeon to the planned orientation of the guide and also provides information about the deviation from the planned orientation. We have found that both the

---

* According to the operative definition of cup alignment.

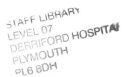

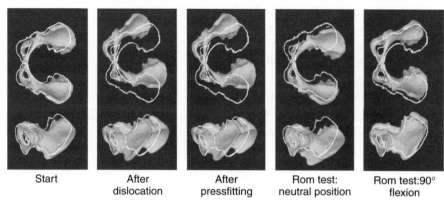

| Start | After dislocation | After pressfitting | Rom test: neutral position | Rom test:90° flexion |

Fig. 10.8 Typical measurements of pelvic orientation during surgery. The white outline represents lateral and AP projections for the theoretically ideal, or 'neutral', pelvic orientation. The full images show actual pelvic orientations measured during a representative HipNav surgery.

process of pressfitting the cup, and the application of screws used to provide additional stability can alter the final orientation of the cup. Therefore, after the insertion of the liner, the final orientation of the cup is measured using an adapter that is attached to the mechanical guide and fits the open face of the acetabular component liner. These final implant measurements can then be used to relate surgical technique and implant alignment directly to patient outcomes.

Pelvic orientation measurements were collected only during the first 40 cases, and complete measurements were available for 33 patients. One example of a patient's initial pelvic alignment on the operating room table and the change of orientation during acetabular preparation and implant alignment is presented in Fig. 10.8. The baseline pelvic orientation is set in the position for which mechanical guides were designed: the anterior plane of the pelvis is parallel to the longitudinal axis and perpendicular to the plane of the operating room table, and the transverse axis perpendicular to the table. This neutral pelvic position is presented as the white outlined pelvis in all subsequent figures and presented in the anteroposterior and lateral projections. If the patient's pelvis was initially aligned in the expected neutral baseline position and there were no changes in pelvic orientation during surgery, the pelvic images would be coincident with the white outlined pelvis.

Pelvic orientation measurements showed a statistically significant variation of the position of the pelvis from the desired neutral alignment on the operating room table. This was evident both initially and during the acetabular alignment phase of surgery for all patients and while using the identical surgical routine.[33,40] Version alignment was widely variable during the acetabular alignment phase of surgery. Pelvic orientation also changed from prior to hip dislocation to the time of acetabular alignment. There was a general trend towards increased flexion and anterior tilting of the pelvis during acetabular alignment with the patient in the lateral decubitus position. This was more pronounced following dislocation of the hip. For all patients, the pelvis was rarely aligned in the assumed neutral position during any phase of surgery. Most importantly, there was not a reliable or reproducible overall pattern of pelvic orientation that potentially could be taken into account by the mechanical guides in assisting surgeons with more accurate cup alignment.

10.4 Clinical trials: less invasive THR surgery

Wide surgical exposures in total hip arthroplasty (THA) provide visualization of the landmarks, accurate fixation and orientation of the implant, but at the same time require large soft tissue dissections, which

(a) (b)

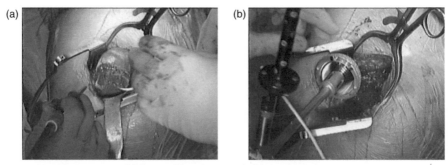

Fig. 10.9 Mini-incision THR surgery: (a) femoral head removal; (b) cup insertion.

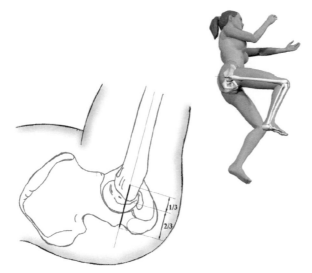

Fig. 10.10 Patient positioning and surgical incision for mini-incision THR procedure.

can increase post-operative complications. We compared in a prospective study the patient's short and early term outcomes using a mini-incision technique (Fig. 10.9) versus the traditional posterior approach for THA.[41] The mini-incision approach is a modification of the traditional posterior (Moore) approach, with significant variation in landmarks for initial skin incision. According to the description by A.H.Crenshaw (modification by Sequeira and Khanuja),[42] a straight incision about 13 cm long is made slightly posterior to the trochanter with the hip adducted and flexed at 90 degrees. The trochanter is at the midpoint of the incision. In contrast to this description, we found that for optimal use of the 'mobile skin window', the hip should be flexed about 70 degrees and two thirds of the incision should be proximal to the tip of the greater trochanter.

General anesthesia was used in all patients. The patient is placed in the lateral decubitus position with the operative side up. To properly align the incision for the surgical approach, the operative leg is positioned at approximately 70–80 degrees of flexion. The greater trochanter is palpated and an eight to twelve centimeter straight incision is then made in line with the femoral shaft with two thirds of the incision carried proximal and one third distal to the tip of the greater trochanter (Fig. 10.10). The skin incision is used as a mobile window in order to permit the visualization of the deeper tissues. The gluteus maximus muscle is split in line with its fibers. The leg is then held in maximum internal rotation and neutral or slight extension. The interval between the pyriformis and gluteus medius muscle is identified and the gluteus medius muscle is carefully retracted superiorly. A posterior flap including the short external rotators and the posterior capsule are then subperiosteally released from the femoral neck. Only standard retractors were used during the surgery. Prior to dislocation of the hip, a one centimeter incision is made over the wing of the ilium allowing application of the pelvic tracking clamp. This clamp has optical tracking targets that enable the navigation system to visualize pelvic position and intra-operative motion. The hip is then dislocated and the neck resection is made with a reciprocating saw.

Registration to the preoperative plan and CT scan is performed using a surface based technique.[33,34] Reaming is performed in a sequential manner. Medialization of the acetabulum is confirmed with the previously planned position. The navigation system allows direct interactive visualization of the medial wall of the acetabulum to determine the amount of bone resected. During acetabular cup impaction, the navigation system continually measures implant orientation, as the cup is pressfit. Supplemental screw fixation is used as necessary. Attention is then turned to the femur. The proximal femur is delivered through the incision by pushing on the knee with simultaneous internal rotation of the femur.

Preparation of the canal is then performed either for a cemented or cementless implant in a routine manner.[43,44] In this particular series, the femoral component was positioned without navigation. The closure is then performed in a routine manner with care taken to repair the posterior structures including the short external rotators and posterior capsule to the femoral neck.[45] All patients had a similar rehabilitation protocol with two sessions of physical therapy per day with weight bearing as tolerated on the first post-operative day.

Thirty-three patients (35 hips) (Group I) were selected out of 121 patients that had undergone a mini-incision THA matched by diagnosis, sex, average age and preoperative Harris Hip Score (HHS) to thirty-three patients (35 hips) (Group II) of 120 patients that had undergone THA using the traditional posterior approach. Both groups were enrolled in the HipNav clinical trial. In Group I, the average age was 65 years (range, 49–80 years old), and in Group II, the average age was 65 years old (range, 49–76 years old) (p > 0.5). In Group I (mini-incision) the average age was 65 years (range, 49–80 years old), in Group II (traditional incision) the average age was 65 years old (range, 49–76 years old) (p > 0.5). The average preoperative HHS was 52.29 (range, 24–74) in Group I and in Group II was 53.44 (range, 22–76) (p > 0.5). The HHS was measured prospectively and by independent observer prior to surgery, 3 months, 6 months and one year post-operatively for all patients.

The length of the skin incisions for Group II (traditional posterior approach) measured on average 20.2 cm (range, 14.8–26.0). The length of the skin incisions for Group I (mini-incision) averaged 11.7 cm (range, 7.3–13.0) (p < 0.001) At the 3 months follow-up, patients in the mini-incision group had significant improvement in limp (p < 0.05) and the ability to climb stairs (p < 0.01) compared to the traditional group. At the 6 month follow-up, the mini-incision group was significantly better in terms of limp (p < 0.05), distance walked (p < 0.001), and stairs (p < 0.001). There was no significant difference between groups in pain, function and range of motion at the one year follow-up.

10.5 **Discussion**

The results of our clinical trial show that mechanical guides currently utilized for acetabular alignment are inadequate in achieving their desired goal. There was significant variation in the range of the cup alignment and variation from optimal practice in abduction and especially in version alignment. The pelvis was not oriented in the assumed neutral location on the operating room table initially or more importantly, during acetabular alignment. For all patients, there were significant changes in pelvic orientation throughout the surgery. There was a general trend toward increased flexion and anterior tilting of the pelvis during acetabular alignment. However, the actual variation from patient to patient, and the magnitude of these differences was variable, leading to the inaccurate and unreliable acetabular implant alignment using the mechanical guides. The significant variability of the orientation of the pelvis on the operating room table implies that surgeons may need to consider the concept of functional cup alignment. As patients move from the supine to standing to sitting position, the orientation of the pelvis changes especially in the direction of flexion and extension. With the cup fixed in the acetabulum, the 'functional' orientation of the cup significantly changes through these positions of daily living. Therefore, functional acetabular implant orientation in addition to anatomic alignment may play a role in instability after total hip replacement and needs to be examined and characterized.

Several clinical series have associated the posterolateral approach with an increased incidence of dislocation compared to the anterolateral approach to the hip[14,46–52] Our results show that one contributing factor to explain this difference is the tendency towards retroversion of the acetabular component if cup alignment is based solely on the mechanical guides which would lead to increased posterior instability for surgeons that utilize the posterolateral approach. These results also show that one obvious strategy to improve acetabular component alignment is to introduce significantly more flexion of the cup than indicated by the mechanical guides during surgery in order to achieve more desirable anatomic anteversion. This adjustment in acetabular alignment is especially important for surgeons who perform a posterolateral approach to the hip with the patient in the lateral decubital position.

One solution may be the utilization of image guided navigation technologies to assist surgeons in obtaining optimal alignment based on individual patient pelvic anatomy. This technology can also inform the surgeon of the orientation of the pelvis during surgery. A secondary benefit of these image guided navigational tools is that alignment strategies, based either on anatomic landmarks or improved mechanical alignment tools, can be validated at clinical test sites using technology such as HipNav. This clinical information could then quickly be passed on to a larger surgical audience. The application of image guided technologies as a validation tool may have a wider clinical impact and improve patient outcomes in a shorter time period then extensive clinical use of the system itself.

Image guided tools for precise implant placement and augmented visualization of the patient's anatomy are also opening the door for significant advances in making the procedure less invasive. In our current trial, we have already been able to reduce the extent of soft tissue dissection by 60–70%, to between 8 and 12 cm skin incisions on a routine basis. Less soft tissue dissection is expected to result in reduced complication rates and speed recoveries of our patients. However, our challenge is to also improve the accuracy of surgical practice, even with less invasive approaches. The assistance of image guided surgical tools will open the doors for broader clinical acceptance and revolutionize our approach to joint reconstructive surgery.

Simulators and image guided surgical navigation systems hold a potential to assist surgeons in providing better care for their patients by optimizing both the surgical plan and the operative technique on a patient-specific basis. Only by coupling simulation based planning with precise surgical placement of implants can we fully take advantage of these new computer assisted tools. We have developed a comprehensive planner, simulator and intra-operative navigation system for THR. In the not too distant future, total joint simulators and planners will examine not only anatomic and kinematic factors, but additional effects such as the mechanical effects of pressfitting, long term levels of polyethylene wear, bone remodeling and resultant joint forces. Inclusion of other simulation variables will eventually allow surgeons to more reliably depend on the predictive capabilities of the planner/simulator and open the possibility of finding the automatically generated optimal solutions with respect to all relevant surgical decisions.

References

1 Dorr LD, Wolf AW, Chandler R, Conaty JP. Classification and treatment of dislocations of total hip arthroplasty. *Clin Orthop* 1983;173:151–8.

2 Eftekhar NS. Dislocation and instability complicating low friction arthroplasty of the hip joint. *Clin Orthop Rel Res* 1976;121(November–December):120–5.

3 Etienne A, Cupic Z, Charnley J. Postoperative dislocation after Charnley low-friction arthroplasty. *Clin Orthop Rel Res* 1978;132:19–23.

4 Turner RS. Postoperative total hip prosthetic femoral head dislocations. *Clin Orthop Rel Res* 1994;301: 196–204.

5 Brien WW, Salvati EA, Wright TM, Burstein AH. Dislocation following THA: comparison of two acetabular component designs. *Orthopedics* 1993;16(8):869–72.

6 Chandler DR, Glousman R, Hull D, *et al.* Prosthetic hip range of motion and impingement. *Clin Orthop Rel Res* 1982;166:284–91.

7 Hedlundh U, Ahnfelt L, Hybbinette C-H, Wallinder L. Dislocations and the femoral head size in primary total hip arthroplasty. *Clin Orthop Rel Res* 1996;333:226–33.

8 Daly PJ, Morrey BF. Operative correction of an unstable total hip arthroplasty. *J Bone Joint Surg* 1992; 74A(9):1334–43.

9 Hedlundh U, Sanzen L, Fredin H. The prognosis and treatment of dislocated total hip arthroplasties with a 22 mm head. *J Bone Joint Surg* 1997;79B(3):374–8.

10 Khan MAA, Brakenbury PH, Reynolds ISR. Dislocation following total hip replacement. *J Bone Joint Surg* 1981;63B:214–18.

11 Ohlin A, Balkfors B. Stability of cemented sockets after 3–14 years. *J Arthroplasty* 1992;7(1):87–92.

12 Ritter MA. A treatment plan for the dislocated total hip arthroplasty. *Clinl Orthop Rel Res* 1980;153(November–December):153–5.

13 Pollard JA, Daum WJ, Uchida T. Can simple radiographs be predictive of total hip dislocation? *J Arthroplasty* 1995;10:800–4.

14 McCollum DE, Gray WJ. Dislocation after total hip arthroplasty: causes and prevention. *Clin Orthop* 1990; 261:159–70.

15 Johnston R, Smidt G. Hip motion measurements for selected activities of daily living. *Clin Orthop* 1970; 72:205–15.

16 Coventry MB, Beckenbaugh RD, Nolan DR, Ilstrup DM. 2,012 Total hip arthroplasties: a study of postoperative course and early complications. *J Bone Joint Surg* 1974;56A:273–84.

17 Herrlin K, Selvik G, Pettersson, *et al.* Position, orientation and component interaction in dislocation of the total hip prosthesis. *Acta Radiologica* 1988;29:441–4.

18 Linberg HO, Carlsson AS, Gentz C-F, Pettersson H. Recurrent and non-recurrent dislocation following total hip arthroplasty. *Acta Orthop Scand* 1982;53:947–52.

19 Paterno SA, Lachiewicz PF, Kelley SS. The influence of patient-related factors and the position of the acetabular component on the rate of dislocation after total hip replacement. *J Bone Joint Surg* 1997; 79A:1202–10.

20 Pierchon F, Pasquier G, Cotten A, *et al.* Causes of dislocation of total hip arthroplasty. *J Bone Joint Surg* 1994;76B:45–8.

21 Fackler CD, Poss R. Dislocation in total hip arthroplasties. *Clin Orthop* 1980;151:169–78.

22 Garcia-Cimbrelo E, Munuera L. Dislocation in low friction arthroplasty. *J Arthroplasty* 1992;7:149–55.

23 Kristiansen B, Jorgensen L, Holmich P. Dislocation following total hip arthroplasty. *Arch Orthop Trauma Surg* 1985;103:375–7.

24 Nolan DR, Fitzgerald RH, Beckenbaugh RD, Coventry MB. Complications of total hip arthroplasty treated by reoperation. *J Bone Joint Surg* 1975;57A:977–81.

25 Lewinnek GE, Lewis JL, Tarr R, *et al.* Dislocations after total hip replacement arthroplasties. *J Bone Joint Surg* 1978;60A:217–20.

26 Pettersson H, Gentz CF, Lindberg HO, Carlsson AS. Radiologic evaluation of the position of the acetabular component of the total hip prosthesis. *Acta Radiol* 1982;23:259–63.

27 Ghelman B. Radiographic localization of the acetabular component of a hip prosthesis. *Radiology* 1979;130:540–2.

28 Ghelman B. Three methods for determining anteversion and retroversion of a total hip prosthesis. *Am J Roentgenol* 1979;133:1127–34.

29 Goergen TG, Resnick D. Evaluation of acetabular anteversion following total hip arthroplasty: necessity of proper centering. *Br J Radiol* 1975;48:259–60.

30 Herrlin K, Pettersson H, Selvik G. Comparison of two- and three-dimensional methods for assessment of orientation of the total hip prosthesis. *Acta Radiol* 1988;29:357–61.

31 Herrlin K, Selvik G, Pettersson H. Space orientation of total hip prosthesis: a method for three-dimensional determination. *Acta Radiol Diagn* 1986;27:619–27.

32 Sellers R, Lyles D, Dorr L. The effect of pelvic rotation on alpha and theta angles in total hip arthroplasty. *Contemp Orthop* 1988;17:67–9.

33 DiGioia AM, Simon D, Jaramaz B, *et al.* Intra-operative measurement of pelvic and acetabular component alignment using an image guided navigational tool. *Trans ORS* 1998;23:198.

34 DiGioia AM, Jaramaz B, Colgan B. Computer assisted orthopaedic surgery: image guided and robotic assistive technologies. *Clin Orthop Rel Res* 1998;354:8.

35 Murray DW. The definition and measurement of acetabular orientation. *J Bone Joint Surg* 1993;75B:228–32.

36 Jaramaz B, Nikou C, DiGioia AM. Effect of cup orientation and neck length in range of motion simulation. *Trans ORS* 1997;22:286.

37 Simon DA, O'Toole RV, Blackwell M, *et al.* Accuracy Validation in image-guided orthopaedic surgery. *Proceedings of the 2nd International Symposium on Medical Robotics and Computer Assisted Surgery*, 1995: 185–92.

38 Simon DA, Kanade T. Geometric constraint analysis and synthesis: methods for improving shape-based registration accuracy. In: Troccaz, Grimson, Mosges eds. *First Joint Conference of Computer Vision, Virtual Reality and Robotics in Medicine and Medical Robotics and Computer Assisted Surgery*, Grenoble, France: Springer, 1997:181–90.

39 Mor AB, Moody JE, LaBarca RS, *et al.* Accuracy assessment framework for surgical navigation systems: an example. *The 15th Annual Symposium of the International Society for Technology in Arthroplasty: ISTA*, 2002. September 25–8. Oxford, England.

40 DiGioia A, Jaramaz B, Plakseychuk A, Moody J, Nikou C, LaBarca R, Levison T, Picard F. Comparison of a mechanical acetabular alignment guide with computer placement of the socket. *J Arthroplasty* 2002;17:359.

41 DiGioia A, Plakseychuk A, Jaramaz B, Levison T. Mini-incision technique for total hip arthroplasty with navigation. *J Arthroplasty*; 2003 Feb;18(2):123–8.

42 Harkess WJ. Arthroplasty of the hip: dislocation and subluxation. In *Campbell's Orthopaedics*, edited by Crenshaw, A.H., 8th, 541–47. St Louis: Mosby, 1992.

43 Bugbee WD, Engh C. Cementless femoral component extensively coated. In: Callaghan J, Rosenberg A, Rubash H, eds. *The adult hip.* vol II. Philadelphia, New York: Lippincott-Raven, 1998:1023–56.

44 Maloney W, Hartford J. The cemented femoral component. In: Callaghan J, Rosenberg A, Rubash H, eds. *The adult hip,* vol. II. Philadelphia, New York: Lippincott-Raven, 1998:959–979.

45 Pellicci P, Bostrom M, Poss R. Posterior approach to total hip replacement using enhanced posterior soft tissue repair. *Clin Orthop Rel Res* 1998;355:224.

46 Gore D, Murray P, Sepic S, Gardner G. Anterolateral compared to posterior approach in total hip arthroplasty: differences in component positioning, hip strength, and hip motion. *Clin Orthop Rel Res* 1982;165:180–7.

47 Horwitz BR, Rockkowitz NL, Goll SR, *et al.* A prospective randomized comparison of two surgical approaches to total hip arthroplasty. *Clin Orthop Rel Res* 1993;291:154–63.

48 Kohn D, Ruhmann O, Wirth C. Dislocation of total hip endoprosthesis with special references to various techniques. *Z Orthop Ihre Grenigeb* 1997;135:40–4.

49 Mostardi R, Askew M, Gradisar I. Comparison of functional outcome of total hip arthroplasties involving four surgical approaches. *J Arthroplasty* 1988;3:279–84.

50 Robinson RP, Robinson HJ, Salvati EA. Comparison of the transtrochanteric and posterior approaches for total hip replacement. *Clin Orthop Rel Res* 1980;147(March/April):143–7.

51 Vicar A, Coleman C. A comparison of the anterolateral, transtrochanteric, and posterior surgical approaches in primary total hip arthroplasty. *Clin Orthop* 1984;188:152–9.

52 Woo RYG, Morrey BF. Dislocation after total hip arthroplasty. *J Bone Joint Surg* 1982;64A(9):1295–306.

Chapter 11

Rationale for computer-assisted orthopaedic knee surgery

Michael A. Rauh and Kenneth A. Krackow

11.1 Introduction

On any given day in our modern world we are intensely exposed to computer technology and methodology—from computer assisted automobile wheel alignment to bar coding and inventory management at the store checkout counter. The medical field is no different. Our anesthesiologists utilize computerized electronics to monitor their tasks, while the nursing staff enter patient and case information into the hospital database. Yet, all of this sophistication happens while orthopaedic surgeons use nothing more than rulers, hammers, screwdrivers, goniometers and power saws. Given that it is our paramount task to be accurate in both planning and execution, there is something wrong with the current situation. It is time for us to step into the modern world and to employ the more sophisticated, accurate, and ultimately convenient features of computer assistance to our cases. Nowhere are these considerations more relevant than in total knee replacement where angular and displacement errors are directly related to both immediate and long-term results.

The newcomer needs to be familiar with different terms and general principles. *Navigation* is used to describe electronic computer associated instrumentation which tracks the positioning of bones, implants, and other instruments. There may be text, numbers, visual displays, screen overlays with radiographic images including computerized axial tomography (CT), and many other visual or audible aides that guide the placement of instruments and implants and assess alignment and overall positioning. The most common equipment in use at the time of this writing relies upon infrared emitting 'lights', which define the position of a rigid body marker and are seen by a lens-camera system whose images and information are processed by an associated computer. As such, the software written for this computer allows other custom written software to assist the surgeon in tracking the position of an instrument, such as the 'pointer' discussed later, within the operative field. This 'labeling' is performed through a similar system of infrared emitters mounted to the particular instrument or anatomical structure.

In the example of total knee arthroplasty (TKA) such markers can be placed on the femur, the tibia, the pelvis, and any pointers or associated knee implantation instrumentation. Thus, the computer navigation system itself can track simultaneously, nearly instantaneously, the positions of all of these things. One can use this information, given proper software within the system computer, to display indications of positions, movement, sizing, alignment, etc. It is also possible to track motion and to solve for center points of rotation and axes of rotation. Systems may make use of diagrams on a monitor screen showing line drawings or artists' renditions of knee elements or may be blended with fluoroscopic or CT images. The CT data would come from a preliminary study of the patient's extremity, while fluoroscopic images would be obtained preliminarily but in the OR directly on the patient's bones with markers in place.

Robots can be brought into the surgical field and directed to perform the basic bone cutting tasks. Current systems make use of CT scans and information input during a preoperative planning session to create a sequence of instructions to the robot defining just where the bone is to be prepared or removed.

It is important to appreciate whether a system requires preoperative planning compared to being a real-time process. In this writer's view, the application of TKA is quite well suited to a completely real-time process because all features of the knee are visible with the exceptions of hip and ankle—both of which are simple enough to locate with the infrared emitters. Others, however, may disagree with this notion and prefer to analyze CT images or work in association with fluoroscopy.

At this point, the concept of *registration* needs to be introduced. Registration is the process by which one brings the image of the bone on the displayed CT into 'agreement' with the bone itself. Ideally, this will enable the operating surgeon to point to an anatomical location on the patient, which corresponds exactly to the radiographic image on the screen. For example, one can imagine working at computer planning station, visualizing a line on the CT scan that has been oriented to pass through the center of the femoral head. This line corresponds to a particular aspect of an instrument in the surgical field designed also to point right at the center of the femoral head. It is essential to understand that there may be errors in the registration process due to the inexactness of the marker position or due to the processing of data by the software. True and accurate *registration* must obtain an accurate correspondence between the CT image and the anatomical structure of interest.

Another limitation of computer assistance relates to 'asking' the computer to solve problems which we surgeons have not yet solved ourselves. I am referring to issues of certain important points and axes used extensively in TKA. And, while considering this point, appreciate that we are looking to computer techniques to give us the most accurate results *all* of the time, not just 99% of the time.

For example, we cannot just 'ask' a computer to find the axis of neutral femoral internal/external rotation if we cannot agree upon what is the best definition of such rotation in essentially *all* cases. Perhaps the issue of tibial bone and tibial component rotation would be an even better example. What objective aspect of the bone itself or even CT cross-sections can be used to define a neutral, antero-posterior (AP), or mediolateral (ML) axis? Furthermore, even if we could agree on the best definition, it would still be necessary to write a program that will gather information using the available equipment to *find* this axis accurately all of the time.

What we can be relatively assured of is our ability to locate a center of rotation, if such a center point truly exists. The best example is the center of the femoral head. In addition, the flexion–extension movement of the knee can be well approximated with a single axis. However, one must appreciate that other axes of rotation are not as well defined. In fact, experienced surgeons attending product design sessions will commonly disagree on the positions of distal femoral and proximal tibial rotation. Therefore, even if we could create software programs to replicate exactly which axis a physician is contemplating in his brain, this may not be a satisfactory method for other surgeons.

To make all of this more concrete we may consider the system shown in Figs 11.1 through 11.14 developed by the senior author of this chapter. The pelvis, femoral, and tibial positions are tracked by the infrared markers which are rigidly attached to the respective bones. The pelvic tracker or marker is used only for the purpose of locating the center of the femoral head. The mathematical algorithm for this is based upon the assumption that functional hip movement occurs as the spherical head moves within a matching spherical cavity, the acetabulum. Any point on the femur tracked during hip rotation will move along the surface of a sphere whose center is coincident with the center of the femoral head. To indicate the relative accuracy of this determination we may consider the 250 different points which are recorded during the location process and construct a ray from the located center to each of these points. We have therefore 250 'rays' of presumably slightly different lengths.

The variance or standard deviation of this set of 250 numbers indicates the accuracy of localization and is typically below 0.5 mm. The localization of the center of the unseen femoral head is therefore as close as the overall accuracy of the detection of tracker position, itself on the order of 0.5 mm. Having determined the femoral head center, the pelvis tracker is moved to become the tracking marker for the tibia.

Next, one inputs points and other information to indicate to the computer program the location of the 'center' of the distal femur, the rotation—internal/external of the distal femur, and the level of the distal femoral condyles as an indicator of the level of the femoral aspect of the knee joint line. All of this is done with the use of a tracked pointer. Similarly, the essential TKA features of the tibia are input. These anatomic structures are the center of the top of the tibia, the level of each tibial plateau, the center of the ankle, and the surgeon's preferred choice for neutral tibial rotation.

At this point it is possible to follow in real-time all six degrees of relative position and motion of the tibia and femur simultaneously. One can display the tibio-femoral angle, flexion angle and internal–external rotation, as well as AP, ML, and proximal–distal distraction. Furthermore, with the trackers in place on the bones these determinations are available without making any alterations in the instruments. That is, we do not need to remove a cutting block and put on an alignment assessor to read an angle. And, with trial or final components in place, all of these values can be appreciated and recorded.

Aside from simply assessing alignment, which most surgeons are fixated upon, we have the ability to gather additional information while ranging the knee. The system can accurately assess the degree of flexion-extension and also ML, AP, and even rotational stability. With the exception of crude assessment of maximum flexion, none of these other determinations have previously been possible.

11.2 Clinical challenges

We look to computer assistance to improve the quality of our TKR results. Improvements are anticipated in the areas of pain relief, range of motion, stability, durability, and alignment as it relates to prosthetic lifespan. In presenting this topic to hundreds of orthopaedic surgeons, many are inclined only to think about potential improvement in overall alignment and to feel that their results in this regard are adequate essentially all of the time. Furthermore, very few routinely obtain, and if so accurately measure, those results. Therefore, practitioners are in no position to conclude that their alignment results are adequate. In addition, Stulberg et al. have shown that long-standing lower extremity films are highly subject to rotational and projectional inaccuracies.[1]

We really ought to look beyond the issue of alignment and recognize the potential for improvements in ligament releasing and assessment of ligamentous stability. In addition, placement of the femoral component in the optimum relationship of extension to the functional axis of flexion can be performed to provide maximum range of motion and stability through out that arc. We can also turn to navigation equipment to indicate proper component sizing as well as placement.

Because of the current relatively high cost of knee navigational systems we are inclined to consider that the major challenge is showing that such an approach is worthwhile in an outcome sense, i.e. whether it really makes a worthwhile difference. At the risk of sounding too self-serving or anti-scientific, let us first be very patient on this point. Currently, we are working with what will probably prove to be crude 'first-generation' computer assistance systems. Allow for the possibility, near certainty, that software and hardware will progress so that systems are more convenient, more informative and also less expensive. This author's personal experience to date suggests that the often-heralded well-controlled prospective studies will be very difficult to complete. First, there are certain quickly apparent and obvious advantages of the computer assistance methodology. As one uses this equipment it becomes immediately clear at multiple points of a case, that one would have accepted an inaccuracy in the absence of using the equipment—an inaccuracy that is unnecessary and at least sometimes significant. Second will be the impracticality of getting patients to agree to participate in a study and being relegated to the noncomputer group. Third will be the related, general patient pressure for the utilization of the high-tech adjunct.

It is critical that the surgeon be provided with and master the complete description of how a chosen system works. Only then will one be able to understand the potential for errors and other problems, be more alert for them and know how to work around them. For example, it is necessary to understand how the system defines bony landmarks and axes and essentially to have a visual appreciation of what is going on.

Again, it is just as important to know the accuracy of the system in its pure function as well as inaccuracies and uncertainties from software computations and the registration process. One needs to assess limitations of marker fixation stability and be able to understand the use of validation tools. As with any new operative technique, it is incumbent upon the surgeon not only to achieve a familiarization but also to practice the use of these devices in mock settings. This will prevent excessive operative, tourniquet, and anesthetic times, thus reducing complications.

11.3 System description

Computer assisted orthopaedic surgery (CAOS) has been developed over the past decade and represents many different systems and concepts. The field can generally be differentiated into simulation devices, preoperative planning systems, robotic assisted surgery, and surgical navigation systems.

Surgical simulators attempt to provide the user with instantaneous feedback through computerized programs and images that test the user's skill and knowledge about particular situations and procedures. These systems are not utilized directly in the operating theater, however, provide the surgeon in training with valuable feedback and information prior to actually performing the procedure on a patient. The success of the simulation depends upon the correlation between 'actual experience' and the simulation.

Preoperative planning systems attempt to utilize available imaging modalities to better assist the surgeon in the operation and lessen the risk of error. An example of this would be the system utilized by Froemel et al.[2]. A preoperative CT scan of the affected leg and knee along with 3D modeling and template utilization, provide the surgeon with the exact planes for osteotomies. In this way, planning systems attempt to reduce operative time and complications while improving clinical results.

Robotic assistive systems such as 'CASPAR' (OrtoMaquet, Rastatt/Germany) as well as the 'ROBODOC®' (Integrated Surgical Systems, Sacramento, CA, USA) have been developed to assist the surgeon in performing more exact bony preparation, typically through assistance in drilling, reaming, and bone cutting. The concepts and particular details of robotic assisted orthopaedic surgery are discussed elsewhere in this text.

Navigation systems involve the utilization of computer instrumentation to intra-operatively track the position of bone, implants, and instruments. Systems such as the 'Hip Nav' developed by DiGioia et al.,[3] and various 'Fluoro-Nav' tools utilize preoperative or intra-operative radiographic images to assist in developing a 3D representation that can be utilized by the surgeon to perform various operative tasks. The 'Stryker Navigation System' (Stryker–Howmedica–Osteonics, Rutherford, NJ, USA), developed by the senior author, is an intra-operative, nonimage based system that utilizes an infrared detector array to determine the axial, rotational, and translational position of the tibia with respect to the femur. Axial deformity about the knee can be determined without preoperative radiographs; however, this system is not intended to replace our current method of care. This system has been developed to allow for better intra-operative alignment of components and hopefully longer implant lifespan.

11.4 **Surgical technique**

A surgeon's first response to the concept of computer assisted orthopaedic surgery is one of loss of autonomy. However, it is our view that a system *need not* and *should not* be designed to this end. For example, the system described here allows the surgeon to utilize the computer to 'see' beyond the human eye and view the knee as having full kinematic dimensions. The best way for the reader to understand what assistance this particular navigation system provides is to actually contemplate a TKA procedure.

An infrared sensor array located at the side of the operating room table is used by this system to localize emitters placed at specific locations on the lower extremity of the patient.

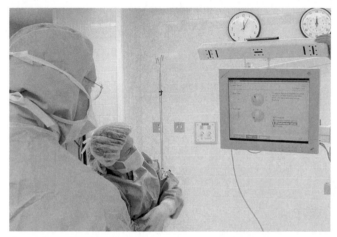

Fig. 11.1 An infrared sensor array.

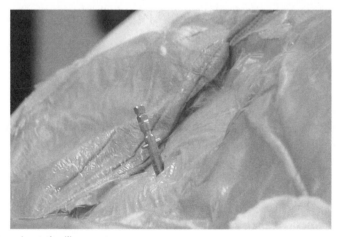

Fig. 11.2 A tracking pin at the iliac crest.

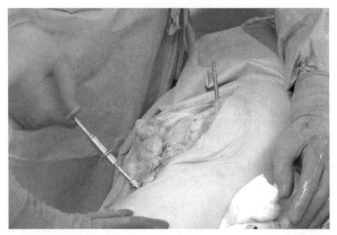

Fig. 11.3 Tracking pins at the distal femur and proximal tibia.

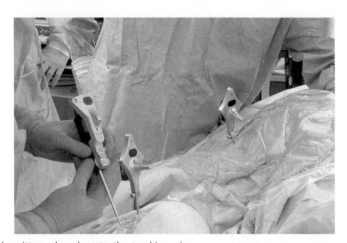

Fig. 11.4 Infrared emitters placed on to the tracking pins.

A tracking pin is placed into the patient's ipsilateral iliac crest for the purpose of identifying the center of the femoral head.

After the surgeon's choice of incision, the distal femur and proximal lateral tibial bony prominences are identified and similar tracking pins can be placed.

With the infrared emitters placed onto the tracking pins, the lower extremity can be manipulated in a circular fashion about the hip. Using an iterative Gauss-Newton algorithm to solve the true non-linear system, the center of the femoral head can be identified by the computer.[4]

Using the pointing device, the geometry of the distal femur is digitized. One must identify the medial and lateral epicondyles, the center of the knee, the AP (anteroposterior) axis of Whiteside,[5] as well as the condylar surfaces.

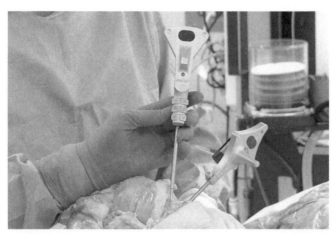

Fig. 11.5 Digitization of the medial epicondyle.

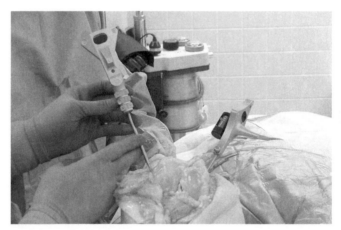

Fig. 11.6 Digitization of the lateral epicondyle.

Using the power of the modern computer, the center of the femoral head is calculated via a subroutine that assumes the head of the femur is spherical. Two-hundred fifty data points are collected in 20 seconds as the surgeon moves the lower extremity about the hip joint in a gentle spherical arc. The method of least squares is used to find the best fit sphere given the data points collected.[6] The center estimate is then determined using an iterative Gauss-Newton algorithm to solve the true nonlinear system. This algorithm runs through 200 iterations to assure convergence. Finally, the center point is transformed into the femoral reference frame.

Likewise, the geometry of the proximal tibia is digitized as the surgeon identifies the sulcus between the tibial spines, the anteroposterior mid-point, as well as the medial and lateral malleoli, along with the center of the ankle.

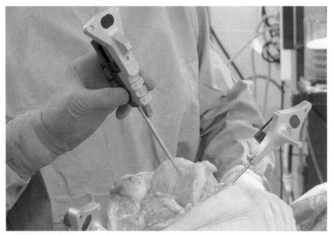

Fig. 11.7 Digitization of the center of the knee.

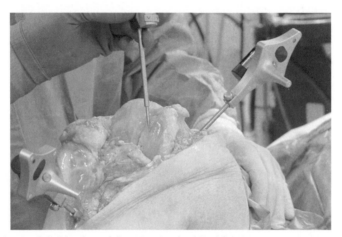

Fig. 11.8 Localization and digitization of the AP axis of Whiteside.

Given all the defined points, the tibiofemoral and mechanical axes can be determined before any bone cuts have been made. This determination then allows accurate depiction of any correction needed to properly align the components. Additionally, this navigation system is able to identify intra-operatively the real-time relative position of the tibia with respect to the femur. That is, one is able to precisely determine tibiofemoral angle, the flexion–extension position, and the amount of relative internal or external rotation of the tibia with respect to the femur. Also, changes in the relative tibiofemoral compression-distraction and mediolateral or antero-posterior displacements can be determined by calculating the change in the directional vector from the tibial to the femoral reference frames.

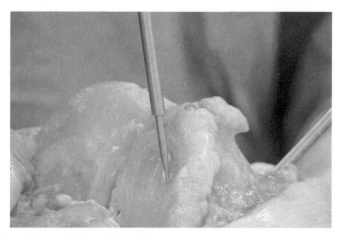

Fig. 11.9 Digitization of the medial condylar surface.

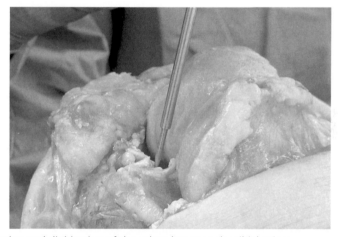

Fig. 11.10 Localization and digitization of the sulcus between the tibial spines.

Armed with this knowledge, the operating surgeon is able to utilize jigs from any specific instrument system to make a more accurate cut. Upon final verification of cuts, one is able to obtain a more accurate alignment of the lower extremity than previously obtained without the use of this device. With more accurate alignment should come a longer lifespan of the given prostheses.

The algorithm for determining the center of the femoral head was tested by three different surgeons on eight different cadaveric hips for inter- and intra-observer consistency. The calculated centers were then compared to a direct measurement made after disarticulating the hip and using the stylus/pointer to digitize the observed center of the femoral head. The dislocated hip, i.e., the femoral head was carefully inspected and an equator drawn free hand. A sagittal saw was then used to cut the femoral head in half, and the midpoint of the remaining surface was digitized in the femoral reference frame.

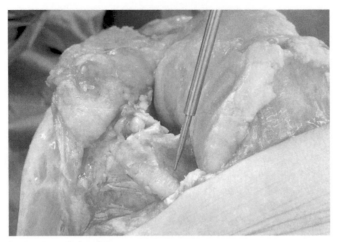

Fig. 11.11 Further digitization of the tibia.

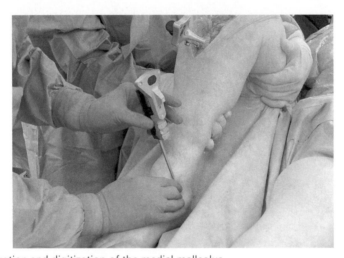

Fig. 11.12 Localization and digitization of the medial malleolus.

The average errors were on the order of two to three mm. These errors applied to a 40-centimeter long femur yielding a potential angular error of <0.55° for the orientation of the mechanical axis. The y-coordinate estimates in the intra-observer calculations were significantly different in both cases between investigators (p = 0.01) using a paired Student's t-test. However, this difference did not lead to a significantly different clinical angular result. Furthermore, these results were obtained in a less accurate setting—one without separate tracking of the pelvis. Tracking true femoral-pelvic motion has brought the variation down to less than one millimeter.[4]

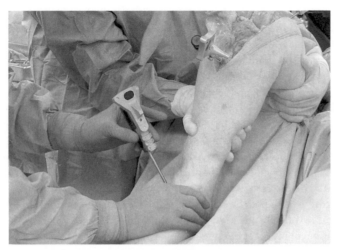

Fig. 11.13 Localization and digitization of the lateral malleolus.

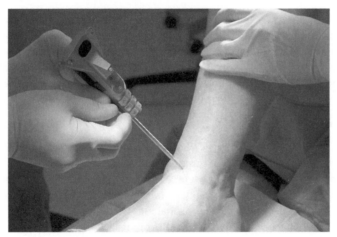

Fig. 11.14 Digitization of the center of the ankle.

11.5 **Comparison with traditional techniques**

When comparing this type of system with traditional techniques, one can easily see that the only 'surgical' difference is the placement of three tracking pins into the iliac crest, distal femur, and proximal tibia. The placement of these pins allows the operating surgeon to utilize the computer's programmed ability to determine alignment and deformity.

A comparison between 'new' and 'old' techniques must always consider issues of blood loss, pain, and operative time. Any increased blood loss or significant lengthening of patient's operative time would be unacceptable and in fact a deterrent from the introduction of a new device. Concerning this issue, the only sites for further bleeding beyond the traditional method for TKA would be the three pin localizing sites which are approximately 3 mm in diameter. These sites of intrusion are easily managed with surgical closure of the overlying tissue and offer no clinically significant blood loss.

The issue of pain is a valid point especially at the site of the iliac crest pin. However, pain from this single pin or screw hole has not presented a clinical problem. In all probability, pain resulting from the TKA itself often is more imposing on the patient.

When contemplating the topic of operative time, one must consider only one question. Familiarity. The operating surgeon, just as he must be 'familiar' with the anatomy of any given procedure, he must also be 'familiar' with his tools. A navigation system is no different than the cutting jigs found in most TKA instrument sets. One must be fully versed in the correct utilization of every piece of equipment.

On 7 August 1997, the first case of computer-assisted total knee arthroplasty was performed in Buffalo, NY, USA with a 'skin-to-skin' operative time of two hours fifteen minutes. It is estimated that the attending surgeon working at the same surgical pace without any of the computer interaction would have taken approximately one hour forty-five minutes. This difference is relatively small, and it must be recalled that these times represented our first clinical case.

Later cadaveric studies illustrated a definite learning curve while using this system. Surgical time differences will be negligible for the patient and the operating room facility, and the potential benefit of having the increased alignment, displacement, and motion information will greatly outweigh any such time differences.

We suggest that every surgeon spend time with sawbones prior to clinical utilization. And, when possible, cadaver work would likely be advantageous. Thus with experience and feedback, it is anticipated that there will be no extra time in the operating room as a result of the utilization of such a navigation system. In fact, it is anticipated that ultimately the utilization of this system would allow for less intra-operative questioning of observed deformity and angulation, and thus less operative time overall.

11.6 **Discussion**

When discussing computer assisted surgery with orthopaedic surgeons, two of the most important concepts for them to grasp are the limits of computer assistance and the specifics of what the computer is doing. These same surgeons often think that because we have a computer and since the system touts 'assistance with knee replacement', it can simply be moved into the room and the operative procedure can proceed with little intra-operative decision making. It is often expected that the computer can replace observation and diligence; however this is far from reality.

The operating surgeon must understand that the computer is only providing information or feedback based upon the computer code that has been specifically programmed. In referring to or locating a point, axis or whatever, we have to be able to program an absolutely reliable method or methodology for determining that point or axis. If the methodology or computer code is not so precise, then the computer cannot be so precise. Expecting the computer to recognize the epicondylar axis when we have no 'iron clad' way ourselves exposes the true limitations of any computer assisted process. Although the computer might be willing to give an 'answer', it cannot be expected to 'just go in and do it'.

We must understand the surgeon's interaction either to directly provide information about where bone is, including the center of the femoral head, end of the femur, proximal tibia, end of the tibia, rotational attitudes, etc, or go through the various routines so that the computer itself can locate these features. Specifically, as mentioned previously, the easiest feature to locate is the center of the femoral head by moving the femur around and solving for the center of the femoral head.[4]

In developing computer assisted surgical techniques, the researchers must be sure of the validity of their measurements, inter-rater reliability, and reproducibility. Prospective users of computer assisted techniques must be sure that each of these issues have been addressed before subjecting real patients to these techniques. The individual steps of the computer assisted process must be evaluated in a step-wise fashion to ensure the expected results. This is especially true when dealing with robotic assisted devices. Imagine the consequences of utilizing the robot to make precise cuts on a distal femur only to realize too late that too much bone had been resected in an incorrect position.

Later, while discussing details of computer assisted total knee arthroplasty, it should become clear that in giving the computer specific information about the femur and tibia, specifically each end of the bone and rotational alignment or orientation of the bone, the computer can instantaneously track the relative positions of those two bones. Varus and valgus angulations, in addition to knee flexion and extension, relative rotation, distraction, and displacement are all available in real time. This is a terribly complicated task that the human mind and eye cannot do. We thus utilize the computer to assist us in providing this type of numerical feedback. This information is essentially what all CAOS systems are attempting to provide.

Any new surgical technique or protocol needs to pass through a period of introspective questioning by the researching surgeon. The questions that must be asked of this new process or technique are if it carries an acceptable level of risk for infection, bleeding, and post-operative pain. Above all, this new process should add to or improve upon the current methodology. With total knee arthroplasty, 'improvements' in technique or prostheses must also address the issues of proper alignment, durability, accuracy, and surgical reproducibility. Computer assisted orthopaedic surgery (CAOS) attempts to achieve an improvement in the quality of the operation performed through the intra-operative feedback to the operating surgeon.

Concerns with appropriate alignment and ligament balancing can be assessed and corrected intra-operatively and with great precision. Whereas previously the operating surgeon relied upon knowledge of deformity corrections with various releases, the process can be monitored with the use of the computer. Exact measurements of flexion extension gaps, varus and valgus deformity, and tibial rotation can be patient specific and observed in real-time.

At the same time, this entire process should be relatively convenient to perform. An additional degree or two of improved alignment need not sacrifice physician and patient comfort. The process should not infringe upon the typical protocol of knee arthroplasty. Instead, it should simply assist the surgeon to perform more efficiently. In summary, a new methodology should improve upon the existing process.

The true clinical challenge posed to the orthopaedic surgeon using computer assisted surgery is one of improving prosthetic lifespan. The ability to reduce implant wear and loosening through better alignment is desired, however can only be confirmed with randomized prospective clinically controlled trials. Only after this comparison can we confirm or deny this statement. It is expected that better alignment and fit obtained through using computer assisted total knee arthroplasty would only lengthen the lifespan of any given prostheses; however, this remains to be proven statistically.

Finally, the new technique needs to be reproducible between different users. One orthopaedic joint surgeon in Europe should be able to obtain the same results as a similarly trained physician in Buffalo, New York. If results are not comparable at different sites, then the new technique cannot be considered useful to all. The need for reproducible results is self-evident and must not be questioned. However, the burden of proof of reproducibility rests with the developers of the system. Individuals utilizing the computerized equipment cannot be held accountable for ensuring the inter-rater reliability of the system. With all of the variables that can be introduced into the process of computer assisted orthopaedic surgery, such as with the patient and with the prostheses, this task becomes rather daunting. The burden of proof on the researcher for clinical reliability and validity is onerous. However, familiarity with the hardware, understanding the software, and knowledge of the system limitations is a responsibility that all operating surgeons share. The operating surgeon must strive to provide postoperative alignment that is not only satisfactory, but also optimal for the prostheses utilized. All who utilize the hardware must understand the intricacies and details of the system being used.

All of these issues must be addressed with whatever system is ultimately chosen by the orthopaedic surgeon. Utilization of critical thinking skills about the individual system must take place prior to the implementation of these computer assisted orthopaedic surgery devices.

11.7 **Summary**

Change is inevitable. To resist change is usually futile. Computer assisted orthopaedic surgery introduces a change in our traditional methods of surgery. Many operating surgeons will oppose the change insisting that it will inevitably lead to loss of autonomy or feel it is not worth the cost or trouble. However, we believe that educating ourselves about new technology will allow us to evolve into better surgeons and provide for better outcomes for our patients.

References

1 Stulberg S, Sarin V, Loan P. The use of computer assisted navigation in TKR: results of an initial experience in 35 patients. *North American Program on Computer Assisted Orthopaedic Surgery*, 2001, July 6–8. Pittsburgh, PA.

2 Froemel M, Portheine F, Ebner M, Radermacher K. Computer assisted template based navigation for total knee replacement. *North American Program on Computer Assisted Orthopaedic Surgery*, 2001, July 6–8. Pittsburgh, PA.

3 DiGioia A, Jaramaz B, Blackwell M, Simon D, *et al.* The Otto Aufranc Award: image guided navigation system to measure intraoperatively acetabular implant alignment. *Clin Orthop Rel Res*, 1998;355:8–22.

4 Krackow K, Mihalko W, Serpe L, Phillips M, Bayers-Thering M. A new technique for determining proper mechanical axis alignment during total knee arthroplasty: progress toward computer assisted TKA. *Orthopaedics*, 1999;22(7):698–702.

5 Whiteside L, Arima J. The anteroposterior axis for femoral rotational alignment in valgus total knee arthroplasty. *Clin Orthop Rel Res*, 1995;321:168–72.

6 Forbes A. Robust circle and sphere fitting by least squares. *Nat Phys Lab Rep*, 1989;153:1–22.

Chapter 12

Total knee replacement: robotic assistive technique

W. Siebert, Sabine Mai, Rudolf Kober, and Peter F. Heeckt

12.1 Clinical challenges

12.1.1 State of the art in traditional total knee replacement

Total knee replacement (TKR) has become the standard procedure in the management of degenerative joint disease after more conservative therapy options have been exhausted. However, despite conscientious planning and carefully performed procedures, surgeons are often unsatisfied with implant alignment. Various authors described significant axial or rotational malalignment, and medio-lateral and ventro-dorsal tilt.[1–4] Seemingly small displacements of 2.5 mm potentially alter the range of motion by as much as 20°.[5] Correct tibiofemoral alignment seems to be particularly important since it is generally agreed that axial deviation and imprecise implantation may lead to early loosening of implant components.[6–9] An axial deviation of more than 3° or Maquet's line not passing through the middle third of the implant is considered the most frequent cause of early TKR failure.[10–13] None of the contemporary improvements in implant design and instrumentation have alleviated these problems.

12.1.2 State of the art of computer assisted orthopaedic surgery for TKR

Computer assisted TKR can be accomplished by image guided or nonimage guided navigation and active or semi-active robotics. Navigation systems that are either based on preoperative CT or MRI images (preoperative model systems) or on computer integrated instrumentation (intra-operative-model systems) have been used clinically.[14–16] First prospective studies show that navigated knee implants seem to yield superior alignment in comparison to traditional technique.[15–17] Navigated TKR still depends on the use of cutting blocks and oscillating jigs which could result in inferior bone resection. To improve the accuracy of implant alignment and bone resection various experimental active and semi-active robotic systems for TKR have been developed.[14,18–20] To our knowledge so far only the commercial active robotic systems ROBODOC® (Integrated Surgical Systems, Sacramento, CA) and CASPAR® (U.R.S.-ortho GmbH & Co. KG, Rastatt, Germany) have been studied clinically in a larger number of consecutive patients.

12.2 System description

12.2.1 Classification

According to the classification for computer assisted knee systems proposed by F. Picard and co-workers[21] the CASPAR® TKR-system used by us would be classified as an active robotic system since the surgical steps are performed autonomously. However, robotic action can be stopped by the surgeon at all times within split seconds.

12.2.2 Important concepts

The CASPAR system is a universal planning and surgical operating system which is currently capable to assist orthopaedic surgeons in total hip replacement, repair of the anterior cruciate ligament and total knee replacement.[22,23] The system consists of an interactive PC planning station based on CT images and a modified industrial robot. By using a combination of computer-assisted preoperative planning and robotic execution of the plan the highest possible level of accuracy in implant positioning can be achieved. For instance in TKR implant position on the femoral and tibial side and all leg axes can be planned in three dimensions according to the surgeon's preferences. The implant can be placed following the classical or anatomical alignment. Even ligament tension and the need for intra-operative soft tissue release can be accounted for preoperatively.

12.2.3 Surgical technique

Robot-assisted TKR consists of the placement of fiducial markers, CT scan, preoperative planning and surgery.

12.2.3.1 Placement of fiducial markers

To facilitate orientation, the robot requires placement of a femoral and a tibial pin that serve as fiducial markers. The pin design is a self-tapping bone screw to which can be affixed a special CT cross which will be detected by later computed tomography. The pins are placed into the femur by an anterior approach and into the tibia via an anteromedial approach (Figs 12.1, 12.2). The stab incisions are positioned in such a way that they can later be incorporated into the primary surgical incision. The robot

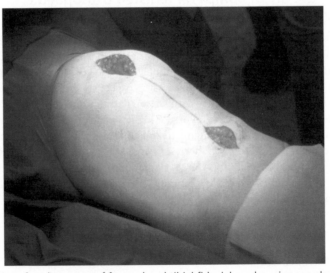

Fig. 12.1 Stab incisions for placement of femoral and tibial fiducial marker pins are placed at the proximal and distal end of the later TKR incision.

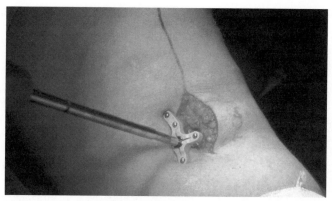

Fig. 12.2 Fastening of the special CT cross on the tibial pin.

uses these pins for spatial orientation and performs geometric calculations based upon their location. To maintain the pins in the required stable position, they are placed bicortically. The incisions are closed over the pins and the main procedure is performed on the same or on the following day.

12.2.3.2 CT scan and preoperative planning

A helical CT scan is obtained immediately after the pins have been placed. Particular attention is paid to the areas of the femoral head, the pins, the knee, and the ankle. A calibration rod is placed next to the extremity. The rod helps to control the quality of the CT scan with respect to motion artifacts. During imaging, all of our patients are maintained under spinal or epidural anesthesia from the pin placement procedure. This greatly reduces the risk for motion artifacts.

The CT data are then transferred into the PC-based planning station. The technical quality of the scan is automatically checked and the pin position is verified. The surgeon identifies specific anatomical landmarks and the anatomical and mechanical axes of the femur and tibia are calculated in the frontal and sagittal planes. The joint line, epicondylar twist (angle between epicondylar line and posterior condylar line), torsion of the tibia (angle between dorsal part of the tibial plateau and a line through the center of the ankle), as well as the relationship of the dorsal part of the tibia and the condylar line serve as additional important parameters. All angles and possible geometric translations are displayed on the video screen at the end of the planning procedure (Fig. 12.3).

The system allows the user to select and position a specific implant size. One needs to decide on the required degree of femoral and tibial external rotation to assure central patellar tracking. Either a classic or an anatomical joint line plus the dorsal slope may be selected. Unintentional notching can easily be avoided. With computer-assisted planning, the strong interdependence of all parameters, including the mechanical axes, becomes quite evident. Implant fit can be accurately assessed by scrolling through the scan, a feature which sometimes makes the surgeon 'pickier' regarding the selection of a specific implant type or size. The system informs the user about the expected change in 'extension' and 'flexion gaps' and the resulting ligament tension.

After positioning the implants, it is important to specify the milling areas in order to avoid redundant cutting and to protect the surrounding soft tissue. As a last step, the system prints out an overview of the final plan. All data are stored on a PC card and transferred to the robot control unit immediately before surgery.

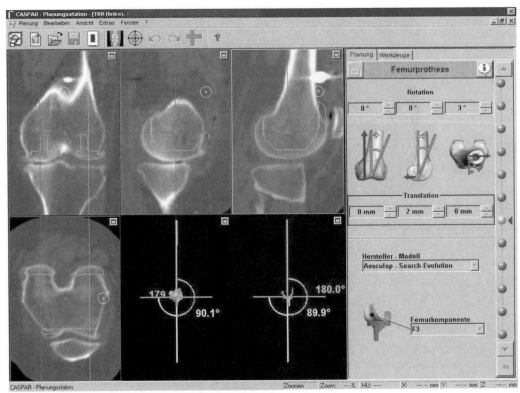

Fig. 12.3 Original screen shot from the planning station showing the PC-based planning of the femoral component and the resulting mechanical leg axis.

12.2.3.3 Robot-assisted surgery

A conventional median incision with parapatellar approach to the knee joint is used. The knee joint is secured by a transfemoral and transtibial self-cutting screw to a specially designed frame. This rigid frame is also used for fixation of self-holding soft-tissue retractors (Fig. 12.4). Sufficient mobility to allow 50° ipsilateral hip flexion is a prerequisite for securing the leg in the fixation frame. Intra-operative difficulties can be caused by a very tight quadriceps muscle or patellar tendon. Since it is necessary to provide sufficient lateral traction on the patella to keep it out of the way when milling the tibial plateau, a temporary release of the tibial tuberosity or a 'quadriceps snip' may be required. In order to control for unwanted micro-movements of the leg during robotic surgery, rigid bodies with light-emitting diodes (LEDs) are firmly attached to the frame. The LED signal is constantly monitored by an infrared camera system, which will automatically shut off the robot in the event of excessive motion (Fig. 12.5). After registration of the fiducial markers, robotic milling is started by the surgeon. As a safety measure, the surgeon is required to constantly depress the robot button on a sterile remote control in order to maintain the cutting action.

The cutting tool is equipped with internal water-cooling and irrigation. A splash-guard helps to keep the operative field and LEDs dry and clean (Fig. 12.6). Milling heads are changed during the procedure depending on the type of cut to be made. Varying with the size of the implant and bone

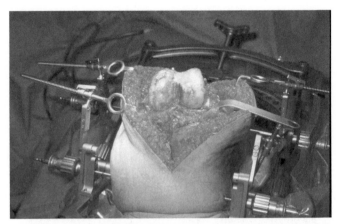

Fig. 12.4 Intra-operative situs before machining of the femoral part. The knee is rigidly fixed in a specially designed frame with self-holding retractors.

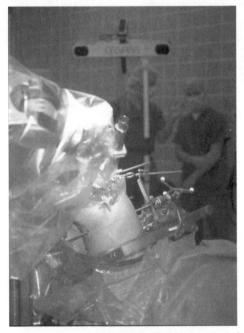

Fig. 12.5 View of the working robot. Unwanted motion is detected by an infrared camera system as seen in the background and corresponding rigid bodies fixed to the frame in the foreground.

density, the entire milling procedure takes approximately 18 minutes. If required, it is possible to revert to conventional manual technique at any point during surgery.

The resulting bone surfaces are accurately shaped and smooth (Fig. 12.7). After the fixation frame and pins are removed, soft tissues are balanced and the components of the implant are inserted.

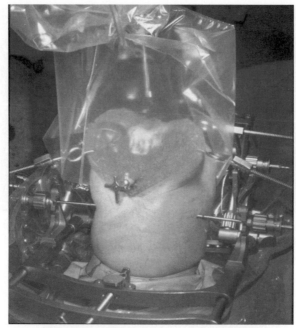

Fig. 12.6 Knee securely fixed with cutting tool and splash guard in place right before femoral milling action commences. The tibial registration cross is still in place at the distal end of the incision.

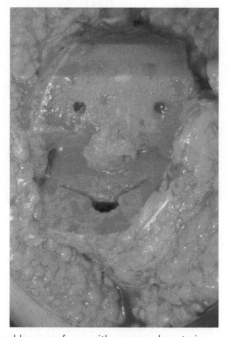

Fig. 12.7 Final tibial and femoral bone surfaces with preserved posterior cruciate ligament.

12.2.4 **Validation**

Experimental studies on phantoms and cadaver bones were done to verify the performance of the robotic system and the information transfer chain between the planning procedure and the robot-assisted intervention. In these tests specifically CT segmentation, robotic precision and total registration of CT and robot were evaluated. A mean error of 1° for the axes and 1 mm for translation with a maximum of 2° and 2 mm respectively were calculated.

12.3 **Comparison with traditional techniques**

Active robotic assistive techniques for TKR differ from traditional and also navigated techniques in many ways. No extra- or intramedullary guides, no cutting blocks and no oscillating jigs are needed. Currently standard knee implants are used but it is conceivable that in the future robotic machining of joint surfaces could allow for different implant geometry. Access to the knee joint and exposure remain traditional. In general the length of the skin incision can be even a little smaller than that of the traditional approach. Alike navigated image guided techniques patients have to be subjected to a CT for preoperative planning. Unfortunately robotic TKR still requires additional surgery for placement of two reference screws. This will be changed when other techniques such as intra-operative surface based registration will be equally precise.

12.4 **Clinical trials**

After a developmental phase in 1999 and a series of successful experiments on phantoms and cadaver bones, a prospective controlled clinical trial was started in March 2000 at the Kassel Orthopedic Clinic. The study was approved by the institutional review board and an independent ethics committee. The first clinical robot-assisted TKR was performed on March 27, 2000. Since then, 62 robot-assisted TKRs have been performed in 61 patients (43 women, 19 men). One female patient received simultaneous, bilateral TKR. The mean age in the robotic group was 67 years (46–87 yrs.) The manually operated control group consisted of 52 patients (40 women, 12 men) with a mean age of 68 years (48–82). The indication for TKR was idiopathic gonarthrosis in all cases. The LC Search Evolution® knee-system (Aesculap, Tuttlingen, Germany) was used for all patients in the robotic group because this was the first knee implant system geometry that was loaded into the planning software. All patients in the manual control group received NexGen® (Zimmer Inc., Warsaw, Indiana, USA) implants.

All complications during surgery and in the post-operative course were recorded. Patients were scored before and after surgery according to the Knee Society Score.[24]

Before and two weeks after surgery, standing long-leg anteroposterior roentgenograms were taken of all patients to control for correct alignment (Figs 12.8, 12.9). The mechanical leg axis was measured on these X-ray films and directly compared to the preoperative plan.

Data were statistically analyzed by using a two-tailed Student's *t*-test. Statistical significance was assumed at a p-value smaller than 0.01.

12.4.1 **Results**

12.4.1.1 General observations and complications

Operating time for the first 62 robotic cases averaged 135 minutes (80–220 min). A learning curve decrease from 220 minutes to approximately 100 minutes was observed.

Soft tissue swelling appeared to be markedly reduced in the early post-operative phase when compared to the traditional technique. Full range of motion also seemed to be regained more quickly

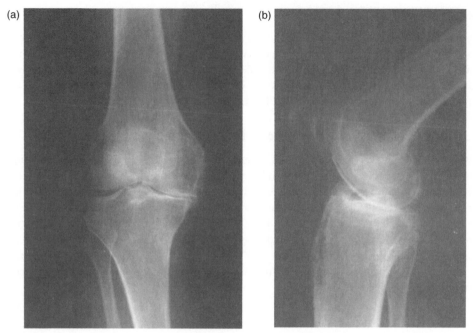

Fig. 12.8 (a, b) Anteroposterior and lateral X-rays of a patient with medial gonarthrosis before robotic TKA.

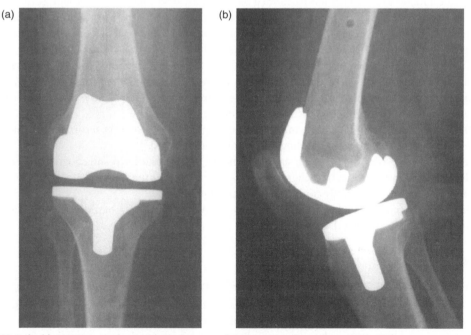

Fig. 12.9 (a, b) Anteroposterior and lateral X-rays of the same patient after robotic TKA.

for the majority of robotic TKR patients. To restore full motion, the knee joints of seven patients in the robotic group and two patients in the manual group had to be mobilized under general anesthesia since it is our general regime to regain full range of motion early. At discharge, all patients had 90° or greater of flexion.

No major adverse events, directly related to the CASPAR system, have been noted. A minor complication occurred in one patient. Due to a defective registration marker, the femoral milling process could not be completed as planned. Full correction was achieved by converting to manual technique. Three patients had superficial infections at one of the pin sites. All resolved under conservative management.

12.4.2 Post-operative tibiofemoral alignment

In the computerized preoperative planning procedure, the mechanical axis was routinely corrected to a tibiofemoral angle of 0°. In the robotic group, one patient with a 20° varus deformation was planned to 3.7° varus in order to avoid too much resection and to maintain sufficient ligamentous tension. The overall mean difference between preoperative plan and post-operative result for tibiofemoral alignment was 0.8° with a standard deviation of 1.0° and a range from 0 to 3°. Only one early patient in the robotic group can be considered a real outlier with a 4° deviation from the planned angle. The mean tibiofemoral angle in the manual group was 2.6° with a standard deviation of 2.2° and a range from 0 to 7°. Eighteen patients (35%) had a deviation greater 3° with a maximum of 7°. The exact distribution of varus and valgus errors of the mechanical axis for both groups is shown in Fig. 12.10. The difference in tibiofemoral alignment was highly significant at $p < 0.0001$.

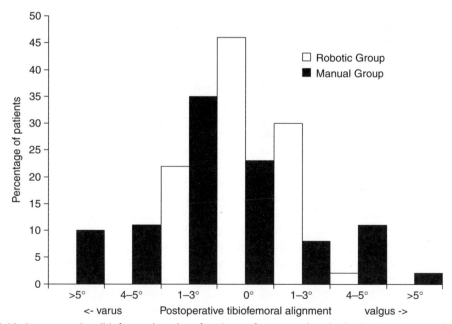

Fig. 12.10 Post-operative tibiofemoral angles of patients after manual and robotic TKA. Measured values show a much broader variation of varus or valgus angles after manual TKA compared to robotic technique ($p < 0.0001$).

The first follow-up examinations at 3 and 6 months did not show any visible change of the initial implant position in either group. Scores at this stage did not significantly differ in patients treated with robotic or manual technique.

12.5 **Discussion**

Various experimental active and semi-active robotic systems have been developed to improve the accuracy of implant alignment. To our knowledge, this is the first clinical report of robotic TKR in a large series of consecutive patients.

Our results clearly demonstrate that, after a short learning period, the CASPAR system allows the surgeon to execute his preoperative plan with an accuracy below 1° and achieve optimum to very good results regarding tibiofemoral alignment in over 95% of the patients as compared to around 65% with manual technique. Aglietti and co-workers reported that the majority of conventionally operated patients end up with a mean valgus angle of 9.6° ranging from 2 to 16°.[25] Correct tibiofemoral alignment seems to be particularly important since it is generally agreed that axial deviation and imprecise implantation may lead to early loosening of implant components.[6–9] The results of alignment after robotic TKR are not only superior to the results of conventional technique, but also to the results of computer-assisted, navigated TKR. Miehlke and co-workers found that 63% of patients had an acceptable tibiofemoral alignment within the 3 degree varus/valgus range after navigated TKR. 30% of the patients had a deviation from ideal alignement of 3–4°. More than 4° of deviation with a maximum of 7° were observed in 7% of the navigated patients.[16]

In a recently presented comparative study Saragaglia and co-workers reported that 84% of navigated patients ended up within the acceptable 3° range versus 75% of the manually operated patients.[17] This indicates that although computer-assisted navigation yields superior results to manual technique it is still inferior to robotic technique regarding orientation of the prosthetic components. In contrast to the CASPAR System, navigation systems for TKR still depend on intramedullary and extramedullary guides, which might be an important cause for potential errors in axial alignment.[26] Another benefit of the robotic technique might be the accurate planning of the milling track and the type of cutting used. This should result in a reduced risk for injury of ligaments, vessels, and nerves, which are undoubtedly endangered by manually directed oscillating saws. The osseous insertion of the posterior cruciate ligament for instance can always be preserved. Implants fit more exactly because the milled surfaces are always precisely flat, a matter of particular importance when cementless systems are used. Finally, the amount of removed bony substance can be minimized which could facilitate later revision surgery.

The design of the fixating frame has been improved already, but we believe that further design improvements and more experience handling the frame will bring additional time savings. We hope that operative times will soon be within the range required for conventional TKRs. Preoperative planning, marker placement, and CT scanning will remain additional time expenditures; but these are the very steps which lead to the higher accuracy achieved with this system and the potential for prolonged implant longevity. Working with a three-dimensional planning system highlights the shortcomings of the various implant systems. Surgeons may want to select the system most suited for a particular patient rather than utilize a single system for all patients. Manufacturers may wish to expand product offerings or to improve the design to make the implant match the high standards defined by this type of planning and operation. Concerns about the best type of coating (hydroxyapatite or porous) for cementless endoprostheses are again becoming a central topic of discussion. The pros and cons need to be assessed in reliable prospective studies which may have to include migration analysis by X-ray stereometric techniques.

We can imagine that surgical robots and navigational systems will be combined in the future. This approach would use the full potential of both computer-assisted systems.

12.6 **Summary**

Total knee replacement (TKR) is a common procedure for treatment of severe gonarthrosis, but the outcome may be unsatisfactory due to primary malalignment of the prosthetic components. In order to improve precision and accuracy of this surgical procedure, a robotic surgical system (CASPAR®) has been adapted to assist the surgeon in preoperative planning and the intra-operative preparation of the tibia and femur.

In a prospective clinical study, 114 patients with idiopathic gonarthrosis were operated on with either a manual (52 patients) or robotic assisted technique (62 patients). No major adverse events related to the use of the robotic system have been observed. The mean difference between preoperatively planned and post-operatively achieved tibiofemoral alignment was 0.8° (0–4.1°) in the robotic group versus 2.6° (0–7°) in the manual group (p < 0.0001).

Clear advantage of robotic assistive TKR is the ability to execute a CT based three dimensional preoperative plan with very high precision. Due to better alignment of the prosthetic components and improved bone-implant fit, we anticipate decreased implant loosening that may be most evident in non-cemented prostheses. Currently clear disadvantages are the need for additional surgery for placement of fiducial markers, increased operating times and higher overall costs.

References

1 Aglietti P, Buzzi R. Posteriorly stabilised total-condylar knee replacement. *J Bone Joint Surg* 1988;70B:211–16.

2 Jeffery RS, Morris RW, Denham RA. Coronal alignment after total knee replacement. *J Bone Joint Surg* 1991;73B:709–14.

3 Petersen TL, Engh GA. Radiographic assessment of knee alignment after total knee arthroplasty. *J Arthroplasty* 1988;3:67–72.

4 Tew M, Waugh W. Tibiofemoral alignment and the results of knee replacement. *J Bone Joint Surg* 1985;67B:551–6.

5 Garg A, Walker PS. Prediction of total knee motion using a three-dimensional computer graphics model. *J Biochem* 1990;23:45–58.

6 Ecker ML, Lotke PA, Sindsor RE, Cella JP. Long-term results after total condylar knee arthroplasty. Significance of radiolucent lines. *Clin Orthop* 1987;216:151–8.

7 Feng EL, Stuhlberg SD, Wixon RL. Progressive subluxation and polyethylene wear in total knee replacements with flat articular surfaces. *Clin Orthop* 1994;299:60–71.

8 Laskin RS. Total condylar knee replacement in patients who have rheumatoid arthritis. A ten year follow-up study. *J Bone Joint Surg* 1990;72A:529–35.

9 Ritter M, Merbst WA, Keating EM, Faris PM. Radiolucency at the bone-cement interface in total knee replacement. *J Bone Joint Surg* 1991;76A:60–5.

10 Goodfellow JW, O'Connor JJ. Clinical results of the Oxford knee. *Clin Orthop* 1986;205:21–4.

11 Insall JN, Ranawat CS, Aglietti P, Shine J. A comparison of four models of total knee-replacement prosthesis. *J Bone Joint Surg* 1976;58A:754–65.

12 Insall JN, Binzzir R, Soudry M, Mestriner LA. Total knee arthroplasty. *Clin Orthop* 1985;192:13–22.

13 Ranawat CS, Boachie-Adjei O. Survivorship analysis and results of total condylar knee arthroplasty. *Clin Orthop* 1988;226:6–13.

14 Delp SL, Stulberg SD, Davies B, Picard F, Leitner F. Computer assisted knee replacement. *Clin Orthop* 1998;354:49–56.

15 Jenny JY, Boeri C. Computer-assisted total knee prosthesis implantation without preoperative imaging. A comparison with classical instrumentation. *Presented at the Fourth Annual North American Programm on Computer Assisted Orthopaedic Surgery*, 2000. Pittsburgh, PA.

16 Miehlke RK, Clemens U, Kershally S. Computer integrated instrumentation in knee arthroplasty—a comparative study of conventional and computerized technique. *Presented at the Fourth Annual North American Programm on Computer Assisted Orthopaedic Surgery*, 2000. Pittsburgh, PA.

17 Saragaglia D, Picard F, Chaussard D, Montbarbon E, Leitner F, Cinquin P. Computer assisted total knee arthroplasty: comparison with a conventional procedure. Results of a 50 cases prospective randomized study. *Presented at the First Annual Meeting of Computer Assisted Orthopedic Surgery*, 2001. Davos, Switzerland.

18 Davies BL, Harris SJ, Lin WJ, Hibberd RD, Middleton R, Cobb JC. Active compliance in robotic surgery—the use of force control as a dynamic restraint. *Proc Instn Mech Eng* 1997;211:285–92.

19 Martelli M, Marcacci M, Nofrini F, *et al.* Computer- and robot-assisted total knee replacement: analysis of a new surgical procedure. *Ann Biomed Eng* 2000;28:1146–53.

20 Kienzle TC, Stulberg SD, Peshkin M, *et al.* A computer-assisted total knee replacement surgical system using a calibrated robot. In RH Taylor *et al.*, eds. *Computer-integrated surgery*. 1995:409–16. Cambridge, MA: MIT Press.

21 Picard F, Moody J, Jaramaz B, DiGioia A, Nikou C, LaBarca RS. A classification proposal for computer-assisted knee systems. *Presented at the Fourth Annual North American Programm on Computer Assisted Orthopaedic Surgery*, 2000. Pittsburgh, PA.

22 Gebhard F, Kinzl L, Arand M. Computerassistierte Chirurgie. *Unfallchirurg* 2000;103:612–17.

23 Petermann J, Kober R, Heinze, R, Frölich JJ, Heeckt PF, Gotzen L. Computer-assisted planning and robot-assisted surgery in anterior cruciate ligament reconstruction. *Oper Techn Orthop* 2000;10:50–5.

24 Insall JN, Dorr LD, Scott R, Scott WN. Rationale of the knee society clinical rating system. *Clin Orthop* 1989;248:13–4.

25 Aglietti P, Buzzi R, Gaudenzi A. Patellofemoral functional results and complications with the posterior stabilized total condylar knee prosthesis. *J Arthroplasty* 1988;3:17–25.

26 Nuño-Siebrecht N, Tanzer M, Bobyn JD. Potential errors in axial alignment using intramedullary instrumentation for total knee arthroplasty. *J Arthroplasty* 2000;15:228–30.

Chapter 13

Knee reconstructive surgery: preoperative model system

F. Picard, James E. Moody, Anthony M. DiGioia III, Branislav Jaramaz, Anton Y. Plakseychuk, and David Sell

13.1 Clinical challenges

13.1.1 State of the art in standard TKR

The first chapter has already reminded us of the rationale of Total Knee Replacement (TKR) and only a few important requirements for the standard TKR surgery have been listed in the following paragraph.

The functional result of a TKR depends on preoperative management, the surgeon's skills, knee kinematics properties, bone quality, soft tissue damages, implant design, and post-operative follow-up.

Longevity of the knee implant depends on material properties (i.e. type of cement or type of polyethylene) and implants positioning. Incorrect positioning, improper alignment and poor soft tissue balance of the limb can lead to accelerated implant wear, loosening, and sub-optimal functional performance.[1,2] Except for the surgical planning and the procedure, other factors, such as polyethylene wear, are out of the surgeon's control.

However, precise intra-operative measurements still remain challenging. Even the most elaborate mechanical instrumentation system relies on visual cues to confirm the accuracy of the limb and implant alignment, particularly rotational orientation, and are subject to significant errors. Thus, the two main challenges facing orthopaedic surgeons during TKR procedure: soft tissue balancing and bone cuts alignment.

13.1.1.1 Soft tissue balancing

Several anatomical components form part of the knee joint soft tissue. Cruciate ligaments and collateral ligaments are the main anatomic factors that need to be balanced during the TKR procedure. In the case of knee varus deformity, the fibular collateral ligament (FCL) becomes lax, and the femur is twisted outward over the tibial plateau. In case of valgus deformity of the knee, the tibial collateral ligament (TCL) also becomes lax, and again traditional clinical and radiological evaluation—even with the use of 'stressed knee X-ray'—underestimates the degree of knee laxity. Authors consider that optimal release for knee balancing of the FCL and TCL is around one centimeter (i.e. 8 degrees in the coronal plane).[3,4]

Actually, the daily challenge for the knee surgeon is to evaluate simultaneously knee laxities, range of motion, medial and lateral joint gaps and patellar motion at any moment of the surgical procedure. Traditional mechanical instrumentation enables the surgeon to measure gaps between the knee in flexion and the knee in extension and surgeons 'eye-ball' to evaluate the tibial polyethylene lift-off.[33] However, accurate measurements of gaps, laxity and tibial-femoral-patellar implants trial need either numerous cumbersome mechanical jigs or considerable surgeon experience.

13.1.1.2 Bone cuts

Three bones (femur, tibia and patella) must be properly cut, in order to secure the knee implants. Bone resections modify ligament tensions and consequently the soft tissue balancing.

Knee anatomy limits the level of bone resections. For instance, only between 18 mm and 22 mm (room for metal back and polyethylene) can be resected between the femur and the tibia on an extended knee.[5] According to the ligament tensions, the size and thickness of the implant, the surgeon defines the ideal bone cut resection. Posterior, anterior and chamfer cuts traditionally depend on the distal femoral cut. However, anterior bone resection influences femoro patellar pressure and stability. Even though several factors have been involved in the patella prosthesis, failures such as vascular factor,[2,6,7] high pressure,[8,9] patellar position,[10] and femoral implants position still remain important issues that the surgeon needs to address.[11]

In addition to the knee anatomic limitations, several bone cut orientations can be performed. For instance, Hungerford[7] and Krackow[12] proposed in the past to perform a three degrees varus femoral cut. Dejour[13] proposed a bone cut perpendicular to the mechanical axis and Insall[2] would rather advise to cut the femur bone in valgus. Several philosophies have also been described for the tibial cut orientation (perpendicular to the mechanical axis, posterior slope, etc.). More recently external femoral knee implant orientation was also emphasized.[14,15]

These are the major issues in standard TKR surgery. Revision knees are still more challenging. This noncomprehensive review of the state of the art in TKR surgery shows us how accurate TKR surgery needs to be. Any surgical tools or devices capable of informing the surgeon accurately and interactively during TKR surgery are very relevant. A precise preoperative plan, immediate and accurate intra-operative feedback information (such as bone resection orientation, alignment, range of motion, and tension) are valuable permitting the surgeon to confidently perform the TKR surgery.

13.1.2 State of the art of related computer assisted orthopaedic surgery (CAOS) applications

13.1.2.1 General considerations

Our objective in this part is to describe the goal of computer assisted systems to address general challenges in TKR. TKR is already a cost effective surgery and represents a good investment for society.[16,17] However, revision cases are growing and unsatisfactory results still remain a daily issue for orthopaedic surgeons, whatever the patient's complaint. The general challenge of computer assisted surgery is to improve the result, to decrease the complications and therefore to be more effective.

Whatever the measure of post-operative TKR outcomes (such as alignment, stiffness, and knee anterior pain), the range of surgical outcomes typically follows a guassian curve (Fig. 13.1). The ordinate axis of the curve is the ideal goal (such as perfect alignment), round the ordinate axis is an area in which the results are estimated as very good and good (red portion of the curve). Then there is a third area around the one just described in which the results are fair or poor (blue portion of the curve). This blue portion represents, for instance, wrong knee implant positioning. The ultimate goal of computer assisted surgery is to reduce variation from best practice and to eliminate the number of outliers.

Our assumption is that by using computer assisted surgical technology surgeons will be able to improve the traditional procedure, avoiding functional and anatomical outliers.

13.1.2.2 Specific considerations

In 1997, Ayers did a comprehensive overview of common complications in TKR.[16] The following table lists the main complications, which occurred after standard TKR. According to current know-how in

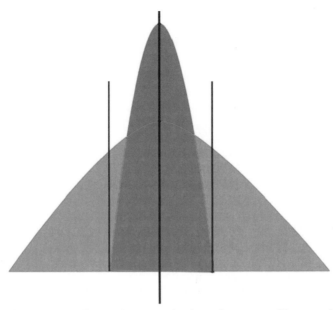

Fig. 13.1 Whatever the post-operative TKR issues are (such as alignment, stiffness, and knee anterior pain), the entire surgical outcomes can be represented with a gaussian curve. (See Plate 3.)

image guided computer assisted technology, we matched the potential ability for this technology to provide tools able to solve complications after TKR. Each time computer assisted technology is able to provide devices for solving or avoiding a complication, we have used a positive sign. Each time computer assisted technology is not currently able to provide any devices for solving or avoiding a complication, we have used a negative sign. Each time we don't know whether or not computer assisted technology will ever be able to provide devices for solving or avoiding a complication we have used a question mark (Table 13.1).

13.2 **System description**

13.2.1 **Classification**

Several image guided TKR navigation systems are now either under development or in clinical use. Image guided navigation for TKR relies on identical principles and we describe below their common concepts. According to the classification, these systems are Surgical Navigation Systems (SNS). There are preoperative-model systems using patient-specific data.

13.2.2 **Important concept**

Image Guided Navigation Technologies for TKR is based on two concepts:

- The first is building a preoperative model on which the surgeon can simulate the surgery such as TKR sizing or implant placement and even simulated range of motion.
- The second is to intra-operatively navigate in order to implement the preoperative planning during the surgical procedure.

Table 13.1 Common complications in TKA

Complications	Classical technique	Computer assisted technique
Wound complication	Vascular investigation Decisional algorithm	?
Neurovascular	Preoperative management	+ (planning)
Infection	Pre-, intra and post-operative management	?
	Vascular investigation Decisional algorithm Antibiotic prophylaxis	+/−
Skin problem	Preoperative management	+ + (planning)
Thrombo-embolic disease	Pre intra and post operative management and pneumatic tourniquet	+ (planning control) − (increased time)*
Problem related to the extensor mechanism		
Patellar instability	Pre and intra operative management	+ (planning and Intra
Patellar fracture	Pre and intraoperative management	Operative (IO) control)
Loosening of Patellar Component	Intraoperative management	+ (planning and (IO) control)
Failure of Patellar Component	Intraoperative management	+ (planning and control)
Patella clunk syndrome	Intraoperative management	+ (planning and control)
Rupture of The Extensor M.	Intraoperative and postoperative management	+/− (planning and control) ?
Stiffness	Intra-operative and post-operative management	+ (planning and control)
Alignment	Pre and intra-operative management	+ + +
Soft-tissue balance	Pre and intra-operative management	+ + +
Supracondylar fracture	Intra-operative management	+ + +

* Duration of the pneumatic tourniquet must be less than two hours. This is a very important requirement in computer assisted surgery.

IO, intra operative.

13.2.3 **Steps**

13.2.3.1 Building a preoperative model

Four major steps must be accomplished during the preoperative model construction:

- taking medical images of the patient;
- surface reconstruction;
- model construction;
- planning and simulation.

Taking medical images. Image guided navigation technology uses medical images to generate an accurate 3D model of the femur, tibia and patella. The current systems use CT scan images, and no current

CAS in clinical use works with MRI images—yet.[18] Ultrasound images have the potential to be more routinely used.

CT protocol

Patient positioning

Most of the image guided systems use pinless registration, meaning that no fiducial markers are fixed in the bone prior to the surgery. However, the robotic assisted systems in current use are image based and need pin fixation prior to the CT scan procedure.[19]

Several steps must be taken before taking CT scan images in order to obtain high quality images. Ensure that the patient has no metal in the leg region which could cause artifact in the scan (i.e. buttons, zippers, etc.) and warn the patient of the procedure especially explaining to him about not moving during it.

Number of slices

The patient is placed in a support fixture on the CT table and is oriented in supine position on the radiological table. The length of the foot cradles are adjusted to fit the patient and all straps and pads are securely fastened. Again, the patient is informed that he needs to remain still during the CT scan. The number of slices is from 75 to 150.[11,20]

Duration of procedure

Images must be continuous, under one exam number, and within the same series. Scouts must be in a separate series than the images. The technician acquires a scout image, which includes the entire femur and tibia. Then, one millimeter selected slice at one millimeter spacing are taken in the crucial area (hip, knee and ankle joints). In metaphyseal areas the selected slices are 1 mm thick and 5 mm spacing. The thickness of the slices in midshaft are 1 mm and spacing 50 mm in noncritical area. The field of view should be as small as possible while ensuring that the entire leg is within the field.

The technician starts the scan and does not adjust the table height or field of view during the scan. At this time the patient must not move at all. If patient motion occurs at anytime during the scan, the procedure should be begun again.

Storage of the images
Downloading to three-dimensional reconstruction station

Surface reconstruction. After receiving the images from the CT scan computer, each slice is then selected and analyzed on the monitor screen in order to perform contour acquisitions. Several algorithms have been implemented to facilitate the process of contour acquisitions.

Model construction. The CT images are transferred from the scanner to a workstation. These images are segmented to obtain contours of the femur, tibia and patella geometry. The segmented image slices are then interpolated between slices in order to generate a full surface and 3D model of the bone geometry (Fig. 13.2).

Once a three-dimensional bone model has been built, a 3D model and slices are downloaded in a software program called planner.

Planning and simulation. Conventional planning for TKR uses biplanar radiographic images and templates. This radiographic planning can approximate implant position and size. Computer assisted

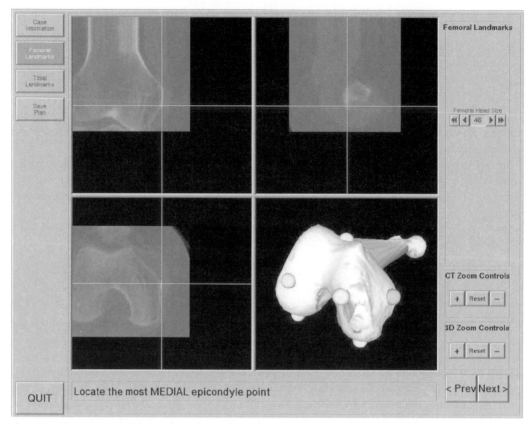

Fig. 13.2 The segmented image slices are then interpolated between slices in order to generate a full surface and 3D model of the bone geometry.

planning permits us to simulate three-dimensional positioning of the implant. Using a series of computer assisted implant models from a data base, the surgeon adjusts as well as is possible the implant in the patient's model. A multitude of features are already available.[4,11,20,21] Graphic software allows the surgeon to simulate cutting, drilling bones, moving implants and bones independently. As a result of this simulation, the surgeon can observe the direct consequences of the surgical procedure such as how much bone should be ideally resected for placing the implants and what the implant orientation is with respect to the anatomical landmarks. Interactive software enables the surgeon to move the bone and the joint in order to appreciate the relationship between implant and bone. In addition to this feature, the computer can simulate the motion of the joint to verify the proper placement of the implant. No image guided TKR preoperative planner is able today to use data based computer gait modeling, or the surgical experience algorithm, yet.

Once the surgeon has optimized the plan and placement of implant components, all relevant parameters are stored for image the guided procedure. The data are then downloaded to a computer in the OR for the intra-operative navigation. Several procedures exist to verify the quality of the data transfer.

13.2.3.2 Intra-operative navigation

The equipment includes. A localizer: optical and electromagnetic. Several models are already in clinical use. One of the most frequently use in the OR is the Optotrak and the Polaris from Northern Digital (Waterloo, Canada). Another alternative is the use of EM (electromagnetic tracking):

—trackers (rigid bodies) containing light emitting diodes or EM tracking;

—coupling mechanical instruments that attach the trackers to the bone (Fig. 13.3);

—a computer;

—a monitor screen;

—a foot pedal control or a virtual keyboard for sterile system control.

Tool calibration. Two options are possible. The first option is to calibrate the traditional surgical device equipped with a tracker. Once the tool calibration is performed, the localizer can follow the assembly in real time. This option has been chosen for some systems (Navitrack, Brainlab). The guides are equipped with a marker and are calibrated for orienting the surgical procedure (Fig. 13.4). The second option is to use traditional untracked instruments and then use a specific tracked tool to measuring their orientation. This option has been chosen for KneeNav-TKR. The traditional jigs were secured

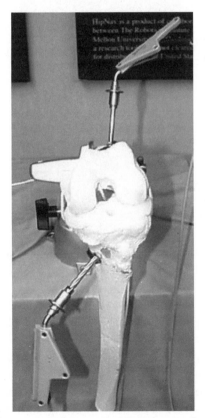

Fig. 13.3 Coupling mechanical instruments that attach the trackers to the bone.

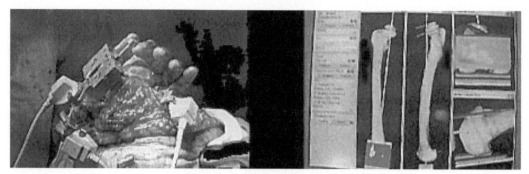

Fig. 13.4 The guides are equipped with a marker and are calibrated for orienting the surgical procedure.

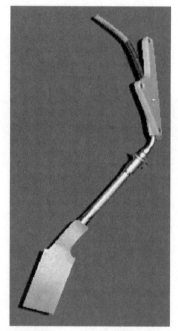

Fig. 13.5 The traditional jigs were secured as usual and a calibrated 'plate-probe' mimicking a traditional saw-blade is used for measuring the jig orientation and predicting saw cuts.

as usual and a calibrated 'plate-probe' mimicking a traditional saw-blade is used for measuring the jig orientation and predicting saw cuts (Fig. 13.5).

Registration. The goal of registration is to establish the proper transformation between the bone model and the CT scan, in essence calibrating the patient. Registration is achieved by minimizing the distance between the intra-operatively acquired cloud of points and the CT based surface model of the bone. Following successful registration, the tibia and femur are independently tracked using the user graphical interface depicted on screen (Fig. 13.6).

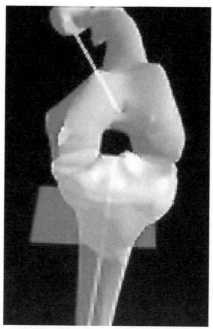

Fig. 13.6 Following successful registration, the tibia and femur are independently tracked using the graphical user interface depicted on-screen.

Verification. Using a calibrated probe on the bone surface, the surgeon verifies that the corresponding point is properly indicated on CT images.

Navigation. Using the preoperative planning data or intra-operative information, the surgeon can obtain immediate feedback on what he is actually surgically performing. Several features have been used, and we listed the most important.

* Soft tissue evaluation

The surgeon can measure laxities in every direction: anterior, posterior and medial, and lateral in each degree of knee flexion and each time he wants to do it. A user interface depicts numbers in degrees (medial/lateral laxity) and in millimeters (anterior/posterior drawer) informing about knee testing.

The surgeon can also be informed about medial and lateral gaps between femur and tibia permanently updated (taking into account the bone resections). This interactive data allows him to adjust and follow the preoperative planning. The surgeon can also control the range of motion of the knee

* Bone cuts

The surgeon can orient cutting guides, jigs, saw-blades, and drilling in real time. Interactive user interfaces represent ideal orientation and tools direction at the same time. Thus, the computer aids to cut the tibia, femur and patella bones in all direction and all planes. According to the preoperative plan and the frame of references—chosen by pointing anatomical landmarks—bone angle cuts and distance measurements inform the surgeon about alignment, implant size, rotational position and relationships between bone and implant (such as anterior femur cortex and implant orientation).

In addition to this information, the surgeon can verify the bone resection height and gaps between bones before trialing implants.

* Documenting

At the end of each case, each surgical step is recorded from the beginning (preoperative planning) to the end (final verification) and can be used to correlate TKR anatomical placement and patient's outcomes.

13.2.4 Surgical technique

13.2.4.1 Patient positioning and surgical exposure

The patient is laid down on the surgical table as for traditional TKR procedure. Pillow, leg holders, lateral holders and pneumatic tourniquets are used as usual.

Draping is performed in a sterilized way excluding the pneumatic tourniquet. No alterations in the surgical incision usually used for TKR surgery need to be made for the computer assisted technique.

Surgical exposure prefers a straight midline skin incision and a medial parapatellar exposure. However, several types of skin and articular incisions are possible as long as the surgeon remembers to leave enough room for trackers and coupling systems.

13.2.4.2 Computer assisted surgical procedure

The next step combines traditional surgery and computer assisted navigation surgery. Most of the image guided navigation systems follow the normal surgical flow, which must be a surgical requirement as important as the sterilization requirements. According to the surgical procedures variability, systems permit to chose the surgical steps such as femur first, tibia second and patella third. Surgical flow and sequences in TKR depend on surgeon preferences. We arbitrarily chose to describe a traditional surgical flow with the tibial cut first, femoral cut second, and patellar cut third. The patellar cut still remains an underdeveloped feature which is not described below. Soft tissue balancing is also an important feature of computer assisted TKR navigation. This feature can be tested before any bone cuts, between tibial and femoral cuts and at any time the surgeon sees fit.

Tibial cut. The surgeon adjusts the mechanical jigs and the tibial cutting block. Both extra- and intramedullary instrumentation can be used. Traditionally, the surgeon places an intramedullary rod inside the tibial canal and secures on the top of it a series of mechanical tools, which serves to orient the actual tibial cutting guide. In addition to the intramedullary rod, extramedullary instrumentation can be used. The monitor screen displays a graphical interface and represents the three dimension orientations with respect to the 3D patient's specific model of the cutting guides equipped with trackers. Several graphical interfaces already exist showing angles and cutting orientations or both.

At this point, there are two possibilities:

- the surgeon adjusts 'free-hand' the cutting block in a satisfactory position using an image guided control or

- he uses an adjustable mechanical instrument for reaching the computer assisted recommended position.

Therefore, the surgeon makes the proximal cut with an oscillating saw. Some image navigation systems also permit the navigation of devices like drill or power bladder. After cutting the bone the cut orientation is measured. Using a plate-probe, the surgeon lays it down on the proximal tibia and can verify the actual cut (Fig. 13.7).

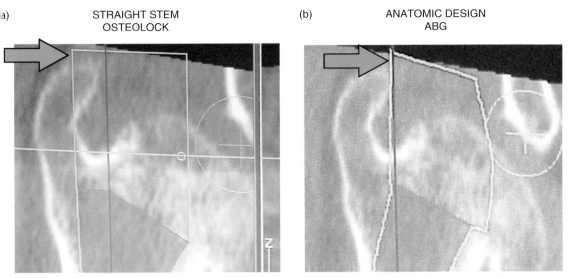

(a) STRAIGHT STEM
OSTEOLOCK

(b) ANATOMIC DESIGN
ABG

Plate 1 Outline of cutting path (green line) in relation to the greater trochanter (arrow) in straight stem design vs. anatomic stem design.

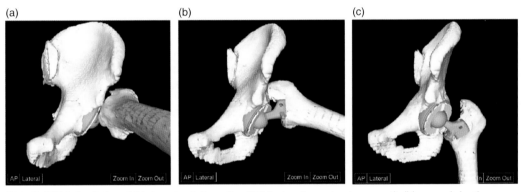

(a) (b) (c)

Plate 2 ROM simulation: (a) internal rotation after 90° flexion (bone impingement); (b) max. abduction; (c) max. external rotation. The red dot indicates the impingement point.

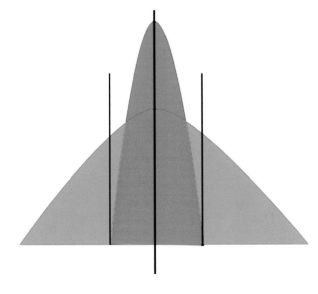

Plate 3 Whatever the post-operative TKR issues are (such as alignment, stiffness, and knee anterior pain), the entire surgical outcomes can be represented with a gaussian curve.

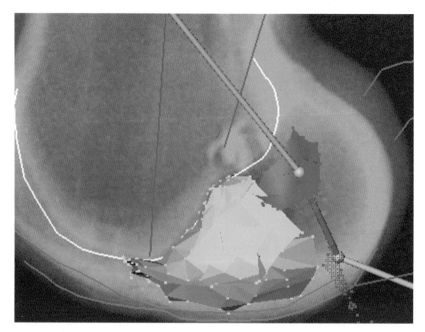

Plate 4 The system can provide the surgeon with feedback on ligament elongation if a *ligament attachment area* has been defined. The **red** zone on the femoral attachment area indicates a region of insertion where elongation exceeds 3 mm. The meaning of these elongation values is, however, controversial.

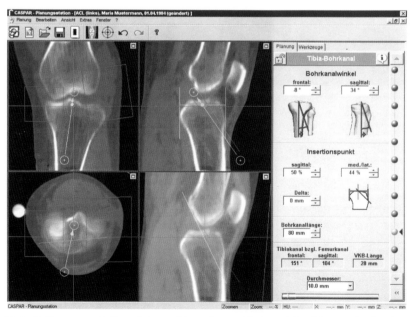

Plate 5 Blumensaat's line of the stable and unstable knee joint (blue and yellow), the planned tibial drill tunnel (yellow) with the chosen diameter (10 mm), and the areas which must not be crossed in order to avoid impingement syndromes are marked.

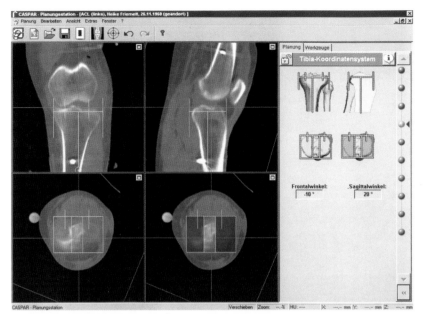

Plate 6
Normalization of the proximal tibia. The tibial axis and the width and depth of the tibia head plateau are marked, and the dimensions of the femoral condyles are the red areas. In this region no tunnel has to be planned to avoid graft impingement syndromes.

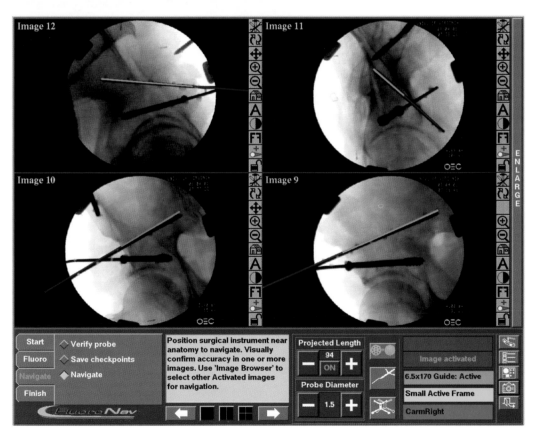

Plate 7 A high anterior column acetabular fracture is reduced intra-operatively with a temporary external fixator. Two screws placed in standard trajectories are then used to stabilize the fracture. In the navigation views for virtual fluoroscopy, the drill guide is represented as a red line, and the predicted trajectory in green is superimposed on the actual position following guide wire placement.

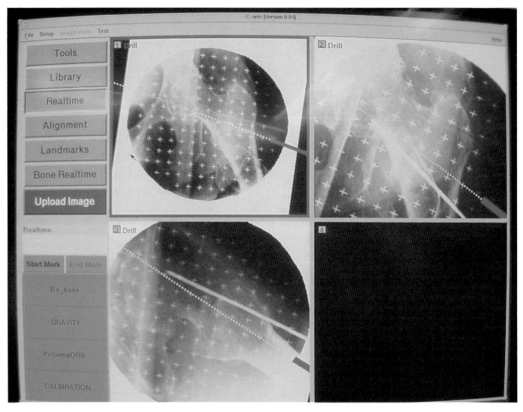

Plate 8 Virtual fluoroscopy for guidewire placement for DHS osteosynthesis of a pertrochanteric femoral fracture. A Kirschner wire was inserted for temporary fracture fixation. Position of the central guidewire is simulated as a red bar and dotted line in an anterior-posterior and axial view simultaneously.

(a)

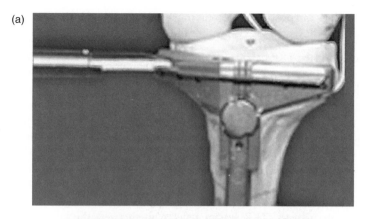

(b)

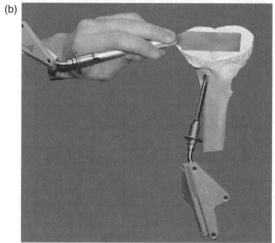

Fig. 13.7 Using a plate-probe, the surgeon controls the cutting guide orientation (a) and lays it down on the proximal tibia and can verify the actual cut. (b)

Femur cut. The surgeon adjusts the mechanical jigs in order to ultimately orient the distal femoral cutting guide. Traditionally the surgeon fits in the femoral canal an intramedullary rod on which a modular block is oriented according to the preoperative planning. Planning determines cut levels, orientations, and relationships between anterior femoral cortex implant sizes.

The series of guides are adjusted until the distal guide is fixed while some graphical interfaces are displayed on the monitor screen in order to improve final instrumentation positioning. Another alternative is to adjust the traditional cutting guides and measure their orientations with the use of a removable device such as a probe.

Afterward, the cut can be verified with the use of tools such as a calibrated plate-probe. The rest of the cuts (anterior/posterior and chamfer cuts) are traditionally performed, or computer oriented.

Patellar cut. Though patellar issues are still among the surgeon's major concerns in TKR. There is currently, no computer assisted image system able to navigate patellar bone cuts or patella balancing, yet.[22,23]

Soft tissue balancing. As explained in a previous chapter soft-tissue balancing remains an open issue in Total Knee Replacement (TKR);[12] poor balancing aggravates with wear, loosening, failure, and revision.

Image guided technology can provide some tools to preoperatively and intra-operatively measure data enabled the surgeon to adjust as well as is possible the TKR balance.

Current computer assisted TKR balancing systems are still at an early stage of development. Ideally, a comprehensive computer-assisted analysis of the soft tissue balancing would establish relationships between knee deformity and soft tissue behaviour preoperatively and intra-operatively.

Current image guided systems can only provide intra-operative information on laxity, range of motion, and the gaps between femur and tibia joints. Computer-assisted image technology gives an opportunity to accurately measure angles, distances, volumes and isometry of the knee joint. Intra-operatively the surgeon tests and evaluates the tension of the collateral ligament in inducing a stress on the knee in varus and valgus in several degrees of flexion. Knee joint manipulations can be made prior to any bone cuts, and at any stage of implant trialing. According to the strength of the surgical manipulations and resultant stress generated on the knee joint, valgus and varus angles are also depicted. In the same way the computer assisted TKR system reflects interactively the knee range of motion and femoro-tibial gaps.

13.3 Validation and accuracy: experimental results

A computer assisted image navigation system KneeNav (Casurgica, Pittsburgh USA) was used to gauge the reliability and repeatability of representative types of mechanical alignment systems.

Two surgeons each performed 20 traditional TKR resections on foambone knee models in a simulated clinical setting. Each surgeon performed ten procedures with intramedullary instrumentation on the femur and ten with extra-medullary instrumentation on the tibia. The goal of the surgery was to perform the femoral and tibial cuts perpendicularly to the mechanical axes (90) and to align the distal femoral cutting guide to the transepicondylar axis. Using computer assisted technology for measuring final cuts, in the frontal plane, the tibia (mean = 89, SD = 0.8) and the femur (89.6 ± 1.3) were repeatedly aligned. In the sagittal plane, tibia (88.2 ± 1.1) was more consistently aligned than the femur (90.8 ± 5.6). The average femoral rotational alignment angle was 2.3 ± 3 with respect to the transepicondylar line. Actual cuts were measured after the cuts were made. But with the tibial slope, no statistical difference between final cutting guide orientations and actual cuts was found (Fig. 13.8).

This computer assisted system was able to evaluate traditional instrumentation, particularly for jig stability and saw slot design.

13.4 Discussion

Using the computer assisted knee system as a measurement tool, we confirmed that traditional instrumentation on sawbone models was reliable and accurate enough for guiding bone cuts especially in the frontal plane. Moreover, using a simple tool called a 'plate-probe' in each measurement step of total knee replacement procedure on sawbones, this computer assisted system collected all angle cuts before and after the surgeons made bone resections with a traditional oscillating saw-blade.

'Total knee arthroplasty is a predictable and durable operation'[8,15] and is also cost effective for society.[9] However, in surgical technique, it has been proven for several years that soft tissue balancing and implant orientation had an important influence upon short and long term results.[24] Poor soft tissue balance and malalignment increase the likelihood of failure. Reducing the number of poor outcomes is an obvious target of this surgery. 'Ad integrum' range of motion (ROM) recovering, painless joint restoration is a common patient and surgeon expectation. Improving long term result from knee

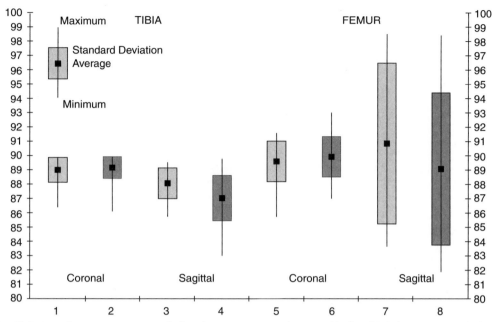

Fig. 13.8 Actual cuts were measured after the cuts were made. But with the tibial slope, no statistical difference between final cutting guide orientations and actual cuts was found.

implants by soft tissue balance control and better alignment also makes sense for limiting polyethylene wear and optimizing knee kinematics.[25]

Our purpose was to evaluate the cutting guide and actual three-dimensional alignments. Frontal and sagittal alignment has been indicated as a traditional concern in the literature.[13] Recent concern is the rotational position of the femoral and tibial components, which influences the patellar tracking.[16,26] Abnormal alignment of the femoral component generates patellar anterior pain, subluxation and even patellar dislocation. Femoro-patellar problems are estimated as one of the main complications of total knee arthroplasty.[27]

The surgeon usually defines the preoperative implant position in a traditional procedure with respect to radiological landmarks.[7,28] The traditional preoperative TKR planning frame is a biplanar X-ray. The surgeon plans on a frontal long leg X-ray the orientation angle of the femoral and tibial intramedullary rod relative to the femoral and tibial mechanical axis. Then, using a set of jigs and guide blocks, the surgeon adjusts the bone cut orientation according to planned templates. This protocol was followed during this experiment. Afterward, using an oscillating saw the surgeon cuts the distal femur, proximal tibia and articular surface of the patella. After trialing the implants, the final components are anchored with or without cement. Each step represents a potential source of error in final component orientation (Fig. 13.9).

Deep landmarks (such as the center of the femoral head), imprecise reference frames (such as epicondyles for the transepicondylar axis reference), and limited accuracy of radiological planning, can generate errors between planning and cutting block orientations.[1,3]

Cutting guide instability, blade quality, bone density variations and unsteady manual sawing can also influence the final orientation of the cut.

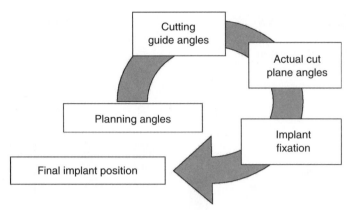

Fig. 13.9 Each step represents a potential source of error in the final component orientation.

Finally irregular cement fixation and asymmetric antero-posterior cuts can prevent an ideal fitting of the component on the actual cut.

Thus cumulative errors can lead to malalignment of the implant and consequently generate poor soft tissue balancing due to asymmetric gaps obtained between extended and flexed knee.[29] Using computer assisted system for measuring each step of alignment allows us to quantify potential error during the implant positioning.

In order to accurately measure the final cutting guides and actual cut angles, a consistent frame of reference must be defined for the femur, the tibia and the patella (which was not analyzed during this experiment). Using identical sawbone models was the strength of this experiment, because the measurements were taken with respect to an identical frame of reference. By definition, a frame is 'an arrangement of structural parts that gives form or support'. The anatomical frame of the femoral and tibial bone is a three-dimensional definitions so that frontal, sagittal and transversal orientations of the bones are included in the definition. We would like to emphasize our discussion on the femoral component, but the rationale concerning other bones is similar.

The femoral mechanical axis is traditionally defined as a line joining the center of the femoral head (center of the sphere) and the center of the radiographic knee (middle of the intercondylar notch).[5] The angle between the intramedullary axis and the mechanical axis measured preoperatively is used to adjust the distal femoral guide (5 was the angle used in our experiment). During the surgical procedure the predefined angle is set on the distal cutting block after the intramedullary rod is placed.[30,31] Because the femoral distal shaft axis (intramedullary axis) does not coincide exactly with the radiographic center of the femoral knee center there is a potential error in the cut orientation.[6,32]

In the sagittal plane, femoral cutting guide orientation is strictly dependent on the intramedullary rod orientation and thus on the distal femoral anatomy. Most of the commercial jigs are made up with a 8 to 12 mm (sometimes greater) diameter intramedullary rod and a support block fixed at 90°. Nevertheless the sagittal intramedullary rod axis does not necessarily align to the femoral mechanical axis due to the anterior-posterior femoral curvature variability (Fig. 13.10).

In our experiment we noticed the discrepancy between the femoral frontal cutting guide orientation (mean = 89.8, SD = ± 1.39) and the femoral sagittal cutting guide orientation (90.8 ± 5.6). Variable directions can be obtained from the 8 mm intramedullary rod relative to the distal femur and can

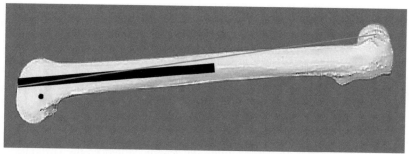

Fig. 13.10 Nevertheless the sagittal intramedullary rod axis does not necessarily align to the femoral mechanical axis due to the anterior-posterior femoral curvature variability.

explain the greater standard deviation. In vivo, bowed femur and variable intramedullary canal morphology can additionally modify the intramedullary rod orientation.[12] Discrepancies in this experiment are due to femoral entry point variation, the small diameter and small length of the intramedullary rod, which modified its orientation. Therefore, it seems better and more logical to use a longer and bigger intramedullary rod in order to eliminate orientation variability. However, a longer and bigger intramedullary rod will increase the fat thromboembolisms.

In routine TKR surgery, CT images are not routinely performed. Biplanar long leg X-rays is the traditional medical image for planning.[33] Radiological planning is supposed to reduce intra-operative mistakes. However, even a standardized rigorous biplanar radiological protocol is unable to take into account the transversal plane. CT (and MRI) scans both offer the advantages of accurate 3D landmarks for transversal implant planning.[19] Accurately define the transversal landmarks help the surgeon to determine the internal/external position of the femoral implant. In addition, orthopaedic surgeons use different intra-operative femoral frames of reference for component placement. At least four frames of reference are established for total knee replacement: the posterior condylar axis, the transepicondylar axis, the Whiteside's line and a systematic 3° external rotation relative to the postcondylar axis using a set of jigs.[2,10] Existence of several frames suggests that no one is undeniably superior to any other. We found a variability of the rotational positioning of the femoral component with a mean angle of 2.3° and significant standard deviation equal to 3°. These results are in agreement with the current concerns in TKR surgery.[16,26,27] All studies published reported an important range of angle distribution for femoral component rotation using an identical surgical protocol and the mechanical tools. These results suggest that an intra-operative navigation tool for component rotation would be useful.

The actual cut can be different with respect to the initial plane orientation as already mentioned. Reasons for changes are instability of the cutting guides, bad blade quality and irregular bone density.[12]

Instability of cutting guides is related to the mechanical play between the cutting blocks and fixture systems (such as pins, nails and threaded wires). The traditional mechanical jigs used in this experiment had pin fixation, which is the most commonly used. The number of pins for fixation and the bone density are also important factors for maintaining an excellent stability during the bone cut. Size and design of the slot in the cutting blocks represent an important factor for blade guidance. Traditionally, the larger the cutting block slot, the less flexible the blade, and consequently, a higher accuracy cut is obtained. On the other hand the larger the slot, the more cumbersome the cutting guide.

In this experiment the slot length of cutting blocks ranged from 10 mm (75% of the slot width) to 20 mm (25% of the block surface) for the tibial cutting block and 15 mm for femoral cutting blocks. No statistical difference was noticed between the frontal tibia cut and the actual cut orientation, whereas a statistical difference was obtained in the sagittal plane (out of degree, p = 0.04).[4] The slot length of a major part of the tibia slot (10 mm) is a reason for this discrepancy, since the orientation of the blade can change due to less mechanical constraints. Concerning the other cutting guides, which are 15 mm thick, no statistical significance was obtained between the distal femoral cutting guide orientation and the actual cut. According to these results we would consider that 15 mm is the minimum length for a reliable cutting guide slot. Thus even with an intramedullary rod, a more stable and more accurate final cut plane depends on cutting guide slot length. Moreover, the sawbones used in our experiment have a consistent texture quality, which is not typical for damaged knees. Osteoarthritic knees, for examples, have different bone density distribution with low bone density in some parts and high bone density elsewhere. Bone density variation and, obviously, the blade quality should also influence the actual cut plane relative to the cutting guide plane that could make a favourable argument for robot utilization. Finally, cement distribution can also modify slightly the final implant position. No cement was used during this experiment. This will be addressed in future work.

This experiment evaluated a mechanical jig system on sawbones, which is one of the main limitations of the study because it was not a real life surgery. The anatomy of the knee is clearly more complex than the sawbone model. Visual cues are more obvious using sawbones and give advantages for mechanical jig adjustment. Moreover, the lack of soft tissue (such as the extensor mechanism of the patella) simplified the jig fixation.

On the other hand, joint damage, and various bone shape and deformities of real knees are more variable than sawbones and would prevent us from having a sound analyze of the result on a perfect and identical base.

This image-guided measurement system enabled us to evaluate the mechanical instrumentation and showed that jig stability and cutting guide design had a significant role in the actual bone cuts.

In addition, this system provides an excellent tool for educational purposes. Junior surgeons would find this device helpful for understanding and practicing TKR in a didactic manner.

References

1 Feng EL, Stulberg SD, Wixson RL. Progressive subluxation and polyethylene wear in total knee replacements with flat articular surfaces. *Clin Orthop Relat Res* 1994;299:60–71.

2 Insall JN. *Surgery of the knee*, 2nd edn. New York: Churchill Livingstone, 1993.

3 Dejour H, Neyret Ph. Les gonarthroses. 7IEME journée Lyonnaise de chirurgie du genou 1991.

4 Delp SL, Stulberg SD, Davies B, Picard F, Leitner F. Computer assisted knee replacement. *Clin Orthop Rel Res* 1998;354:49–56.

5 Figgie HE, Golberg VM, Figgie MP, *et al.* The effect of alignment of the implant on fractures of the patella after condylar total knee arthroplasty. *J Bone Joint Surg* 1989;71A:1031–9.

6 Goutallier D, Hernigou Ph. L'arthroplastie unicompartimentale (type Lotus) dans le traitement de la gonarthrose latéralisée du sujet âgé. *Rev Chir Orthop* 1985;71:213–18.

7 Hungerford DS, Krackow KA, Kema RV. Total knee Arthroplasty: a comprehensive approach—Baltimore-Williams and Wilkins. 1984;167–178.

8 Incavo SJ, Johnson CC, Beynnon BD. Posterior cruciate ligament strain biomechanics in total knee arthroplasty. *Clin Orthop* 1994;309:88–93.

9 Jiang CC, Insall JN. Effect of rotation on the axial alignment of the femur. *Clin Orthop Rel Res* 1989;248:50–6.

10 Kahler DE, Lyttle D. Surgical interruption of the patellar blood supply by total knee arthroplasty. *Clin Orthop* 1988;221–7, 229.

11 Kienzle TC, Stulberg SD, Peshkin M, *et al.* (1995) A computer-assisted total knee replacement surgical system. In: Taylor R, Lavallee S, Burdea G, Mosges R, eds. *Computer-integrated surgery.* Cambridge MA: MIT Press, 1995.

12 Freeman MAR, Todd RC, Bamert TP, Day WH. ICLH arthroplasty of the knee. *J Bone Joint Surg* 1978; 60-B(3):339–44.

13 Dejour H, Deschamps G. Technique opératoire de la prothèse totale à glissement du genou. *Prothèses totales du genou. Cahier d'enseignement de la SOFCOT* 1989;35:13–24.

14 Berger RA, Crosset LS, Jacobs JJ, *et al.* Malrotation causing patellofemoral complications after total knee arthroplasty. *Clin Orthop Rel Res* 1998;356:144–53.

15 Heegaard J, Leyvraz F, Curnier A, *et al.* The biomechanics of the human patella during passive knee flexion. *J Biomech* 1995;28:1265–79.

16 Ayers DC, Dennis DA, Johnson NA *et al.* Common complications of total knee arthroplasty. *J Bone Joint Surg* 1997;79-A(2):278–311.

17 Rorabeck CH, Murray P. The cost benefit of total knee arthroplasty. *Orthopedics* 1996;19(9):777–9.

18 Pagetti C, Ciucci T, Papa E, Allota B, Dario P. A system for computer assisted arthroscopy. *Springer Verlag. CVR Med-MRCAS'97,* 1997;653–62.

19 Bauer A. Robot assisted total hip replacement in primary and revision cases. Techniques. *Orthopaedics* 2000;10(1) (January):9–13.

20 Fadda M, Bertelli D, Martelli S, Marcacci M, *et al.* Computer assisted planning for total knee arthroplasty. *First Joint Conference of CVRMed and MRCAS,* 1997, 619–28. Grenoble, France: Springer.

21 Muller ME, Elminger B. Jahresergebnisse mit der sog. *Setzholz Totalprothese. Orthopadie* 1979;8:73–4.

22 Ritter MA, Campbell ED. Postoperative patellar complications with or without lateral release during total knee arthroplasty. *Clin Orthop* 1987;219:163–8.

23 Tria AJ, Harwood DA, Alice JA, *et al.* Patellar fractures in posterior stabilized knee arthroplasties. *Clin Orthop* 1994;131–8, 299.

24 Corses A, Lotke PA, Williams JL. Strain characteristics of the posterior cruciate ligament in the total knee replacement. *Orthop Trans* 1989;13(3):527.

25 Pagano MW, Cushner FC, Scott WN. Role of the posterior cruciate ligament in total knee arthroplasty. *J Am Aca Orthop Surg* 1998;6:176–87.

26 Alback S. Osteoarthritis of the knee: a radiological investigation. *Acta Radiol* 1968;(Suppl. 277).

27 Aglietti P, Rinonapoli E. Total condylar knee arthoplasty. A five-year follow-up study of 33 knees. *Clin Orthop* 1984;186:104–11.

28 Laskin RS. Alignment of the total knee components. *Orthopaedics* 1984;7:62.

29 Miyasaka KC, Ranawat CS, Mullaji A. Total knee arthroplasty in the valgus knee: intermediate term results and technique for ligament balancing. *J Arthroplasty* 1997;12(2):220.

30 Krackow KA. Proximal realignment during total knee arthroplasty of the valgus knee. *Clin Orthop* 1991;273:9–18.

31 Krackow KA. (1984) Management of fixed deformity on total joint arthroplasty. In: Hungerford, Krackow, Kenna B, eds. *Total knee arthroplasty.* Baltimore: Aspen, 1984:163–78.

32 Golberg VM, Figgie HE, Inglis AE, *et al.* Patella fracture type and prognosis in total condylar total knee arthroplasty. *Clin Orthop* 1988;236:115–22.

33 Scuderi GR. Knee balance in flexion. In: Laskin RS ed. *Contreversies in total knee arthroplasty.* Oxford University Press (in press). January 2001.

Chapter 14

Total knee replacement: navigation technique intra-operative model system

S. David Stulberg, Dominique Saragaglia, and Rolf Miehlke

14.1 Introduction

The success of total knee replacement surgery depends on several factors, including proper patient selection, appropriate implant design, correct surgical technique, and effective peri-operative care. The outcome of total knee replacement surgery is particularly sensitive to variations in surgical technique.[1–8] Incorrect positioning or orientation of implants and improper alignment of the limb can lead to accelerated implant wear and loosening and suboptimal functional performance. A number of studies have suggested that alignment errors of greater than three degrees are associated with more rapid failure and less satisfactory functional results of total knee arthroplasties.[1,9–19] Recent studies have also emphasized that the most common cause for revision of TKR is error in surgical technique.

Mechanical alignment guides have improved the accuracy with which implants can be inserted. Although mechanical alignment systems are continually being refined, errors in implant and limb alignment continue to occur. It has been estimated that errors in tibial and femoral alignment of more than three degrees occur in at least ten percent of total knee arthroplasties, even when performed by experienced surgeons using mechanical alignment systems of modern design. Mechanical alignment systems have fundamental limitations that limit their ultimate accuracy. The accuracy of preoperative planning is limited by the errors inherent to standard radiographs. It is difficult to determine accurately, with standard instrumentation, the correct location of crucial alignment landmarks (e.g., the center of the femoral head, the center of the ankle). Moreover, mechanical alignment and sizing devices presume a standardized bone geometry that may not apply to a specific patient. Even the most elaborate mechanical instrumentation systems rely on visual inspection to confirm the accuracy of the limb and implant alignment and stability at the conclusion of the TKR procedure.

Computer based alignment systems have been developed to address the limitations inherent in mechanical total knee instrumentation.[20–26] Three types of computer based TKR systems are currently in various stages of development: (1) image-free navigation systems (also referred to as intra-operative models); (2) image-based navigation systems; and (3) robotic systems. Navigation systems augment mechanical instrumentation through the addition of measurement probes that can be used to locate joint centers, track surgical tools and align prosthetic components. Image-free navigation systems utilize information that is acquired in the operating room, during the performance of the total knee replacement. Image-guided navigation systems utilize three-dimensional preoperative plans, derived from CT scans, or fluoroscopy based images obtained in the operating room, that guide the placement of TKR components. Robotic TKR systems use machines that guide or replace the surgeon during portions of the TKR procedure.

The image-free navigation technique described in this chapter is an example of an intra-operative model system. All of the information that the computer system requires to guide the positioning of the total knee replacement cutting blocks is acquired in the operating room during the performance of the TKR.

The technique that is described:

(1) incorporates the use of standard mechanical cutting blocks that have been adapted for use with the navigation system;

(2) uses commonly available, relatively inexpensive computer equipment (e.g. desk-top computer, low-end optical localizer);

(3) is currently in clinical use;

(4) has available multicenter clinical results comparing its use with mechanical systems.[25,27-29]

Because a computer-based surgical technique introduces concepts and equipment not currently familiar to a large proportion of surgeons who perform TKR surgery, we will compare the steps of the navigation technique with the corresponding steps of conventional, intramedullary manual systems. It is important to understand that the goal of computer-based navigation systems is to increase the accuracy and reproducibility with which the **objectives of mechanical intramedullary alignment systems** are achieved.

After describing the computer assisted surgical technique, we will summarize the results that have been obtained with this approach. We will also compare these results with those achieved using conventional intramedullary systems.

14.2 **Surgical technique**

14.2.1 **Preoperative planning**

Image-free TKR techniques reduce the importance of preoperative planning. Conventional mechanical instrumentation systems that utilize intramedullary femoral alignment guides require that the surgeon determine the desired anatomic alignment (femoral-tibial angle) on a full length (including hip, knee, and ankle joints) standing anterior-posterior (AP) radiograph. In addition, many surgeons also determine the desired posterior slope of the tibial cut using a lateral radiograph. The desired size of the femoral and tibial components can also be estimated by holding scaled templates of the implants against AP and lateral radiographs of the knee joint.

Mechanical systems use the information obtained during preoperative templating to determine the appropriate setting on the femoral intramedullary alignment guide (anatomic axis) that will correct the preoperative medial-lateral deformity to a mechanical axis of zero. Image-free navigation systems use the information obtained during intra-operative registration to align the cutting blocks to correct the preoperative medial-lateral and anterior-posterior deformities to mechanical axes of zero. Image-free computer assisted techniques locate the center of the hip, knee and ankle joint during the surgical procedure. In addition, the image-free navigation system allows the surgeon to determine intra-operatively the desired posterior slope of the tibia and correct sizes of the femoral and tibial implants. Image-free navigation systems eliminate the need to acquire this information preoperatively.

14.2.2 **Patient positioning and surgical exposure**

The mechanical alignment and computer-assisted surgical techniques use similar approaches for patient positioning and surgical exposure. Leg holders and pneumatic tourniquets, routinely used with mechanical instrumentation, can also be used for the computer-assisted technique.

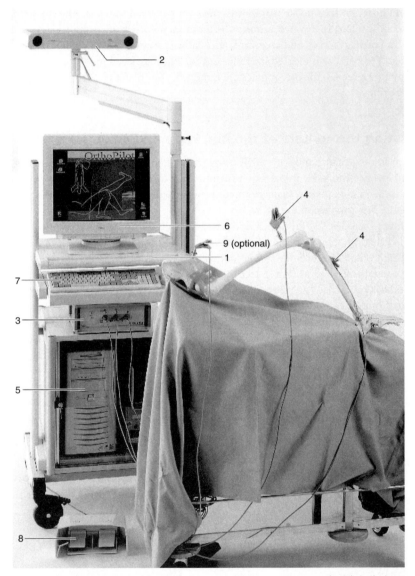

Fig. 14.1 The image-free navigation system components: (1) instrument stand with isolation transformer; (2–3) camera system and control unit; (4(a)) infrared transmitters (rigid bodies); (5) Workstation; (6) computer monitor; (7) keyboard and mouse; (8) foot control.

No alterations in the surgical incision usually used for TKR surgery need to be made for the computer-assisted technique. Although this procedure will require the placement of screws to hold diode containing rigid bodies in the proximal tibia and distal femur, the sites for these screws can be reached through a conventional incision and exposure.

We prefer a straight midline skin incision and a medial parapatellar exposure of the knee. This exposure extends distally along the medial-most edge of the quadriceps tendon and patella to a point just medial and distal to the patellar tendon insertion on the tibial tubercle. The superficial and deep medial collateral ligament is elevated around the anterior medial half of the tibia. The ligamentum mucosum, infra-patellar fat pad, and anterior lateral capsule are elevated from the anterior-lateral surface of the tibia. The patellar is everted laterally, and the knee is placed in 90° of flexion. The anterior cruciate ligament is resected, the osteophytes are removed, and the fat pad trimmed to allow adequate exposure of the tibia.

14.2.3 Locating the centers of the hip, knee and ankle joint

The initial step in the performance of a TKR using image-free navigation is the determination of the centers of the hip, knee and ankle joints. Equipment unique to computer-assisted surgery must be used to determine these joint centers. This equipment is also used to guide the positioning of the cutting blocks during the performance of the TKR.

The equipment includes: (1) an optical localizer; (2) rigid bodies containing diodes; (3) 3.5-mm stainless steel bicortical screws specifically designed to hold one of the rigid bodies on the bone; (4) a metal plate to hold a rigid body to the foot; and (5) a computer, a monitor, and a foot control. The localizer consists of cameras that detect the infrared radiation emitted by the diodes contained in the rigid bodies (Fig. 14.1). The rigid bodies are securely affixed to the bones by using the bicortical screws so that they do not move relative to the bones when the leg is flexed, extended, and rotated. The localizer is connected to the computer and the monitor. The position of the leg and bones can be seen on the computer screen when the surgeon activates the foot control. The localizer is positioned at the level of the knee joint on the side opposite to the extremity on which the TKR is to be performed.

The screws that hold the rigid bodies are inserted at the beginning of the surgical procedure. Femoral and tibial screws are placed immediately after making the skin incision and exposing the knee joint. The femoral screw is inserted into the medial cortex approximately four inches proximal to the knee joint. The tibial screw is inserted into the anterior-medial cortex approximately 8 cm below

(a)

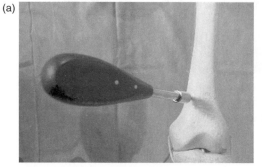

(b)

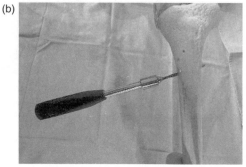

Fig. 14.2 Placement of screws and attachment of transmitters. (a, b) 4.5 mm cortical screws are placed in the distal femur and proximal tibia with adapters that allow the infrared transmitters to be attached. The screws must be positioned so that the transmitters are visible to the camera. The screws must also be rigidly fixed to the bones so that they do not move during surgery.

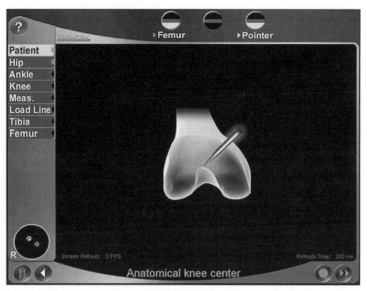

Fig. 14.3 The anatomic center of the knee is palpated to determine the optimal motion for registering the center of the femoral head.

the tibial plateau (Fig. 14.2). The heads of these screws have been specially designed to hold the rigid bodies.

The center of the femoral head is determined first using a kinematic registration technique. This requires that the femur be flexed, extended, abducted, adducted and rotated. This movement generates a cloud of points on a sphere. The center of the sphere (i.e. the femoral head) that created this array of points can then be computed (Fig. 14.4). The technique used to move the femur is important for accurately determining the center of the femoral head. Excessive hip motion will cause the pelvis to move. Inadequate motion will not generate adequate information to allow a calculation of the femoral head center. Therefore, visual cues are displayed upon the computer screen to guide the surgeon during the acquisition of the information (Fig. 14.3–14.16). Once the registration is completed, the surgeon is instructed to proceed to the next step, kinematic registration of the center of the ankle joint.

The center of the ankle joint is determined by attaching a metal plate containing an adapter to hold a rigid body to the foot with a rubber band. The rigid body is then attached to this plate (Fig. 14.6a). The ankle joint is then flexed and extended. Visual cues to guide the movement of the ankle joint during registration are displayed on the computer screen (Fig. 14.6b). Once adequate information has been obtained to permit calculation of the center of the ankle joint, the surgeon is instructed to proceed to the next step, kinematic registration of the center of the knee joint.

The kinematic center of the knee joint is determined by slowly flexing and extending the knee from zero to 90°. As with hip and ankle joint registration, the surgeon is provided with visual cues on the computer screen (Fig. 14.7). Although not essential, the accuracy of the registration may be increased by rotating the tibia on the femur with the knee flexed 90°.

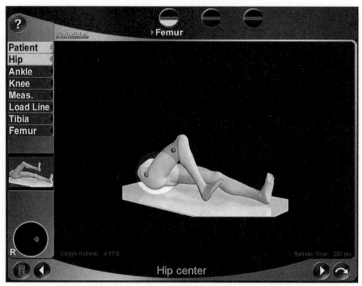

Fig. 14.4 Positioning the limb to determine the kinematic center of the femoral head. This screen shows the surgeon how to position the leg and confirms that the transmitter on the femur is visible to the camera.

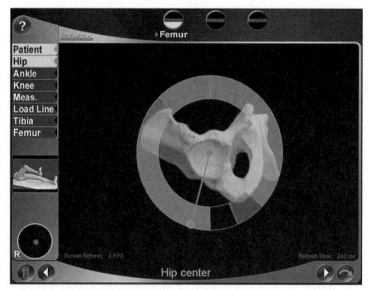

Fig. 14.5 Registering the center of the femoral head: The point on the screen guides the movement of the leg and assures that registration of the center of the femoral head is accurate.

Kinematic registration of the hip, knee and ankle joints makes it possible to determine the mechanical axes of the extremity in the frontal and sagittal planes. However, in order to: (1) determine the level from the knee joint line of the femoral and tibial resections, (2) calculate the size of the femoral component, (3) place the femoral and tibial cutting blocks in correct medial/lateral position; and

(a)

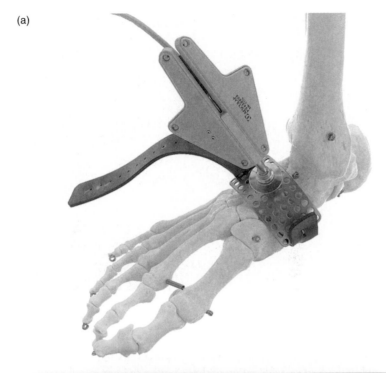

(b)

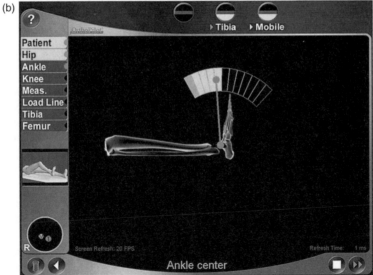

Fig. 14.6 Kinematic registration of the center of the ankle joint: (a) The transmitter is mounted on the adapter to the foot in such a way that the diodes in the front of the transmitter point toward the camera; (b) The movement of the ankle joint is guided by the pointer to assure accurate registration of the center of the ankle joint.

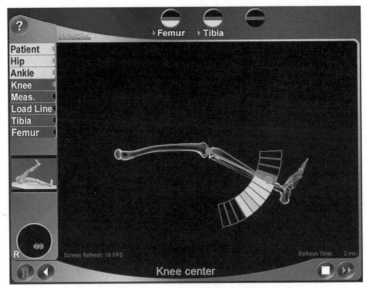

Fig. 14.7 Kinematic registration of the center of the knee joint: The pointer guides the movement of the knee joint to assure accurate registration.

(4) orient the femoral cutting block in proper rotation, it is necessary to perform a surface registration of the knee and ankle joint. Surface registration of these joints also increases the accuracy of the calculation of the joint centers established initially using kinematic registration.

14.2.4 **Establishing the tibial and femoral reference points**

To determine the level of the tibial resection, a pointer to which a diode containing rigid body is attached, is placed on the point on the tibial plateau from which the depth of the tibial resection is to be measured. This is usually the deepest point on the least damaged side of the plateau (Figs 14.8, 14.9).

To determine the size and rotation of the femoral component, the rigid body containing pointer is placed on the posterior medial and lateral femoral condyles at the points farthest from the anterior femoral cortex (Figs 14.10a-c). The anterior femoral cortex is then palpated with the pointer directly above the center of the trochlea (Fig. 14.10d).

Although rotation of the femoral component is usually determined using the posterior condylar axis, it is also possible to use the epicondylar axis by using the pointer to locate the medial and lateral epiconcyles (Fig. 14.11). This axis is compared to the posterior condylar axis measured using an orientation block that abuts against the distal and posterior condyles (Fig. 14.13).

The palpation registration step is completed by using the pointer to locate the medial and lateral malleoli and midpoint of the ankle joint in the frontal plane (Fig. 14.12). This information is used to confirm the determination of the center of the ankle joint originally calculated using kinematic registration.

Once the registration process has been completed, it is possible to orientate the femoral and tibial cutting blocks and position them to guide the levels of resection. Prior to positioning the cutting blocks, however, the presurgical alignment in the frontal and sagittal planes, the medial-lateral stability in extension and the range of motion are measured and recorded (Fig. 14.14).

(a)

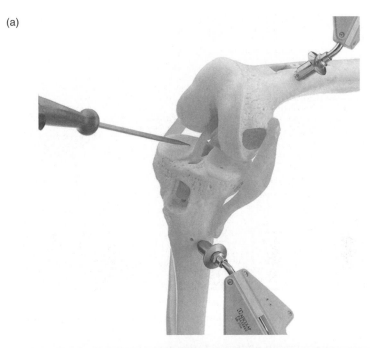

(b)

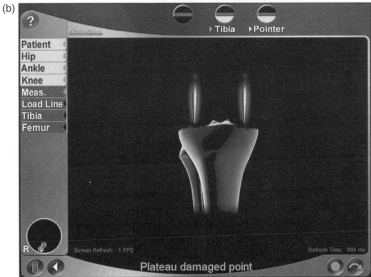

Fig. 14.8 Establishing the level of tibia resection: (a) the tip of the pointer is placed on the point on the tibial plateau from which the depth of the tibial resection is to be measured. This is usually the deepest point on the least damaged side of the plateau; (b) the monitor directs the placement of the pointer on the plateau.

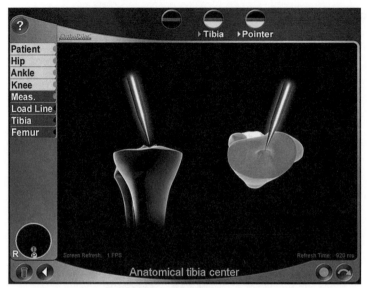

Fig. 14.9 Surface registration of the center of the intercondylar eminence of the tibia. This information is used with the kinematic information to optimize the determination of the center of the knee joint.

14.2.5 Preparation of the tibia

A rigid body is placed on the tibial cutting block, which is then attached to a tibial orientation instrument. This device is analogous to the external tibial alignment guide of conventional manual instruments (Fig. 14.15a). The orientation instrument is secured to the tibia with pins.

The frontal and sagittal orientation of the cutting block and the level of tibial resection are then determined. The location and orientation of the cutting block are displayed on the computer screen (Fig. 14.15b). The desired orientation of the tibial cutting block is exactly perpendicular to the frontal and sagittal mechanical axes of the tibia. The amount of tibial resection can be directly determined from the computer screen.

Once the tibial cutting block is in the desired position, it is fixed to the tibia with pins. The tibial orientation instrument is removed. The position of the cutting block is checked using the navigation equipment. The tibia resection is then performed.

Conventional manual tibial instrumentation is quite similar to the jig used with the navigation system. The manual instrumentation requires the surgeon to visually locate the center of the knee joint (tibial spine) and center of the ankle joint. The surgeon must also visually align the extramedullary tibial rod parallel to the sagittal longitudinal axis of the tibia. The cutting block is then placed perpendicular to the visually determined frontal and sagittal axes of the tibia. The tibial manual instrumentation technique is analogous to using the palpation registration sequence in the computer-assisted technique. The level of tibial resection in the manual technique is determined using a stylus. The level in the computer technique is a direct measurement from the point at which a stylus would be placed. In both techniques, the tibial instrumentation is rotated until it points to the medial third of the tibial plateau.

(a)

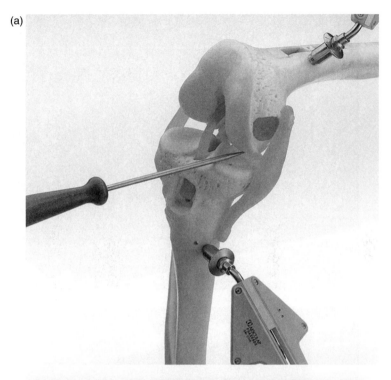

(b)

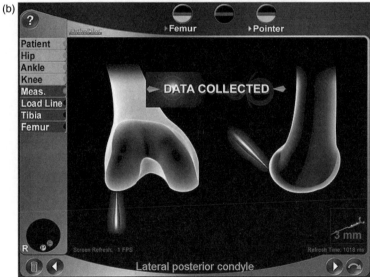

Fig. 14.10 (*Continued*).

(c)

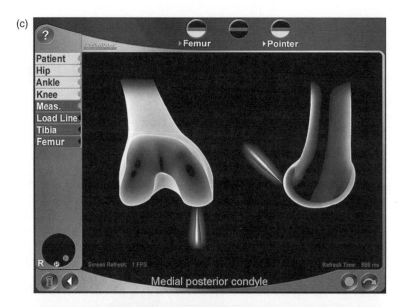

(d)

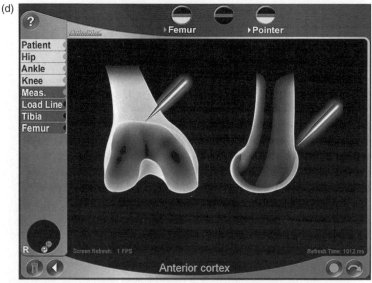

Fig. 14.10 Surface registration of the femur: this step accomplishes 3 goals: (1) optimizes the center of the knee joint with the previously acquired kinematic data; (2) determines the size of the femoral component; (3) establishes the rotation of the femoral implant. (a, b, c) Palpation of the dorsal midpoints of the medial and lateral femoral condyles; (d) palpation of the anterior cortical surface of the femur.

14.2.6 **Preparation of the femur**

A rigid body is attached to the femur cutting block. This block is attached to the femoral orientation guide and placed on the distal femur (Fig. 14.16a). The orientation and level of the block are then adjusted until the desired position as seen on the computer screen is obtained (Fig. 14.16b). The block

(a)
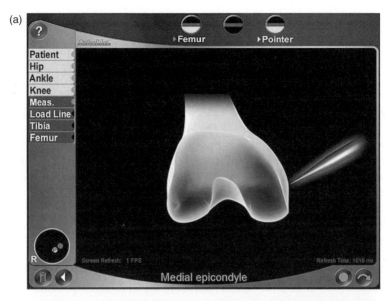
Medial epicondyle

(b)
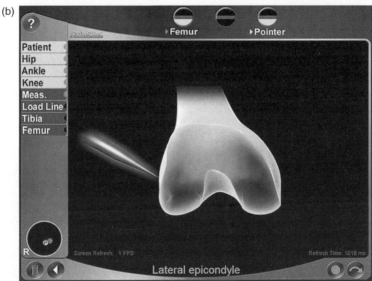
Lateral epicondyle

Fig. 14.11 Determination of the epicondylar axis: (a, b) palpation of the medial and lateral epicondyles with the pointer establishes the epicondylar axis. This information can be used to aid in the rotational positioning of the femoral component.

is then fixed to the femur with pins and the orientation guide removed. The position of the cutting block is checked. The distal femur is then resected.

The femoral orientation guide with a rigid body attached is then repositioned against the resected distal femoral surface. The posterior plates of the guide are placed against the posterior surfaces of the medial and lateral femoral condyles. The rotation of the femoral component in relation to the posterior condyles can then be established (Fig. 14.16c). If desired, the epicondylar axis can also be used to determine the rotational positioning of the orientation guide. Holes for the femoral cutting block are then drilled through the orientation guide. The cutting block for the femoral component whose size has been previously determined is then secured to the distal femur. The position of the block is checked and the anterior-posterior and chamfer resections are performed.

Conventional manual instrumentation is similar in many ways to that used in the navigation technique. However, there is one important difference. Manual instrumentation of the femur relies upon the use of an intramedullary rod (i.e. anatomic axis) to establish the frontal and sagittal resection planes. Because the navigation technique determines the locations of the centers of the hip and knee joints, it is able to align the cutting blocks with the mechanical axis using extramedullary instruments. Many investigators have suggested that this use of extramedullary instruments may be associated with a decreased amount of bleeding and a reduced incidence of fat embolization.

Manual instrumentation systems use referencing guides off of the posterior femoral condyles and/or anterior femoral cortex to establish the size of the femoral component. The navigation system determines the size of the femur during the palpation registration process.

Both the manual and navigation systems use the posterior condylar line or the epicondylar line to establish femoral component rotation. Both systems can also use the anterior-posterior intercondylar line (Whitesides line) to determine the correct rotation of the femoral component.

14.2.7 Trial reduction

Once the femoral and tibial resections are completed, a trial reduction is carried out. The polyethylene insert that best balances the knee in flexion and extension is selected. The navigation system is used to measure the final alignment of the extremity, the amount of medial-lateral laxity in extension and the final range of motion. The system can be used to guide the release of tight soft tissues medially, laterally and posteriorly.

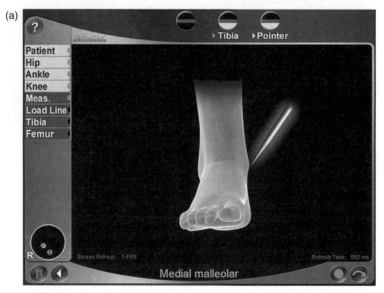

Fig. 14.12 (Continued).

(b)

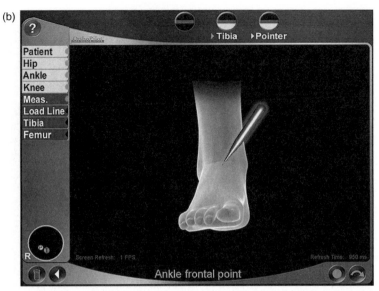

Fig. 14.12 (a–b) The medial and lateral malleoli and the mid-point of the tibia in the frontal plane are palpitated to determine the center of the ankle joint. These data are integrated with the previously acquired kinematic data to optimize the registration of the ankle joint center.

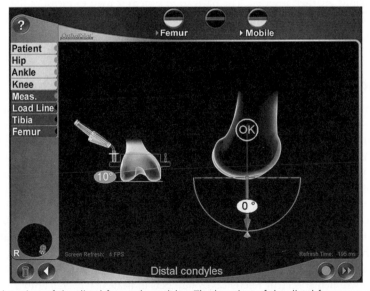

Fig. 14.13 Registration of the distal femoral condyles: The location of the distal femora condyles is determined. This permits the measured resection of the distal femur.

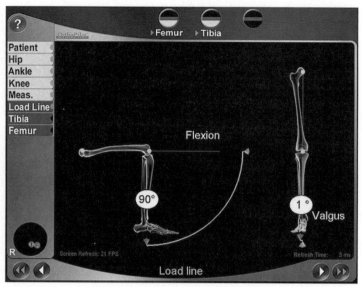

Fig. 14.14 Determination of the pre-operative alignment. Once the centers of the hip, knee and ankle joint are determined, the pre-operative alignment of the leg, the range-of-motion of the knee and the pre-operative stability of the knee joint can be measured and recorded.

14.2.8 **Completion of the procedure**

The actual implants are then inserted. The navigation system is used to measure the final frontal and sagittal alignment of the extremity, the final medial-lateral stability and the final range of motion. These measurements are recorded in the computer.

The fixation screws for the rigid bodies are then removed. Closure is carried out in routine fashion.

14.3 **Clinical results**

The OrthoPilot™ system described in this chapter has been used in more than 5000 total knee replacement cases. Most of these have been performed in France and Germany, the countries where the device was first introduced. Consequently, the results of the initial experience with the OrthoPilot™ have been published in French and German periodicals.

These reports indicate that the Navigation System is safe. There have been no reports of complications specifically associated with the use of the device. Moreover, clinical outcomes have not been adversely affected by the use of the OrthoPilot™. The early versions of the OrthoPilot™ system required that a pin be placed in the rim of the iliam to allow monitoring of pelvic motion to registration of the hip joint. Many navigation systems still require this pin placement. No complications have been associated with the use of these pins.

The reports which compare the alignment results obtained with the OrthoPilot™ to results obtained using manual instrumentation (site references by number) indicate that overall limb alignment achieved with the Navigation System is equal to or better than that achieved with manual instrumentation. If the

(a)

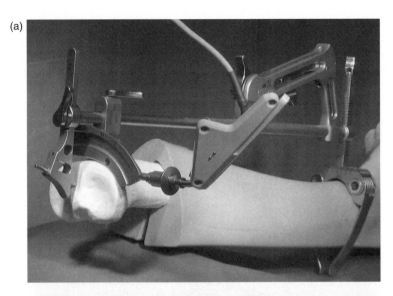

(b)

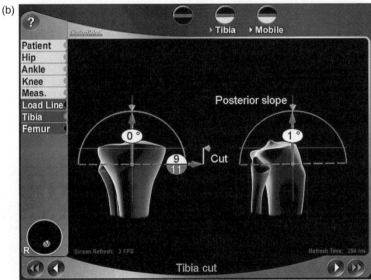

Fig. 14.15 (a) The tibial instrumentation with attached transmitters is positioned on the tibia; (b) The depth and alignment of the tibial resection is displayed on the monitor.

alignment in all planes of the femoral and tibial components are compared, the OrthoPilot™ achieved perfect alignment much more frequently than manual instrumentation (Jenny, Kiefer).

One of the goals of computer assisted TKR systems is to increase the reliability and reproducibility of the procedure. The initial experience with the OrthoPilot™ indicates that this goal is being achieved. There are fewer alignment 'outliers' when the navigation system is used.

Navigation systems also make it possible to determine the accuracy of evaluation tools that are currently being used to determine the outcome of total knee replacement. The OrthoPilot™ system has been used to demonstrate that pre and post-operative radiographs are not accurate methods for determining implant and limb alignment. The system has also been used to determine pre and

(a)

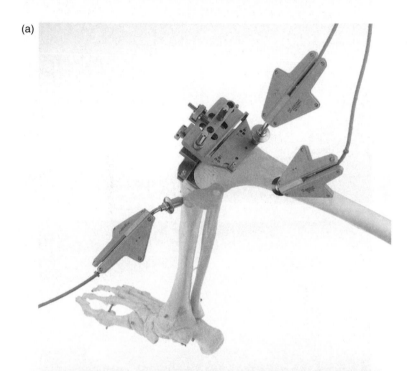

(b)

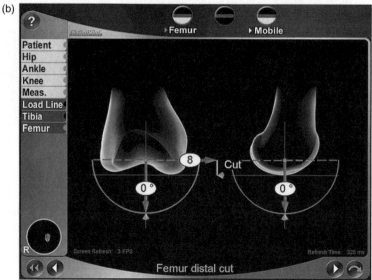

Fig. 14.16 (*Continued*).

(c)

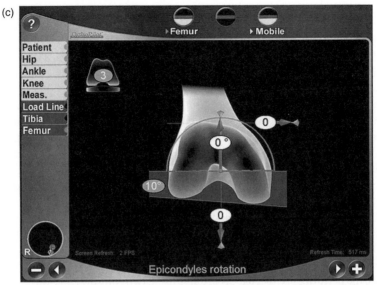

Fig. 14.16 (a) The femoral orientation and cutting blocks with attached transmitters are placed on the distal femur; (b) The depth and alignment of the distal femoral resection is displayed on the monitor; (c) The rotation and anterior-posterior position of the cutting block is displayed on the monitor and guides the anterior and posterior femoral resectors.

post-operative medial-lateral ligament laxity and range of motion. It has been possible to correlate post-operative range of motion with post-operative medial lateral stability and establish that knees that are 'tight' medial-laterally achieve the same degree of flexion as those which are less tight. (SDS)

Finally, navigation systems, including the OrthoPilot™, have been used to determine the accuracy and reproducibility of currently available manual instrumentation systems. It has been shown that manual intramedullary systems are capable of producing accurate and reproducible alignment in the frontal plane. However, these systems are less reliable in reestablishing the mechanical axis in the sagittal plane. There is a tendency for the surgeon to leave a knee in slight flexion if a manual system and visual confirmation of final alignment are used (Stulberg, Picard).

14.4 **Summary**

Computer assisted navigation systems have been developed for use in total knee replacement surgery to address the inherent limitations of mechanical instrumentation. Both image-free and image-based computer assisted systems are now being used to implant total knees. As has been emphasized in this chapter, the alignment objectives which these computer assisted systems attempt to optimize are the identical alignment goals that mechanical systems seek to achieve. It is anticipated that by improving the accuracy and reliability with which the frontal, sagittal axes are restored, the correct femoral and tibial implant rotation and size are achieved, and the correct medial-lateral and anterior-posterior ligament stability are established, the functional results of TKR will be improved, morbidity of TKR surgery will be decreased, and longevity of TKR will be increased. Longer term follow-up studies of TKR performed using computer assisted techniques will have to become available before it can be determined whether these goals have been achieved.

There are other, perhaps equally important, potential benefits of using currently available computer assisted total knee replacement systems. The designs of mechanical instruments can be improved with the information that is gathered by computer based instrumentation systems. For example, it is clear from the initial use of computer-based systems that it is difficult for a surgeon to determine if the sagittal mechanical axis has been correctly restored. There is a tendency for surgeons to leave knees with slight flexion contractures. This tendency can be reduced if mechanical systems use pins in the femoral and tibial trials that are parallel when the knee is in full extension (assuming the implants are correctly aligned with the bones). The use of computer-assisted systems indicates that a number of relatively small changes in currently available mechanical instruments could improve the accuracy of these devices.

In addition, currently available computer assisted systems are likely to influence the design of the next generation of total knee implants. The information obtained through the use of these systems is likely to influence the size distributions and dimensions of implants, the orientation of the patellar tracking mechanisms, and the location of the cam and post on posterior stabilized designs.

The use of currently available computer assisted systems will also influence the ways in which total knee implants are inserted. For example, computer assisted systems allow a surgeon to determine how much medial-lateral laxity is present at the end of the TKR procedure. This laxity can be related to other outcomes, e.g. range of motion. Thus computer-assisted systems can help surgeons determine how to optimize the performance of TKR procedures using currently available implants.

However, the real appeal of computer assisted TKR systems lies in their ability to help surgeons optimize TKR procedures for individual patients. Computer systems are likely to become available in the near future which allow the surgeon to individualize alignment to at patient's specific anatomy. The computer systems of the near future, by utilizing information about individual patient's specific anatomy, will also lead us to re-examine the alignment goals of TKR surgery.

Finally, computer-assisted systems of the near future will have the capability of integrating information about human gait and knee function that is currently being obtained. This information can further increase the accuracy with which TKRs are performed and improve the quality of the outcome of those procedures.

References

1 Dorr LD, Boiardo RA. Technical considerations in total knee arthroplasty. *Clin Orthop* 1997;205:5–11.

2 Figgie HE, Goldberg VM, Heiple KG, Moller HS, Gordon NH. The influence of tibial-pallellofemoral location on function of the knee in patients with posterior stabilized condylar knee prosthesis. *J Bone Joint Surg* 1986;68A:1035–40.

3 Freeman MAR, Todd RC, Bamert P, *et al.* ICLH-arthroplasty of the knee: 1968–1977. *J Bone Joint Surg* 1978;60B:339–44.

4 Goodfellow JW, O'Connor JJ. Clinical results of the Oxford knee. *Clin Orthop* 1986;205:21–42.

5 Insall JN, Binazzi R, Soudry M, *et al.* Total knee arthroplasty. *Clin Orthop* 1985;192:13–22.

6 Insall JN, Ranawat CS, Aglietti P, *et al.* A comparison of four models of total knee-replacement prostheses. *J Bone Joint Surg Am* 1976;58:754–65.

7 Insall J, Scott WN, Ranawat CS. The total condylar prosthesis. A report of the hundred cases. *J Bone Joint Surg Am* 1979;61:173–9.

8 Stulberg SD, Picard F, Saragaglia D. Computer-assisted total knee replacement arthroplasty. *Oper Techn Orthop* 2000;10(1):25–39.

9 Ecker ML, Lotke PA, Windsor RE, *et al.* Long-term results after total condylar knee arthroplasty. Significance of radiolucent lines. *Clin Orthop* 1987;216:151–8.

10 Feng EL, Stulberg SD, Wixson RL. Progressive subluxation and polyethylene wear in total knee replacements with flat articular surfaces. *Clin Orthop* 1994;229:60–71.

11 Garg A, Walker PS. Prediction of total knee motion using a three-dimensional computer-graphics model. *J Biomech* 1990;23:45–58.

12 Jeffery RS, Morris RW, Denham RA. Coronal alignment after total knee replacement. *J Bone Joint Surg Br* 1991;73:709–14.

13 Laskin RS. Total condylar knee replacement in patients who have rheumatoid arthritis. A ten-year follow-up study. *J Bone Joint Surg Am* 1990;72:529–35.

14 Oswald MH, Jacob RP, Schneider E, Hoogewoud H. Radiological analysis of normal axial alignment of femur and tibia in view of total knee arthroplasty. *J Arthroplasty* 1993;8:419–26.

15 Piazza SJ, Delp SL, Stulberg SD, Stern SH. Posterior tilting of the tibial component decreases femoral rollback in posterior-substituting knee replacement. *J Orthop Res* 1998;16:264–70.

16 Ranawat CS, Adjei OB. Survivorship analysis and results of total condylar knee arthroplasty. *Clin Orthop* 1988;226:6–13.

17 Ritter MA, Faris PM, Keating EM, Meding JB. Post-operative alignment of total knee replacement: its effect on survival. *Clin Orthop* 1994;299:153–6.

18 Ritter MA, Herbst SA, Keating EM, *et al.* Radiolucency at the bone-cement interface in total knee replacement. *J Bone Joint Surg Am* 1994;76:60–5.

19 Stulberg SD, Sarin V, Loan P. X-ray vs. Computer assisted measurement techniques to determine pre and post-operative limb alignment in TKR surgery. *Proceedings of the Fourth Annual American CAOS Meeting*, July 2001. Pittsburgh, PA.

20 Davies BL, Harris SJ, Lin WJ, Hibberd RD, Cobb JC. Active compliance in robotic surgery—The use of force control as a dynamic constraint. *J Eng Med Proc H Inst Mech Engs* 1997;211:H4.

21 Delp SL, Stulberg SD, Davies B, *et al.* Computer assisted knee replacement. *Clin Orthop* 1998;354:49–56.

22 Fadda M, Bertelli D, Martelli S, *et al.* Computer assisted planning for total knee arthroplasty. *Proceedings of the First Joint Conference on Computer Vision, Virtual Reality and Robotics in Medicine and Medical Robotics and Computer Assisted Surgery*, 1997:619–28. Grenoble, France: Springer.

23 Leitner F, Picard F, Minfelde R, *et al.* Computer assisted knee surgical total replacement. *Proceedings of the First Joint Conference on Computer Vision, Virtual Reality and Robotics in Medicine and Medical Robotics and Computer Assisted Surgery*, 1997:630–8. Grenoble, France: Springer.

24 Matsen FA III, Garbini JL, Sidles JA, *et al.* Robotic assistance in orthopaedic surgery: a proof of principle using distal femoral arthroplasty. *Clin Orthop* 1993;296:178–86.

25 Picard F, Leitner F, Raoult O, Saragaglia D, Cinquin P. Clinical evaluation of computer assisted total knee arthroplasty. *Second Annual North American Program on Computer Assisted Orthopaedic Surgery*, 1998; 239–49. Pittsburgh, PA.

26 Stern SH, Insall JN. Posterior stabilized prosthesis: results after follow-up of 9–12 years. *J Bone Joint Surg* 1992;74A:980–6.

27 Jenny JY, Boeri C. Computer-assisted total knee prosthesis implantation without preoperative imaging: a comparison with classical instrumentation. *Fourth Annual North American Program on Computer Assisted Orthopaedic Surgery*, 2000:97–8. Pittsburgh, PA.

28 Miehlke RK, Clemens U, Kershally S. Computer integrated instrumentation in knee arthroplasty: a comparative study of conventional and computerized technique. *Fourth Annual North American Program on Computer Assisted Orthopaedic Surgery*, 2000:93–6. Pittsburgh, PA.

29 Orthopilot® Users Meeting, Tuttlinger, Germany; 2000.

30 Stulberg SD, Sarin V. The use of a navigation system to assist ligament balancing in TKR. *Proceedings of the Fourth Annual American CAOS Meeting*, July 2001. Pittsburgh, PA.

Chapter 15

Unicompartmental knee prosthesis implantation with a non-image-based navigation system

Jean-Yves Jenny and Cyril Boeri

15.1 Clinical challenge

The accuracy of implantation is an accepted prognostic factor for the long term survival of unicompartmental knee prostheses (UKP).[1–3] However, most UKP systems offer a limited and potentially inaccurate instrumentation that rely on substantial surgeon judgment for prosthesis placement. Rates of inaccurate implantation as high as 30 per cent have been reported with conventional, free hand instrumentation.[4] The intramedullary femoral guiding device can improve these results,[5,6] but does not allow reproducible optimal implantation.

Computer assisted systems have been developed for total knee prosthesis implantation, and should allow a higher precision of implantation for such implants in comparison to conventional instruments. Most of them are currently only experimental;[7] only one system has been clinically validated by a prospective, randomized, controlled study[8] and a subsequent case-control study.[9] This system is considered as non image based, because it only relies on a pre-operative kinematic analysis of the lower limb. We developed an adaptation of this technique for UKP implantation, without any extramedullary or intramedullary guiding device. We hypothetized that the navigation system will allow to place the prosthesis in a different and better position than the conventional technique, and that the radiological results will be different based on the type of instruments used. The present study reports the early and radiological results of two paired groups of patients in whom a UKP was implanted with either conventional or navigated instrumentations.

15.2 Operative techniques

15.2.1 Conventional instrumentation (Fig. 15.1)

After a medial parapatellar approach, the tibial resection guide was fixed on an extramedullary rod, which was visually aligned with the tibial axis on both coronal and sagittal planes. The height of resection was measured with a stylus according to the preoperative X-ray planning. The guide was pinned on the tibia, and proximal tibial resection was performed with an oscillating saw, preserving the tibial attachment of both cruciates.

The femoral canal was entered at the most proximal point of the intercondylar notch, and an intramedullary rod was fixed in the femoral canal, representing the femoral coronal and sagittal anatomical axes. The distal femoral resection guide was fixed on this rod with a coronal orientation defined on preoperative long lex X-rays according to the angle between the mechanical and the

(a)

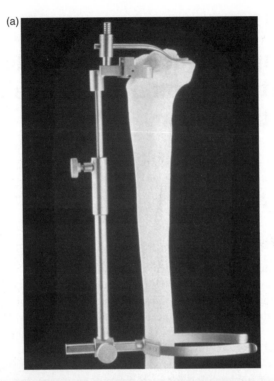

(b)

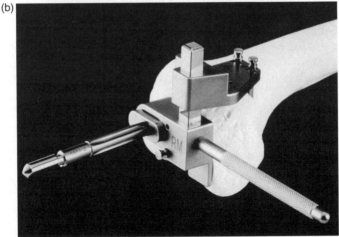

Fig. 15.1 Conventional operative technique: proximal tibial resection with extramedullary alignment (a), distal femoral resection with intramedullary alignment (b).

anatomical axes of the femur, and distal femoral resections were performed with an oscillating saw. A second femoral guide was applied on this distal resection to perform the dorsal femoral resection and the chamfer resection.

The trial implants were tested, and the definitive prosthesis (Search® prosthesis, AESCULAP, Chaumont, France) was cemented if the test was satisfactory.

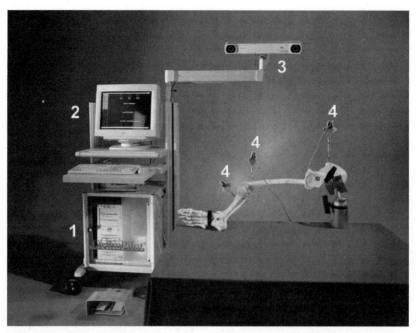

Fig. 15.2 Navigation system: computer (1); monitor (2); infrared camera (3); localizers (4).

15.2.2 Navigated technique (Figs 15.2 and 15.3)

The used navigation system is an intra-operative non-image-based one. Four infrared localizers were implanted on screws in the anterior iliac crest, in the distal femur and in the proximal tibia, and strapped on the dorsal part of the foot. The relative motion of two adjacent localizers was observed by an infrared camera (Polaris®, Northern Digital, Toronto, Canada). The dedicated software calculated the center of rotation of this movement, and so defined the respective centers of rotation of the hip, knee and ankle joints. With these centers were calculated the mechanical axes of both femur and tibia on both coronal and sagittal planes. A localizer was then fixed on tibial or femoral resection blocks, and the software displayed on-line the orientation of this block in comparison to the mechanical axes of the bone. The surgeon could fix the block with the desired orientation before performing the bony resection with a classical motorized saw blade. The trial implants were tested, and the definitive prosthesis (Search® prosthesis, AESCULAP, Chaumont, France) was cemented if the test was satisfactory.

15.3 Material and methods

286 patients have been operated on for a medial gonarthrosis at the authors' institution from January 1996 to December 2000 with implantation of a UKP (SEARCH® unicompartmental prosthesis, AESCULAP, Tuttlingen, FRG) with either conventional (256 cases) or navigated (30 cases) instrumentation. The prosthesis was designed to be implanted as follows (see Fig. 15.4): coronal femorotibial mechanical angle of 0–5 degrees, coronal orientation of the femoral component of 90 ± 2 degrees, sagittal orientation of the femoral component of 90 ± 2 degrees, coronal orientation of the tibial component of 90 ± 2 degrees, and sagittal orientation of the tibial component of 88 ± 2 degrees. All patients had a

complete radiological examination in the first three months after the index procedure, with AP and lateral plain knee X-rays and AP and lateral long leg X-rays.

The 30 patients operated with the navigation system (group A) were matched to 30 patients operated with the conventional technique (group B) using age (with intervals of 5 years), sex, body mass index (with intervals of 5 units), preoperative coronal mechanical femorotibial angle (with intervals of 5 degrees) and severity of the preoperative degenerative changes according to Ahlback.[10] By the selected patients, the following angles were measured on long leg X-rays (Fig. 15.4) by a unique observer (JYJ) who was unable to be blinded to the type of instruments used as the presence or

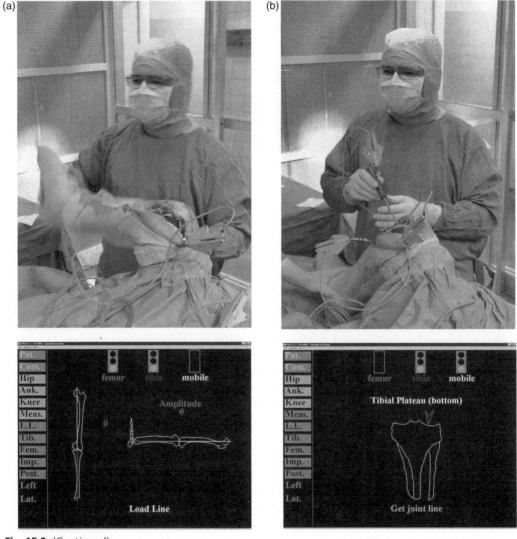

Fig. 15.3 (Continued)

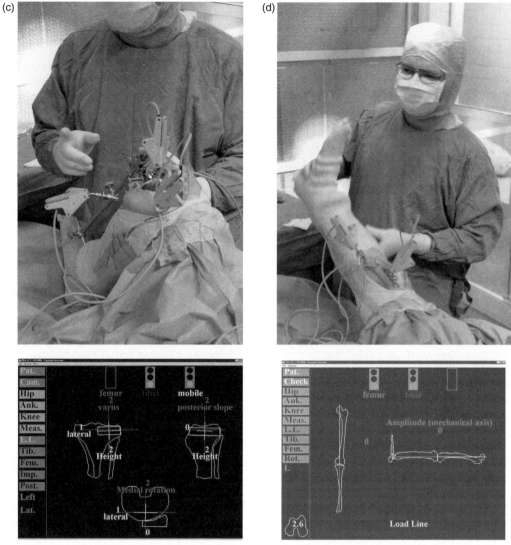

Fig. 15.3 Navigated operative technique: registrations of joint centers of motion (a); registration of bony landmarks (b); orientation of the resection blocks (c); control with the trial implants (d).

absence of the rigid bodies fixation holes was evident:[11]

(1) mechanical femorotibial angle (desired range: 0–5 degrees);

(2) coronal orientation of the femoral component in comparison to the mechanical femoral axis (desired range: 88–92 degrees);

(3) sagittal orientation of the femoral component in comparison to the anterior femoral cortex (desired range: 88–92 degrees);

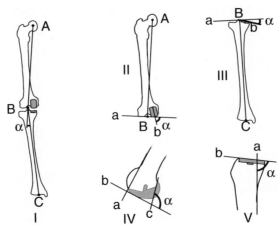

Fig. 15.4 Radiographic measurements of the prosthesis orientation. **I:** Coronal femorotibial mechanical angle (α): A = center of the femoral head, B = center of the knee (center of the tibial eminentia), C = center of the ankle joint. **II:** Coronal orientation of the femoral component (α): A = center of the femoral head, B = center of the knee (center of the tibial eminentia), a = line perpendicular to AB through A, b = vertical axis of the femoral component. **III:** Coronal orientation of the tibial component (α): B = center of the knee (center of the tibial eminentia), C = center of the ankle joint, a = line perpendicular to BC through B, b = coronal horizontal axis of the tibial component. **IV:** Sagittal orientation of the femoral component (α): a = anterior femoral cortex, b = line perpendicular to a and tangent to the lowest point of the femoral component, c = posterior femoral resection. **V:** Sagittal orientation of the tibial component (α): a = posterior tibial cortex, b = sagittal horizontal axis of the tibial component.

(4) coronal orientation of the tibial component in comparison to the mechanical tibial axis (desired range: 88–92 degrees);

(5) sagittal orientation of the tibial component in comparison to the posterior tibial cortex (desired range: 88–92 degrees).

Mean angular values in both groups were compared for each criterion with a Student *t*-test. Prosthesis implantation was considered as satisfactory when all X-rays angles were within the desired range by a given patient on early long leg X-rays. The rate of satisfactory implanted prostheses was compared in both groups with a chi-square test. The rate of prostheses implanted within the desired range for each criterion was also compared in both groups with a chi-square test. All statistical tests were performed with a 0.05 limit of significance.

15.4 Results

Sixty patients met the eligibility criteria, 30 in each group: 36 men and 24 women, with a mean age of 67 years (range 47–82 years). The mean body mass index was 29.5 (range 20.1–44.2). The mean preoperative coronal femorotibial mechanical angle was 8 degrees (range 4–15 degrees). There were 28 grade 2 and 32 grade 3 degenerative changes according to Ahlback.[10]

Radiographic results at the early follow-up are reported in the Tables 15.1 and 15.2. The mean mechanical femorotibial angle was 1.5 degrees (range: −4 to 5 degrees, standard deviation = 2.2 degrees)

Table 15.1 Radiographic results (mean, maximum, minimum, standard deviation)

	Group A (N = 30)	Group B (N = 30)	
Coronal femorotibial mechanical angle	1.5	0.7	p = 0.42
	5	10	
	−4	−10	
	2.2	3.9	
Coronal orientation of the femoral component	89.1	88.1	p = 0.13
	90	94	
	85	80	
	1.3	2.8	
Sagittal orientation of the femoral component	89.7	89.4	p = 0.70
	92	95	
	86	80	
	1.5	2.8	
Coronal orientation of the tibial component	89.2	88.1	p = 0.07
	90	94	
	87	80	
	1.2	2.5	
Sagittal orientation of the tibial component	89.9	86.4	p < 0.01
	93	97	
	88	78	
	1.0	3.0	

Table 15.2 Radiographic results: number of prostheses in the desired angular range

	Group A (N = 30)	Group B (N = 30)	
Coronal femorotibial mechanical angle	26	20	p > 0.05
Coronal orientation of the femoral component	27	19	p < 0.02
Sagittal orientation of the femoral component	27	19	p < 0.02
Coronal orientation of the tibial component	26	19	p < 0.05
Sagittal orientation of the tibial component	28	21	p < 0.02
Satisfactory implanted prosthesis	18	6	p < 0.01

in group A and 0.7 degrees (range: −10 to 10 degrees, standard deviation = 3.9 degrees) in group B (p = 0.42). The mean coronal orientation of the femoral component was 89.1 degrees (range: 85 to 90 degrees, standard deviation = 1.3 degrees) in group A and 88.1 degrees (range: 80 to 94 degrees, standard deviation = 2.8 degrees) in group B (p = 0.13). The mean sagittal orientation of the femoral component was 89.7 degrees (range: 86 to 92 degrees, standard deviation = 1.5 degrees) in group A and 89.4 degrees (range: 80 to 95 degrees, standard deviation = 2.8 degrees) in group B (p = 0.70). The mean coronal orientation of the tibial component was 89.2 degrees (range: 87 to 90 degrees, standard deviation = 1.2 degrees) in group A and 88.1 degrees (range: 80 to 94 degrees, standard deviation = 2.5 degrees) in group B (p = 0.07). The mean sagittal orientation of the tibial component was 89.9 degrees (range: 88 to 93 degrees, standard deviation = 1.0 degrees) in group A and 86.4 degrees (range: 78 to 97 degrees, standard deviation = 3.0 degrees) in group B (p < 0.01).

An optimal mechanical femorotibial angle was obtained by 26 cases in group A and 20 cases in group B ($p > 0.05$). An optimal coronal orientation of the femoral component was obtained by 27 cases in group A and 19 cases in group B ($p < 0.02$). An optimal sagittal orientation of the femoral component was obtained by 27 cases in group A and 19 cases in group B ($p < 0.02$). An optimal coronal orientation of the tibial component was obtained by 26 cases in group A and 19 cases in group B ($p < 0.05$). An optimal sagittal orientation of the tibial component was obtained by 28 cases in group A and 21 cases in group B ($p < 0.02$). An optimal implantation with all optimal items was obtained by 18 cases in group A and 6 cases in group B ($p < 0.01$).

No complication occurred in relation to the navigation system, either with software or hardware. All navigated procedures could be completely performed, and no conversion to the conventional technique was necessary. The mean operative time increased from 67 to 86 minutes because of the use of the navigation system.

15.5 Discussion

UKP is a valuable alternative to high tibial osteotomy[12] or total knee prosthesis for the treatment of isolated medial gonarthrosis.[13–17] However the exact indications are still controversial, as some authors have reported a low survival rate of such implants.[18] Inaccurate implantation is an accepted factor for early failure.[1,3] Most instrumentations offer unprecise guiding systems, which mainly rely on the surgeon's skill.[5] Even intramedullary guiding systems do not offer reproducible optimal implantation technique.[6] The navigated instrumentation used in this study is similar to that used for total knee prosthesis implantation. It allowed to get a significant higher rate of implantation into the desired angular range on postoperative X-rays for all criteria. It also allowed a significantly higher rate of global satisfactory implantation, with all measured angles within the desired range by one given patient: 60% of the instrumented prostheses had a satisfactory implantation, compared with 20% with the classical instruments.

The used system of navigation can be compared to a measuring instrument. In a general way, the measuring instruments are affected of two error types. Systematic error is a deviation of constant value and direction of the measurement provided by the system compared to reality. Random error is a deviation of random value and direction of this measurement compared to reality. These two errors are strictly independent of each other. In other words, a system generating a systematic error shifts the maximum of the curve distribution of the values measured by the system, supposed to be a normal distribution if the number of measured values is sufficient, compared to the real mean, without interfering over the width of the curve. A system generating a random error widens the curve distribution, without changing the place of its maximum. It is thus necessary, to study the validity of a system of measurement, to study the systematic error by a suitable test of mean comparison (the maximum of the curve), and the random error by a test of distribution (the width of the curve).

In the present study, the suited test of comparison of means, taking into account the sample size, is the Student t-test. No significant difference in the measured mean angular values was observed, with the exception of the sagittal orientation of the tibial component. The absence of significant difference between the observed means in the two groups is not surprising, because the required goal for each criterion was the same. This is not an argument against the superiority of one system compared to the other. This absence of significant difference expresses only the fact that there is no systematic error on radiological implantation quality between the two groups with or without navigation.

For the study of random error, the tests of comparison of variance are not very sensitive, and are only seldom suitable. In the present study, the most suitable test is the chi-square test, comparing in the two groups the number of optimal implantations and the number of errors related to the used instrumentation system, which well represents an evaluation of the dispersion of the observed values around the desired mean. The presence of a significant difference between the rates of optimal implantation between the two groups in favor of the computer-assisted implantation thus expresses the fact that the dispersion of the angular values is less broad with this system. In other words, there is a significant improvement of the quality of implantation of the prostheses with computer assisted implantation, characterized by a less great frequency of the nonoptimal implantation for all the studied criteria, with the exception of the global mechanical femorotibial axis.

The precision of the used system was experimentally calculated to be of 1° for angle measurements and of 1 mm for distance measurements.[7] Only slight modifications of the well known classical operative technique and instruments are necessary. The system works with a completely intra-operative analysis of the lower limb kinematics, without any additional imaging, and consequently with lower costs than other, image guided systems. The surgeon decides himself and without any limitation the optimal orientations of the bony resections according to the intra-operative displayed information, and he can at any time switch back to the classical instruments if necessary.

The surgeons' acceptance was high in this study. The software user's interface is friendly. There are few modifications between the classical and the navigated operative techniques, and specially the resection blocks are only slightly modified. The mean operative time was 20 minutes higher with the navigated technique than with the classical one, but this increase was felt acceptable in comparison to the relevant displayed informations. No navigated procedure had to be interrupted.

Allmost all cases seem to be fitted to the navigated technique. Even very big coronal deformations had been succesfully treated. The only contra-indications to this navigated technique are hip and/or ankle arthrodesis, as the kinematic analysis cannot be performed. These cases are however very rare. This system could offer the best cost-effectiveness ratio of the currently available computer assisted systems for total knee prosthesis implantation.

Geometrical femoral resections have the theoretical disadvantage of removing more subchondral bone than resurfacing ones. As a consequence, the femoral component could be implanted on soft cancellous bone,[2] with a higher risk of loosening. An angled bone-prosthesis interface with straight arms has been reported to enhance the shearing stresses.[19] However, no early complication related to the new instrumentation and the related prosthesis has been observed. Specially, no early femoral loosening in relation to the geometrical distal femoral resection occurred.

The follow-up of the navigated prostheses is currently too short to know if clinical outcome or survival rates will be improved. Longer follow-up is required to determine the respective advantages and disadvantages of both techniques.

15.6 Conclusion

Navigated implantation of a UKP with the used, non-image-based system allowed to improve the accuracy of the radiological implantation without any significant inconvenience and with little change in the conventional operative technique. This improvement could be related to a longer survival of such implanted prostheses.

References

1 Cartier P, Sanouillier JL, Grelsamer RP. Unicompartmental knee arthroplasty surgery. 10-year minimum follow-up period. *J Arthroplasty* 1996;11:782–8.

2 Hernigou P, Deschamps G. Prothèses unicompartimentales du genou. *Rev Chir Orthop* 1996;82(Suppl. 1):23.

3   Lootvoet L, Burton P, Himmer O, Piot L, Ghosez JP. Prothèses unicompartimentales de genou: influence du positionnement du plateau tibial sur les résultats fonctionnels. *Acta Orthop Belg* 1997;63:94–101.

4   Voss F, Sheinkop MB, Galante JO, Barden RM, Rosenberg AG. Miller-Galante unicompartmental knee arthroplasty at 2- to 5-year follow-up evaluations. *J Arthroplasty* 1995;10:764–71.

5   Argenson JN, Chevrol-Benkeddache Y, Aubaniac JM. Modern cemented metalbacked unicompartmental knee arthroplasty: a 3 to 10 year follow-up study. *Poster Presentation, 68th Annual Meeting of the American Academy of Orthopaedic Surgeons*, 2001. San Francisco.

6   Jenny JY, Boeri C. Unicompartmental knee prosthesis. A case-control comparative study of two types of instrumentation with a five year follow-up. Proposed for publication in *J Arthroplasty* 2002;17:1016–20.

7   Delp SL, Stulberg SD, Davies B, Picard F, Leitner F. Computer assisted knee replacement. *Clin Orthop* 1998;354:49–56.

8   Saragaglia D, Picard F, Chaussard C, Montbarbon E, Leitner F, Cinquin P. Mise en place des prothèses totales du genou assistée par ordinateur: comparaison avec la technique conventionelle. *Rev Chir Orthop* 2001;87:18–28.

9   Jenny JY, Boeri C. Implantation d'une prothèse totale de genou assistée par ordinateur. Etude comparative cas-témoin avec une instrumentation traditionnelle. *Rev Chir Orthop* 2001;87:645–52.

10 Ahlback S. Osteoarthrosis of the knee. A radiographic investigation. *Acta Radiol Diagn* 1968;(Suppl. 277):1–72.

11 Epinette JA, Edidin AA. Hydroxyapatite-coated unicompartmental knee replacement. A report of five to six years' follow-up of the HA Unix tibial component. In: Cartier P, Epinette JA, Deschamps G, Hernigou P, eds. *Unicompartmental knee arthroplasty*. Paris: Expansion Scientifique Française, 1997:243–59.

12 Schai PA, Suh JT, Thornhill TS, Scott RD. Unicompartmental knee arthroplasty in middle-aged patients: a 2- to 6-year follow-up evaluation. *J Arthroplasty* 1998;13:365–72.

13 Newman JH, Ackroyd CE, Shah NA. Unicompartmental or total knee replacement? Five-year results of a prospective, randomised trial of 102 osteoarthritic knees with unicompartmental arthritis. *J Bone Joint Surg* 1998;80B:862–5.

14 Robertsson O, Borgquist L, Knuston K, Lewold S, Lidgren L. Use of unicompartmental instead of tricompartmental prostheses for unicompartmental arthrosis in the knee is a cost-effective alternative. 14,437 primary tricompartmental prostheses were compared with 10,624 primary medial or lateral unicompartmental prostheses. *Acta Orthop Scand* 1999;70:170–5.

15 Robertsson O, Dunbar M, Pehrsson T, Knutson K, Lidgren L. Patient satisfaction after knee arthroplasty: a report on 27,372 knees operated on between 1981 and 1995 in Sweden. *Acta Orthop Scand* 2000;71:262–7.

16 Squire MV, Callaghan JJ, Goetz DD, Sullivan PM, Johnston RC. Unicompartmental knee replacement. A minimum 15 year follow-up study. *Clin Orthop* 1999;367:61–72.

17 Tabor OB Jr, Tabor OB. Unicompartmental arthroplasty: a long-term follow-up study. *J Arthroplasty* 1998;13:373–9.

18 Bert JM. 10-year survivorship of metal-backed, unicompartmental arthroplasty. *J Arthroplasty* 1998;13:901–5.

19 Riebel GD, Werner FW, Ayers DC, Bromka J, Murray DG. Early failure of the femoral component in unicompartmental knee arthroplasty. *J Arthroplasty* 1995;10:615–21.

Chapter 16

Hip and pelvic osteotomies

Frank Langlotz, Andreas F. Hinsche, and R.M. Smith

16.1 Introduction

Dysplasia of the hip joint is characterized by an insufficient coverage of the femoral head by the acetabular cup. As a result loading of the joint is increased,[1] and early joint degeneration is expected. Women are affected more often than men.[2] Although total hip replacement has been reported for the treatment of dysplastic hips,[3] osteotomy of the pelvis with reorientation and subsequent internal fixation of the acetabulum is the preferred treatment method whenever possible. In 1955 Chiari described a pelvic osteotomy to improve the deficient femoral coverage,[4] though satisfactory results are dependent on well-defined indications.[5] Salter[6] introduced a single osteotomy of the innominate bone for the treatment of dysplastic hips in children. Since the center of the hip joint is shifted considerably by Salter's osteotomy, adverse effects on the biomechanics of the joint could be demonstrated.[7] To overcome these problems and to allow treatment of a larger variety of hip dysplasia especially in older patients, triple osteotomies were developed. Two of the earliest techniques were described by Steel[8] and Tönnis.[9] Both authors proposed osteotomies of the pubis, ischium, and ilium in order to allow for larger correction of the completely mobilized acetabulum, normally performed through two incisions. Ganz et al.[10] introduced a periacetabular osteotomy (PAO). The principle of this operation is to place all osteotomies at minimum distances form the hip joint to provide a maximum of corrective potential with improved biomechanics. In contrast to Steel's and Tönnis' techniques, the posterior column and therefore the sacropelvic connection remains intact, enabling fragment fixation by only two screws and permitting early mobilization of the patient.[10] Moreover, the ability for normal child delivery following pelvic surgery remains.[11] This is an important factor, considering that girls and young women are the majority of those patients receiving operative treatment for hip dysplasia.

16.2 Preoperative computer assistance

Pelvic osteotomies are technically challenging interventions. Important steps of the procedures are complex three-dimensional tasks such as placing and guiding the surgical chisels for the osteotomies and the re-orientation and fixation of the detached acetabular fragment. Consequently, three-dimensional computed tomography (CT) data sets have been used for the planning and preparation of these complex operations. There is an ongoing discussion about whether it is sufficient to look at the problem of dysplasia from a purely geometrical view or how much biomechanical consideration such as joint contact pressure should be given.[12] More recently, the diagnostic of hip dysplasia has been challenged and new means to assess the acetabular deficiency have been described. Nakamura et al. proposed a specific CT processing method for a better inspection of the pelvis.[13] Using a 'top view of the hip' to visually assess femoral coverage, the authors recommended this view as a reliable measure to determine hip deficiency. Roach et al.[14] proposed a more quantitative approach by using a best-fit sphere, allowing evaluation of joint congruency as well as the measurement of the distance between joint surfaces. As a result, force concentrations in the hip could be identified and better surgical planning was facilitated. However, the determination of optimal acetabular correction was completely in the surgeon's responsibility and was not eased by the author's planning software.

Other groups developed specific software packages not only for the preoperative analysis of pelvic anatomy but also to simulate post-operative changes or suggest optimal correction parameters for pelvic osteotomies. Klaue *et al.* described a simplified planning and simulation program, in which manual digitization of CT films creates a set of bone contours, which are reconstructed three-dimensionally to make separate models of femur and acetabulum.[15] Automatic calculation of femoral head coverage was used as a feedback to evaluate the potential post-operative correction by successive trials of rotations and shifts about the three coordinate axes. The resulting optimal reorientation of the acetabulum was then used during the surgical procedure for periacetabular osteotomy.

Hip *et al.* presented a method to calculate joint contact pressures in an individual mathematical model, generated from the patient's CT scan.[16] Segmentation and manual determination of the acetabular joint surface gave a precise representation of the load-bearing zone. In addition, their software could predict an acetabular correction producing a minimum pressure distribution. The authors performed an in-vitro study on cadaveric specimens and measured contact pressures by means of Fuji pressure-sensitive film. In two thirds of all cases, the simulation software predicted correctly the measured values.

Mittelmeier *et al.* evaluated the method of rapid prototyping for operation planning and simulation in the context of pelvic osteotomies.[17] Through segmentation of CT data a three-dimensional surface model of the dysplastic hip was created. The data were further processed to generate input parameters for a computerized numerical control (CNC) milling machine that manufactured a 1:1 model of the pelvis from a polyurethane block. This model then provided a realistic hands-on representation of the patient's pelvis and could be used to plan and simulate various intra-operative steps. The authors reported their experiences gained during 28 cases of pelvic tumors, 55 triple osteotomies, and four total hip arthroplasty revisions after implant loosening. They concluded that the rapid prototyping technique offers a valuable instrument to facilitate complex and three-dimensional preoperative planning especially in difficult cases, but increased costs and logistic demands are disadvantageous.

Dahlen *et al.* reported experiences with a multipurpose planning system for orthopaedic surgery that runs on a standard PC.[18] Initially developed for reconstructive foot surgery, the authors recommended the software also for applications in other anatomical regions. Moreover, they specifically mentioned its applicability for the planning of pelvic osteotomies. Various processing tools allowed segmentation of the three-dimensional CT or MRI data and simulation of osteotomies, fragment manipulation as well as the precise measurement of geometric values. For realistic interaction with the software, virtual reality devices such as shutter glasses and a 3D computer mouse were used.

16.3 Intra-operative computer assistance

Limited access and visibility during pelvic osteotomies increases the surgical technical demands during such complex procedures. Consequently, computer applications have been developed to allow not only sophisticated planning and simulation, but also precise intra-operative realization of the required surgical intervention. During pelvic osteotomies this often includes delicate bone cuts, usually performed with specifically shaped chisels and the reorientation of the acetabular fragment. Most of the guidance systems have been described for the complex triple osteotomies. In 1995, Sato *et al.* presented a laboratory study, in which an optical 3D localizer had been used to trace an osteotome, cutting through a foam block.[19] Subsequently, the motion of this free-cut fragment could be visualized. Three years later the authors reported on their first clinical experience using the described system.[20] A preoperative data set was used to define the osteotomization plane. Intra-operatively the system visualized the predetermined target plane as well as the current location of a tracked osteotome and displayed graphically the deviation between the two. In a similar manner, acetabular correction could be aligned following a preoperative plan. Nishii *et al.* described this as 'a promising modality to improve accuracy and reproducibility' during pelvic osteotomies.

In 1998 Radermacher *et al.* chose a different approach.[21] They used the patient's CT data to plan preoperatively the osteotomy cuts for a Tönnis' osteotomy with the help of specific planning software. This allowed preoperatively the simulation of planned osteotomies and realignment of the acetabulum. As a special feature, the system automatically determined a set of osteotomization planes permitting maximum mobility of the detached fragment. The quality of potential post-operative configurations could be assessed by online calculation of several angles. In order to realize the planning result intra-operatively, rapid prototyping technology was used. Using a CNC milling machine negative molds were manufactured, representing the shape of the bone in the region of the planned cuts. In addition, mechanical chiseling guides were milled into the molds. Intra-operatively these templates were attached to the pelvic bone. The precise representation of the bony surface allowed fixation of the devices only at their appropriate positions. Each osteotomy was carried out exactly as planned with the help of these mechanical cutting guides. The authors reported good accuracy and highlighted the fact that intra-operatively no specific tracking or navigation technology was required.

In 1997 Langlotz *et al.* presented the results of a series of twelve patients, in which periacetabular osteotomy had been performed with assistance of a navigation system.[22] This system used a preoperative CT scan for the definition of the fragment to be detached and for the visualization of all intra-operative steps. An optoelectronic camera (OPTOTRAK®, Northern Digital Inc., Waterloo, Canada) traced the loca-

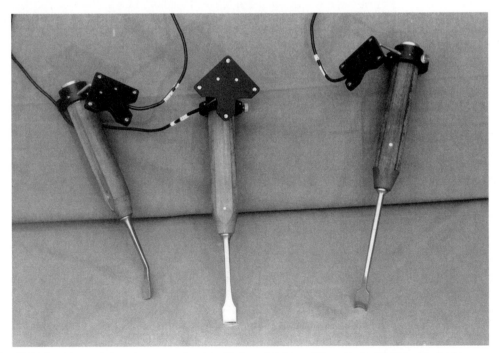

Fig. 16.1 A probe each housing a quadruplet of infrared light emitting diodes (LED) is attached to every osteotome. It allows intra-operative real-time tracking of the instrument by means of an optoelectronic camera.

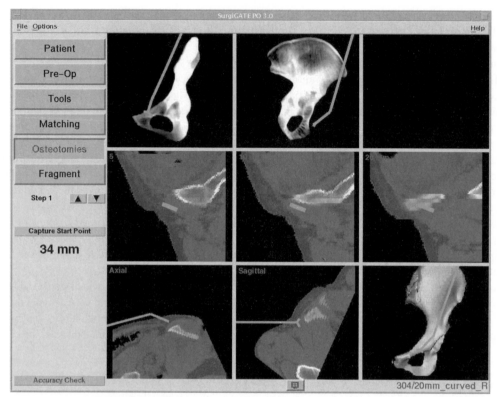

Fig. 16.2 Intra-operative surgical action (here: osteotomization of the pubic bone) is visualized in two- and three-dimensional CT reconstructions.

tion and orientation of four different osteotomes by means of shields, which were attached to each of the chisels and equipped with infrared light emitting diodes (LEDs) (Fig. 16.1). In order to relate these tool-data to the patient's anatomy, a modular dynamic reference base[23] was fixed to the ipsi- or contralateral iliac crest. Following a combined paired-points and surface-matching algorithm[24] to correlate the patient's anatomy with the CT data set, all chisels were displayed relatively to the dynamic reference base without the need for preoperatively fixed fiducial markers such as screws or pins. Subsequently, all surgical action performed with any of the tracked osteotomes was visualized in real-time in two- and three-dimensional reconstructions of the patient's CT data (Fig. 16.2). Once the acetabulum was mobilized, its motion in space was followed with a second reference base, enabling on-screen visualization of the correction maneuvers in progress. Although the surgical technique of periacetabular osteotomy had been conventionally established, the use of this surgical navigation system proved to be a valuable assistance, particularly during the final osteotomy and the realignment of the acetabular fragment.[24] Since introduction, the system has been also used and described for other triple osteotomies and posttraumatic malunion of the pelvis. Hüfner *et al.* described the case of a young woman, in which a severely malunited post-traumatic pelvic ring and acetabular injury had been precisely reconstructed with the assistance of the above described navigation system (SurgiGATE®).[25]

With the introduction of fluoroscopy-based navigation,[26] computer guidance became available for a variety of additional orthopedic applications. Based on images acquired with a standard image

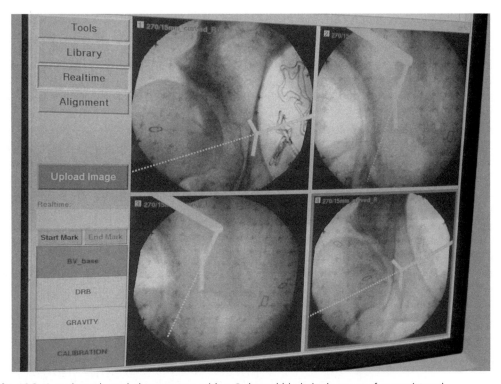

Fig. 16.3 A navigated, angled osteotome with a C-shaped blade is shown on four registered fluoroscopic images. The working direction of the instrument is indicated by a dotted line.

intensifier calibrated for the image guidance system, there is no need for preoperative CT-scanning and a sometimes time-consuming intra-operative registration (matching) procedure. Most surgeons are used to two-dimensional images from the image intensifier within the operating room and therefore only minor adjustments to the usual theater set-up are necessary. Up to four c-arm images can be displayed simultaneously on the computer screen, and the image intensifier can then be removed from the operating field to give the surgeon more operating space. During the procedure further images can be acquired and the immediate intra-operative image 'up-dating' enables the surgeon to follow and check individual steps of the procedure. Following experiences for pelvic screw insertion, first satisfactory experiences with the application of such a method during periacetabular osteotomies were presented.[27] The authors described the use of the fluoroscopy-based navigation system (SurgiGATE®, Medivision, Oberdorf, Switzerland) in a series of four cases of late congenital hip dysplasia (Fig. 16.3). It was highlighted that following the initial acquisition of several C-arm images displaying the relevant acetabulum and hemipelvis, the operation could be performed faster and with significantly reduced radiation exposure for patient and surgical staff. However, three-dimensional planning of the intervention and realignment of the acetabular fragment was impossible in the absence of a three-dimensional data set.

16.4 **Discussion and conclusion**

Osteotomies of the pelvis are complex procedures. Although endoscopic treatment of hip dysplasia has been recently reported,[28] the open approach is necessary in the majority of cases. A variety of conceptually different solutions for preoperative planning, simulation, intra-operative guidance, and post-operative assessment have been described over the years. CT scans provide the preferred means to represent the complex three-dimensional problem. Approaches to improve intra-operative precision using rapid prototyping concepts[17,21] seem to lack acceptance due to the increased planning demands and the logistical setup obligatory for the production of the models. The remarkable method of using fluoroscopy-based navigation for pelvic osteotomies[27] offers image guidance without the necessity of any preoperative data preparation and allows intra-operative image updating. CT-based image guided surgery systems with optoelectronic tool tracking have been proposed[20,24] and provide precise real-time feedback about surgical action within a realistic three-dimensional representation of the operated anatomy.

To date, no system for computer assisted pelvic osteotomy is available covering the complete course of treatment, from preoperative planning to intra-operative therapy. Such a system would have to allow for planning of bone cuts, fragment reorientation, intra-operative image updating and the appropriate way of fragment re-fixation respecting both geometrical and biomechanical considerations. Intra-operatively, the surgeon would be guided to perform all steps (osteotomization, correction, fixation) according to the plan. The combination or fusion of different image modalities, e.g., CT, MRI, US, and fluoroscopy might help the development of such a system. Relatively small numbers of cases as well as the complex demands make the development of such a planning and navigation tool a difficult and complex task but the experiences with the existing systems so far are encouraging and confirm clearly the potential for further developments in the future.

References

1 Gillingham BL, Sanchez AA, Wegner DR. Pelvic osteotomies for the treatment of hip dysplasia in children and young adults. *J Am Acad Orthop Surg* 1999;7:325–37.

2 Hefti F. *Kinderorthopödie in der Praxis*. Berlin, Heidelberg, New York: Springer; 1998.

3 Korovessis PG, Stamatakis M, Baikousis A, Petsinis G. Treatment of dysplastic and congenitally dislocated hips with the Zweymüller total hip prosthesis. *Orthopaedics* 2001;24:465–71.

4 Chiari K. Ergebnisse mit der Beckenosteotomie als Pfannendachplastik. *Z Orthop* 1955;87:14–26.

5 Reynolds DA. Chiari innominate osteotomy in adults. *J Bone Joint Surg Br* 1986;68B:45–54.

6 Salter RB. Innominate osteotomy in the treatment of congenital dislocation and subluxation of the hip. *J Bone Joint Surg Br* 1961;43B:518–39.

7 Rab GT. Biomechanical aspects of Salter osteotomy. *Clin Orthop* 1978;132:82–7.

8 Steel HH. Triple osteotomy of the innominate bone. *J Bone Joint Surg Am* 1973;55A:343–50.

9 Tönnis D. Eine neue Form derr Hüftpfannenschwenkung durch Dreifachosteotomie zur Ermöglichung späterer Hüftprothesenversorgung. *Orthop Praxis* 1973;15:1003–5.

10 Ganz R, Klaue K, Vinh TS, Mast JW. A new periacetabular osteotomy for the treatment of hip dysplasias. *Clin Orthop* 1988;232:26–36.

11 Flückiger G, Eggli S, Kosina J, Ganz R. Geburt nach periazetabulärer Osteotomie. *Orthopäde* 2000;29:63–7.

12 de Kleuver M, Kapitein PJ, Kooijman MA, van Limbeek J, Pavlov PW, Veth RP. Acetabular coverage of the femoral head after triple pelvic osteotomy: no relation to outcome in 51 hips followed for 8–15 years. *Acta Orthop Scand* 1999;70:583–8.

13 Nakamura S, Yorikawa J, Otsuka K, Takeshita K, Harasawa A, Matsushita T. Evaluation of acetabular dysplasia using a top view of the hip on three-dimensional CT. *J Orthop Sci* 2000;5:533–9.

14 Roach JW, Hobatho MC, Baker KJ, Ashman RB. Three-dimensional computer analysis of complex acetabular insufficiency. *J Pediatr Orthop* 1997;17:158–64.

15 Klaue K, Wallin A, Ganz R. CT evaluation of coverage and congruency of the hip prior to osteotomy. *Clin Orthop* 1988;232:15–25.

16 Hip JA, Michaeli DA, Murphy SB. An integrated approach to acetabular osteotomies. In: Nolte L-P, Ganz R, eds. *Computer assisted orthopedic surgery (CAOS)*. Seattle, Toronto, Bern, Göttingen: Hogrefe and Huber 1999;121–7.

17 Mittelmeier W, Peters P, Ascherl R, Gradinger R. Rapid prototyping—Modellherstellung zur präoperativen Planung von rekonstruktiven Beckeneingriffen. *Orthopäde* 1997;26:273–9.

18 Dahlen C, Zwipp H. Computer-assistierte OP-Planung—3D-Software für den PC. *Unfallchirurg* 2001;6:466–79.

19 Sato Y, Nakajima Y, Nishii T, Tamura S. Image guided orthopaedic surgery using osteotome with 3D localizer. *Int Soc Comput Aided Surg* 1995;2(Suppl. 1):26–7.

20 Nishii T, Sugano N, Sato Y, Sasama T, Nakajima Y, Tamura S, Ochi T. Computer navigation system for rotational acetabular osteotomy in the hip joint. In: Lemke HU, Vannier MW, Inamura K, Farman AG, eds. *Computer assisted radiology and surgery*. Amsterdam, Lausanne, New York: Elsevier, 1998;913.

21 Radermacher K, Portheine F, Anton M, Zimolong A, Kaspers G, Rau G, Staudte HW. Computer assisted orthopaedic surgery with image based individual templates. *Clin Orthop* 1998;354:28–38.

22 Langlotz F, Stucki M, Bächler R, Scheer C, Ganz R, Berlemann U, Nolte L-P. The first twelve cases of computer assisted periacetabular osteotomy. *Comput Aided Surg* 1997;2:317–26.

23 Nolte L-P, Zamorano L, Visarius H, Berlemann U, Langlotz F, Arm E, Schwarzenbach O. Clinical evaluation of a system for precision enhancement in spine surgery. *Clin Biomech* 1995;10:293–303.

24 Langlotz F, Bächler R, Berlemann U, Nolte L-P, Ganz R. Computer assistance for pelvic osteotomies. *Clin Orthop* 1998;354:92–102.

25 Hüfner T, Pohlemann T, Gänsslen A, Geerling J, Krettek C, Tscherne H. Computer assisted surgery (CAS) for correction of a malhealed pelvic ring fracture in a young female patient. *Comput Aided Surg* 1999;4:154.

26 Hofstetter R, Slomczykowski M, Sati M, Nolte L-P. Fluoroscopy as an imaging means for computer assisted surgical navigation. *Comput Aided Surg* 1999;4:65–76.

27 Hinsche AF, Giannoudis PV, Smith RM. Fluoroscopy-based multiplanar guidance for periacetabular osteotomy. *Comput Aided Surg* 2001;6:57.

28 Wall EJ, Kolata R, Roy DR, Mehlman CT, Crawford AH. Endoscopic pelvic osteotomy for the treatment of hip dysplasia. *J Am Acad Orthop Surg* 2001;9:150–6.

Chapter 17

Computer-assisted high tibial osteotomies

Randy E. Ellis, John F. Rudan, and M.M. Harrison

17.1 **Introduction**

A high tibial osteotomy (HTO) is indicated for the relatively young and active patient who has painful unicompartmental knee arthrosis, especially an arthrosis due to an early stage of osteoarthritis. The intended outcome of the surgical procedure is to realign a bone in order to change the biomechanics of the knee joint, especially to change the force transmission through the joint. Such a procedure must be performed accurately, not only to create the desired geometries but also to provide biological environments for rapid and effective healing. The most common forms of HTO for addressing medial-compartment arthrosis are (a) the closing wedge osteotomy, in which the realignment is achieved by removing a lateral wedge of bone from the proximal tibia; (b) the opening-wedge osteotomy, in which the realignment is achieved by opening a medial cut and grafting a wedge of bone or bone substitute into the defect; and (c) a barrel-vault osteotomy, in which a circular arc is cut into the proximal tibia and the distal fragment is rotated about the pivot axis of the arc. In opening-wedge and barrel-vault osteotomies, the tibiofibular joint is commonly disrupted in order to avoid excessive stresses during the realignment that can lead to pain or fracture. Figure 17.1 shows a plain X-ray film of a typical patient suffering from medial-compartment arthrosis.

The most common surgical alternative to the procedure is a total knee arthroplasty or unicompartmental arthroplasty. Total knee arthroplasty has a typical survival rate of 90% at 15 years after the procedure, but the polyethylene articulating surfaces generate wear particles that lead to loosening or failure and subsequent revision of the prosthesis. By contrast, HTO preserves the joint's original cartilagenous surfaces and corrects the fundamental mechanical problem of the knee. This advantage of HTO is especially important to the young active patient, for whom an arthroplasty has a greater probability of earlier failure than is likely for an older inactive patient. In North America at the time of writing, the cost of an osteotomy is approximately 1/3 that of an arthroplasty.

The major difficulty with HTO is that the outcome is not predictable, and the major suspected reason for the unpredictability in patients who meet the indications is that it is difficult to attain the desired correction angle. Numerous long-term clinical studies have shown that osteotomy results are improved if the femoral-tibial alignment angle is between 7° and 13° of varus alignment.[1,2] Immediate post-operative results show a large variability—by averaging the variances of reported results for closing-wedge osteotomy, calculation shows that the overall standard deviation of angular correction is 2.5° for HTO performed with jig systems and 5.6° for those without the use of jigs.[3–9] Significant changes in the angle of correction after operation can be observed, which can be attributed to fragment mobility. Recent results have suggested that proper patient selection, more careful planning, and more precise execution of the osteotomy can produce a longer-lasting HTO.[10,11] For example, an extensive clinical review[10] reports on 128 knees that were studied for up to 15 years, finding a revision rate was only 10.9%.

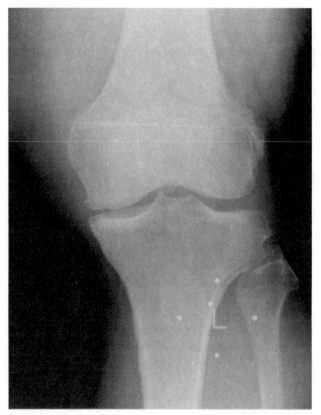

Fig. 17.1 A plain X-ray film of the left knee of a typical patient. Note the loss of medial joint space, varus angulation, and increased medial cortical bone density. The circular markers are fiducials for correcting the X-ray perspective distortion.

17.1.1 Traditional techniques for high tibial osteotomy

The most common form of HTO is the closing wedge osteotomy, popularized by Coventry in 1973.[2] The wedge is first planned on a frontal-plane standing X-ray by drawing a wedge of the desired correction angle, where the wedge's upper plane is parallel to the tibial plateau and the lower plane is above the tibial tubercle. Ideally, the wedge will produce a hinge of cortical bone approximately 2–5 mm in thickness. Surgical technique uses one of several incisions (mid-line, 'hockey-stick', or transverse) to expose the anterolateral tibia. The medial half of the proximal tibial-fibular joint is then excised to mobilize the fibula. One or more Kirschner wires are drilled, usually under fluoroscopic guidance, to act as guides for resection. The wedge is removed, the defect is reduced with the remaining medial cortex acting as a hinge, and fixation is achieved with step-staples, plates, or wires.

For opening-wedge osteotomy only the resection plane and angle are planned. Intra-operatively, the tibia is resected and distracted to the desired correction angle. Surgical technique is similar to that for the opening wedge, but works on the anteromedial tibia. After resection the tibia is opened using the lateral cortical hinge. The resulting defect is filled, most often by viable autologous bone graft from the iliac crest and alternatively by heterologous bone or an artificial bone substitute.

A barrel-vault osteotomy is indicated for a large correction in the femoral-tibial alignment (greater than 14°). (This would require a wedge correction of 19°, which would be excessive for a closing or opening wedge osteotomy.) For this osteotomy the rotational axis, radius of the barrel, and desired correction angle must be planned. Surgical technique uses a midline skin incision centered over the tibial tubercle followed by excision of the medial half of the proximal tibial-fibular joint. An extended tibial tubercle osteotomy, approximately 6–8 centimeters in length, leaves a medial soft-tissue hinge. The barrel vault osteotomy is marked on the proximal tibial metaphysis, and the osteotomy is completed using multiple drill holes and resecting the remaining bone with small osteotomes. The barrel-vault osteotomy is typically fixed with a buttress plate and screws, and the tibial tubercle osteotomy with screws only.

For all of these osteotomies, technical difficulties often arise from the use of fluoroscopy, such as image-intensifier nonlinearities and distortions that compromise accuracy. Also, parallax errors can provide misleading angular and positional guidance. Because planning and guidance are performed from plain X-ray images, axial alignment and correction are usually disregarded.

17.1.2 A computer technique for high tibial osteotomy

The major contribution of computer assisted surgery to HTO has so far been in preoperative planning, whereby the surgeon is provided with a prediction of post-operative alignment or loading. One such system, developed by the Tsumura group[12] for closing-wedge osteotomy, used a two-dimensional static biomechanical model originally proposed by Coventry and Insall.[13,14] The other preoperative planner, also for closing-wedge osteotomy, was developed by Chao *et al.* and used a two-dimensional rigid-body spring model to simulate the forces across the articular surfaces.[15–17] It also attempted to account for ligamentous effects, and simulated two-dimensional dynamic loading.

A drawback of these approaches is that planning and simulation of the three-dimensional osteotomy are carried out in only two dimensions. There are many inherent problems in executing a two-dimensional plan in three-dimensional space. For example, tilting of the saw blade in the anterior/posterior direction is not controlled by the traditional technique. Further, if the axis for closing the osteotomy is not perpendicular to the frontal plane, an unintended internal/external rotation of the foot is induced: if the hinge is located on the posteromedial aspect then internal rotation of the foot occurs, and vice versa for anteromedial location of the hinge.

We submit that, in addition to inappropriate patient selection, the premature failures and large variability in HTO are due to: (1) the inability of current planning methods to address the fact that HTO is a three-dimensional procedure; and (2) the incapability of manual surgeries to produce the planned amount of axis shift accurately. Our approach to solving these problems is to achieve accurate and reproducible three-dimensional corrections using computer assistance. A surgical enhancement system has been developed that facilitates preoperative planning in three-dimensional space. This three-dimensional plan can then be executed in an image-guided surgery system. The inherent precision in the image-guided surgery system is expected to lead to better reliability, consistency and reduced operative time in HTO than can be achieved by the traditional techniques.

The goal was to reduce the incidence of the common post-operative problems. With a three-dimensional guidance and planning system it should be possible to eliminate, or greatly reduce the probability of (a) incorrect valgus alignment, (b) incorrect proximal/distal location of the osteotomy, and (c) inadvertent internal/external foot rotation. If proximal-fragment fracture is due to proximity of the osteotomy to the joint, especially because of inadvertent anterior/posterior sloping of the proximal resection, then the probability of fracture should be reduced. Finally, if the post-osteotomy fixation is also planned and guided, the danger of fixation into the joint articulation should also be reduced.

17.2 Computer-assisted technique

All three types of high tibial osteotomies can be performed using a computer-assisted technique. We performed ours in eight steps:

1. CT images of the knee were acquired from the femoral condyles to below the tibial tubercle, using axial-mode slices of 3 mm width spaced 2 mm apart. Five axial-mode slices of the ankle were also acquired, to determine the anatomical axis of the tibia. (Helical scans also produce acceptable images.)

2. A three-dimensional surface model of the tibia was reconstructed from the CT images by isosurface extraction.

3. With the isosurface model, and data from standardized weight-bearing radiographs, the surgeon used preoperative planning software to plan the procedure. Given the desired correction in the sagittal and frontal planes, the planner simulated the results of the osteotomy. The surgeon could visually inspect the three-dimensional position of the resection planes, assess the rotational corrections computed by the planning software, and adjust the planes as desired.

4. Intra-operatively, an optically tracked target was attached to the bone that was to be cut. The coordinate system common to the CT scan, the computerized tibia model, and the planned osteotomy were mapped onto the coordinate system of the patient by means of a robust surface registration algorithm.[17]

5. The osteotomy guidance aids were implanted. A full-screen, real-time computer animation displayed the relative positions of surgical instruments superimposed on the plan, the model, and in orthogonal reformats of the CT volume. The guidance aids varied depending on the procedure type:

   - For an opening-wedge osteotomy, a single Kirschner wire was implanted so that its distal surface grazed the planned osteotomy plane. An additional point on the plane was identified with a tracked pointer and marked, to provide full control of the resection.

   - For a closing-wedge osteotomy, a second K-wire was implanted so that its proximal surface grazed the inferior planned osteotomy plane.

   - For a barrel-vault osteotomy, a Schantz pin was implanted along the planned barrel-vault axis. The guidance was represented as a pair of orthogonal intersecting planes.

6. A tracking pin was installed on the bone opposite to the furthest osteotomy site, and the orientation of the pin with respect to a guidance plane was noted.

7. For opening-wedge and closing-wedge osteotomy, the wire(s) were then used as saw guide(s) to perform the osteotomy as per traditional technique[18] and osteoclasis was used to complete the formation of a hinge (for a closing-wedge osteotomy, the wedge fragment was also removed). For a barrel-vault osteotomy, the guide pin was used as a pivot; a plate was used to drill holes parallel to the axis at a desired radius, then saws and osteotomes were used to complete the barrel vault.

8. The orientation of the guide pin was tracked with respect to its original orientation to ensure that the desired angulation was achieved. After the tibia adjusted to the new angulation, staples or plates were used to immobilize the fragments and the surgical field was closed.

We used two distinct planning systems, one for closing-wedge and opening-wedge osteotomy, and the other for barrel-vault osteotomies. The reason is purely historical: the wedge planner was developed first, specifically for only that procedure, and we subsequently developed the more general second planner by building on our experiences.

17.2.1 Planning closing-wedge and opening-wedge osteotomies

The closing-wedge and opening-wedge osteotomies produce a rotation about a cortical bone hinge (medially and laterally, respectively). The procedures are particularly suited to computer-assisted planning because the reduction can be modeled as a rotation about an axis in space. Such a planning process is linear and well structured, so the planner was implemented as a *wizard-based* system in which each window had text describing the step and a graphical interface for effecting that step. The preoperative planning system was implemented in X/Motif, and its major function was to allow the surgeon to specify two resection planes on a graphical model of a tibia.

The reconstructed CT slice images were electronically transferred from a HiSpeed CT scanner (General Electric, Milwaukee WI) to a UNIX workstation (SUN Microsystems, Sunnyvale, CA). Custom software was used by a research assistant to extract an isosurface model of the proximal tibia, a process that required approximately 30 minutes. The tibial eminence and ankle were located on individual CT slices, as was the tibial tubercle. Three noncollinear points of subchondral bone of the tibial plateau were located. The anatomical axis, the frontal axis, and the plateau plane were calculated from these locations.

The triangulated isosurface model of the tibia, plus numerical definitions of the anatomical and frontal axes, were loaded and displayed by the planning system. The surgeon who performed the planning verified that the tibial anatomical axis frontal axis were correctly defined. The second step was selection of the tibial plateau, which was rendered as a plane that could obscure or be obscured by the proximal tibial surface. The user had control over the varus/valgus tilt, the anterior/posterior tilt, and the proximal/distal placement of where the plateau plane intersected the anatomical axis. Typically, the surgeon viewed the superimposed axes and plateau carefully to ensure full understanding of the anatomy of the individual patient. Preoperative planning required approximately 10 minutes. Figure 17.2 shows a conventional plan drawn upon a plain X-ray film, and a computer-enhanced method of identifying the tibial axis and tibial plateau in three dimensions.

The third and final step was selection of the resection plane or planes. The user moved the proximal plane down to an appropriate level (usually 12–16 mm). For closing-wedge osteotomy, the user also specified the correction angle of the wedge as measured from a preoperative plain X-ray film or as an adjustment to the tibial-plateau/tibial-shaft angle that is automatically calculated by the system. The user could translate the hinge axis in proximal/distal and medial/lateral directions, and could rotate it about the internal/external axis. Figure 17.3 shows a planned closing wedge from two different viewpoints. Note that, for either procedure, the surgeon can clearly visualize the amount of medial cortical margin that constitutes the medial hinge of the osteotomy.

The original tibia—with superimposed resection planes—was displayed on one side of the monitor, and on the other side was the predicted result including preoperative and predicted post-operative axes. The images could be visualized from any viewpoint, to facilitate understanding of the full three-dimensional consequences of the osteotomy. Because the tibial cortex was modeled as a triangular mesh, a desktop UNIX workstation running OpenGL could render each virtual surgery very rapidly. Figure 17.4 shows a typical completed plan for an example patient.

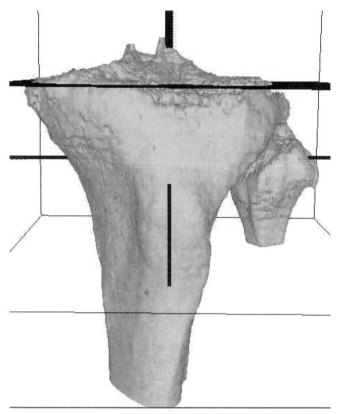

Fig. 17.2 Preoperative determination of the tibial axis and tibial plateau. The traditional surgical procedures require determining the tibial axis and tibial plateau from a frontal X-ray film. A computer-enhanced procedure uses a three-dimensional surface mesh in establishing the anatomical features.

(a)   (b)

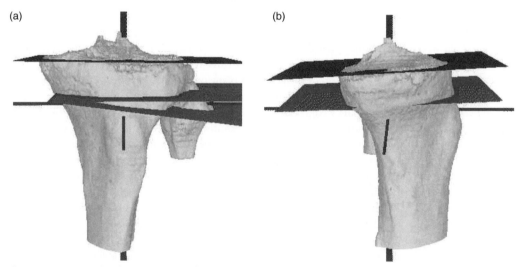

Fig. 17.3 Preoperative determination of the wedge to be removed. The wedge can be reviewed from various viewpoints, to ascertain its three-dimensional relationship to the tibia and to examine the planned geometry of the medial hinge.

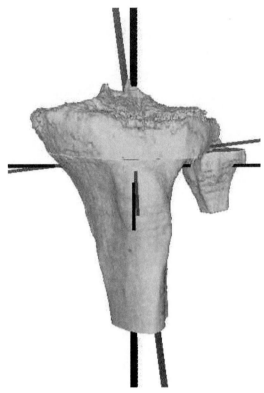

Fig. 17.4 A preoperative planning system for closing-wedge tibial osteotomy. The system displays the predicted post-operative result of the surgical procedure, as well as the three anatomical angles that might be changed by the procedure. The large dark lines are the preoperative anatomical axes, and the large light lines are the predicted post-operative axes. (On the computer screen, these axes are color-coded to aid in their identification.)

The software program guided the user through the steps of preoperative planning. Object motion in three dimensions was controlled mainly by means of mouse motion, with transformations smoothly rendered by interpolating rotations as quaternions.[19–21] The osteotomy's geometry was rendered visually and the rotational parameters were displayed as the Grood–Suntay parameters of valgus/varus, internal/external rotation, and flexion/extension.[22] The user could adjust the osteotomy's correction via a mouse, or enter values via a keyboard, to achieve the desired correction.

17.2.2 Planning a barrel-vault osteotomy

A barrel-vault osteotomy is used to achieve pure rotation about an axis. Thus, the plan must at minimum include the location and orientation of the rotational axis. In addition, the surgeon must choose a radial distance away from the axis where the bone is eventually to be resected.

One can thus think of a barrel-vault osteotomy as a *cylinder*. The axis of rotation is the axis of the cylinder, and the distance from the axis is the radius of the cylinder. We plan the osteotomy by 'flying' a semi-cylinder onto the CT-based model of the patient. The surgeon first places the axis, typically perpendicular to the tibial axis and aligned with the AP axis. Next, the surgeon selects the desired cylindrical radius; the system displays the resulting plan, as shown in Fig. 17.5.

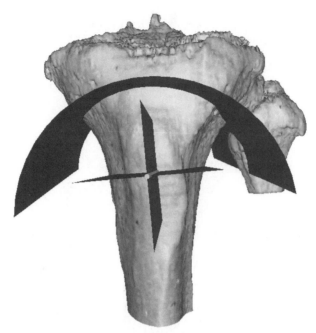

Fig. 17.5 A preoperative planning system for barrel-vault tibial osteotomy. The plan includes the location and orientation of the barrel axis, and the vault created by intersecting part of a cylinder with the model of the patient. In this case, only the tibia would be resected surgically.

The planner exports two perpendicular planes that intersect on the cylindrical axis. Intra-operatively, the surgeon can either drill a pin along the cylindrical axis and apply a mechanical jig or can drill a sequence of pilot holes that are at a fixed distance from the axis and are parallel to both planes (as described above for traditional surgical technique).

Thus, the intra-operative guidance system needs to understand only *two* planes in order to guide closing-wedge, opening-wedge, and barrel-vault osteotomies.

17.2.3 An image-based guidance system

The image-based guidance system was composed of software running on a desktop UNIX workstation (SUN Microsystems, Sunnyvale CA) and either a mechanical localizer (FARO Technologies, Lake Mary, FL) or an optical localizer (Northern Digital, Inc., Waterloo, Canada). For optical localization a dynamic reference base was attached to the tibia, distal to the planned osteotomy site, in order to track leg motion. Registration for mechanical localization used pre-implanted fiducials; for optical localization, it was accomplished by touching three or more anatomical regions on the tibia ('spotlights') with a tracked surgical probe, then calculating the rigid transformation between localizer coordinates and CT coordinates using a mathematically robust estimation algorithm.[23]

With registration accomplished, it was possible to transform any model or action represented in one coordinate system to the other coordinate system. The surgeons found that the most helpful information was (a) rendering transverse, frontal, and sagittal planes from CT volumetric data, with the location and orientation of the surgical instrument superimposed in color on the gray-scale images, and (b) using solid modeling to render the three-dimensional surface model of the tibia, models of the

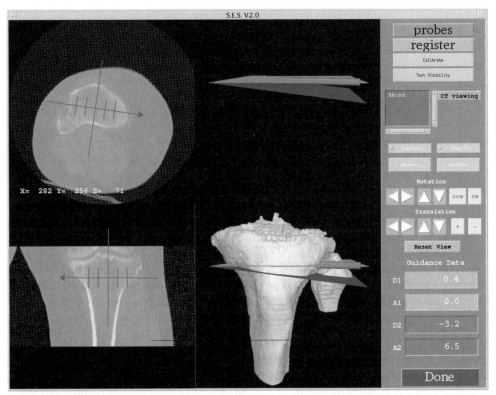

Fig. 17.6 An image-based guidance system for orthopedic surgery. The surgery software displays the position and orientation of the surgical instrument in axial and frontal planes, as well as the tibial model, the planned resection planes, and a virtual surgical instrument. It also numerically displays the distance to each resection plane in millimeters (D1 and D2), and the angle in degrees between the instrument and the resection plane (A1 and A2). It is useful to display only the plan and the virtual instrument, as in the upper right pane, because the 3D model of the tibia can obscure the virtual instrument as drilling proceeds.

resection planes, and a three-dimensional model of a virtual surgical instrument. Additional guidance information was available digitally, as required by the surgeon, by means of simple queries to the software. Figure 17.6 shows the screen layout for tracking a drill during implantation of a proximal guide wire in a closing-wedge osteotomy.

17.3 A laboratory study of closing-wedge osteotomy

Laboratory tests were surgical simulations of closing-wedge osteotomies, performed on plastic bone models (Pacific Research Laboratories, WA). Prior to testing, the bone models were prepared for registration and scanned with CT. Four registration markers were inserted into accurately milled holes on the anterolateral surface of each model. The positions were selected so that the markers would be within a realistic surgical exposure and would also be located only on the distal fragment of the tibia after osteotomy.

To facilitate resection, each bone model was fixed in a special jig that held the tibia model at a 45° angle from the horizontal. Black closed-cell foam masked the proximal part of the bone model, to simulate the visual obstructions created by soft tissue that appear clinically. After the wedge was removed, the distal and proximal fragments of the tibia were held together by strong adhesive (Shoe Goo) and with woodworking staples delivered from a staple gun so that the reduced osteotomy could be assessed.

Thirty surgical simulations were performed, with intended corrections of 9°, 14°, and 19°. The tasks were to (a) perform the osteotomy with fluoroscopic guidance of the saw blade followed by conventional cutting and osteoclasis, and (b) perform the osteotomy by computer-enhanced planning and guidance of pin placement followed by conventional cutting and osteoclasis. For each task each angular correction was performed five times in a randomized sequence, alternating tasks (a) and (b).

Subsequently, the wedge angles were measured. These measurements took advantage of the presence in the models of a transverse hole approximately 15 mm inferior to the tibial plateau; this hole is parallel to the Cartesian X axis of the Grood–Suntay[22] coordinate system. The wedges were placed in a jig that fixed the wedges via the transverse hole and surface points were collected from the superior wedge surface using a precision mechanical arm (FARO Technologies, Lake Mary, FL). Varus/valgus angulations were calculated as the total rotation about the Cartesian Y axis of the Grood–Suntay coordinate system of the tibia. The differences between the intended varus/valgus angle and the achieved varus/valgus angle were computed, tabulated, and statistically assessed.

17.3.1 Laboratory results

The surgeons found that the two major pieces of software—the three-dimensional preoperative planner and image-based guidance system—provided an appropriately user-friendly interface. The modeling of preoperative and post-operative alignment gave the surgeon an unprecedented control and preview of the surgical procedure. The information provided by the image-based guidance system was very useful to the surgeon, in that the guide wires were easily installed by looking solely at the screen.

The mean, standard deviations, and total ranges of error are shown in Table 17.1. According to the classic F-test, the reductions in standard deviations and total ranges are significant to a 95% confidence level. Differences in the mean errors are not statistically significant, and in both sets the errors are essentially of zero mean.

There were no training effects observed in the trials, i.e. the errors were evenly distributed through time. The errors increased as the correction angle increased, which is not a surprising result. A particularly interesting observation was the formation of the osteotomy hinge when the surgeon operated with computer assistance. In every trial the hinge was between 1 mm and 3 mm in thickness. When the surgeon operated in the traditional way, with fluoroscopic guidance of the saw blade, the hinge could be non-existent (totally mobile fragments) or up to 5 mm in thickness.

Table 17.1 Summary of laboratory test results. Errors are the difference between the measured varus/valgus angle and the intended angle. The range is the difference between the largest and smallest error

	Wedge errors		
	Mean	Std. dev.	Range
Traditional	−0.4°	2.3°	8.4°
Computer-enhanced	0.1°	1.4°	3.7°

17.4 **A pilot clinical study of closing-wedge osteotomy**

Clinical tests involved sixteen patients, all having arthrosis confined to the medial compartment and otherwise meeting indications for high tibial osteotomy. For the first six patients, registration was accomplished with fiducial markers and guidance was performed with a mechanical localizer; for the next ten patients, registration was accomplished by robust estimation and guidance was performed with an optical localizer. The markers were implanted by an interventional radiologist, and two surgeons (authors MMH and JFR) operated. The study was approved by the Research Ethics Board of Kingston General Hospital, and the patients provided free informed consent prior to their participation.

For the first six patients, four markers were implanted and images were acquired at two to five working days prior to surgery; for the subsequent ten patients only CT scanning was required. Each patient was preoperatively instrumented with titanium-alloy markers 1.9 mm diameter, 3.5 mm length, which were the screws of soft-tissue anchors (Wright Medical). Local anesthesia was applied, and each marker was inserted percutaneously into the anterolateral aspect of the proximal tibia under fluoroscopic guidance. Instrumentation required approximately five minutes per marker, and each marker was tested for secure implantation by tugging on the suture of the screw prior to removing the suture. The small wounds were closed with Steri-strips. Each patient was then imaged with Roentgen stereogrammetric analysis (to validate the absolute accuracy of the intra-operative registration), with standardized radiographs (to establish the clinical axes in a weight-bearing stance), and with axial-mode computed tomography (to provide three-dimensional images of the anatomy and the markers).

Image preparation and preoperative planning were conducted in a manner similar to the methods used in the laboratory trials. For mechanical localization, the patient's lower affected leg was held in a specially constructed holder that could rigidly hold the leg in angles from full extension to over 90° flexion. To reduce tibial motion intra-operatively, the patient's calf was padded posteriorly, medially, and laterally with cloth towels and then clamped to the holder with Velcro-fastened straps. Marker identification was simple, and little preparation of the bone surface or surrounding soft tissues was required to expose the tiny markers. For optical localization, a dynamic reference body was attached to the tibia by means of external-fixation devices.

Intra-operative registration and drilling of the two guide wires required a maximum of 6 minutes, compared to a minimum of 12 minutes for typical fluoroscopically guided wire insertion. Resection, reduction, and fixation with step-staples were conducted in the traditional manner, and the markers were removed prior to closing the wound in layers. Typical operative time was 42 minutes ('skin to skin'). Figure 17.7 shows implantation of the first (proximal) guide wire.

Post-operative plain X-ray films were taken to assess the osteotomy and to ensure that the staples did not intrude into joint. These films were then measured by one of the surgeons (MMH) who was familiar with radiological assessment and who was unaware of the desired correction angle to be achieved. (The use of markers, even though they had been removed, left radiological clues to the use of computer-assisted technique.) The preoperative and post-operative tibial-plateau/tibial-shaft angles were calculated, and their differences were compared to the intended corrections that had been established using the preoperative planning system.

17.4.1 **Clinical results**

No infection arose from the marker implantation and the patients reported only minor discomfort from this procedure. In two of the six cases, one marker had loosened and only three were available for use in registration; in both cases the marker was found to have been secured into thick anterior

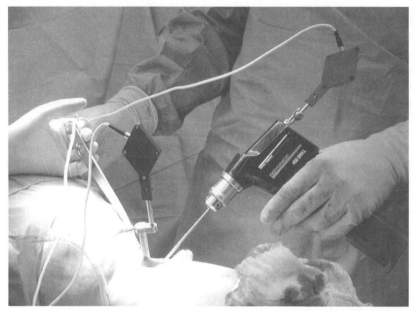

Fig. 17.7 Intra-operative guidance with optically tracked instruments. One optical target is attached to the tibia, and the other is attached to a battery-operated drill.

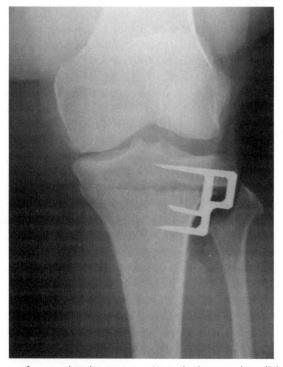

Fig. 17.8 Plain X-ray image of a completed osteotomy. Note the increased medial gap, due to more load being carried through the lateral compartment.

Table 17.2 Post-operative valgus error, in degrees, measured from frontal X-ray films

Patient number	Error (degrees)
1	+1
2	−4
3	+3
4	0
5	−2
6	−5
7	−1
8	+1
9	−3
10	−4
11	0
12	−4
13	+6
14	0
15	−6
16	0

Statistic	Value (degrees)
Mean	+1.0
Std.Dev.	3.3
Min	−6.0
Max	+6.0

periosteum rather than into cortical bone. Intra-operative motion of the tibia was negligible in the superior/inferior direction, and less than 1 mm in the medial/lateral and anterior/posterior directions. Because registration and drilling of K-wires were both performed with the tibia compressed from the lateral aspect, it is unlikely that significant tibial motion occurred.

For each patient, the intra-operative evaluation of the procedure was that the medial hinge was correctly placed and of the correct thickness. The resected bone surfaces were, in each case, visually smooth and flat. Technically each osteotomy was not only acceptable but was judged to be between very good and excellent. The post-operative radiographic examination in each case showed very good to excellent bone-surface contact and no fixation problems. Figure 17.8 shows a plain X-ray film of a reduced and stapled osteotomy, which has excellent mating of the cut surfaces.

Table 17.2 summarizes the results. Two of the sixteen patients had post-operative results that fell outside the expected ±4° error, but both reported noticeable decrease of pain and a return to normal activities of daily living.

17.5 Clinical observations of opening-wedge and barrel-vault osteotomies

We have performed a preliminary clinical trial on opening-wedge and barrel-vault osteotomies (three patients for each kind). The guidance is similar, in manner and time, to the guidance for closing-wedge osteotomy. We have also developed a method for intra-operatively monitoring the angular correction as the bone fragments are manipulated.

The monitoring is done with two optical tracker devices. In order to achieve a registration, we need to place an optical tracker placed on the tibia. After osteotomy, this tracker remains attached to one of the two tibial fragments; for the purposes of description, suppose it is on the proximal fragment. Prior to resection, we also guide a pin or screw into the tibia on a site that is distal to the planned osteotomy. After resection, a second optical tracker is reattached to the distal pin. The guidance system can then report the actual angular change between the fragments, and the surgeon can 'dial in' the desired correction angle. (This method can also be used with the closing-wedge technique, to ensure that the desired correction angle is actually achieved.)

17.6 **Discussion**

The major contribution of this work has been the development of software that supports preoperative planning of high tibial osteotomies in three dimensions, and accompanying software that guides the surgeon to achieve the desired result. Work by other investigators, even with the use of computers, described planning in only two dimensions and thus the three-dimensional consequences of the osteotomy were not correctly modeled.

If, as is common, the surgical plan for an opening-wedge or closing-wedge osteotomy is derived from only a frontal-plane film then there is an implicit assumption that the hinge axis is always perpendicular to the frontal plane. The intended kinematics of this plan will be reproduced in the patient only if this hinge is truly accomplished. Should the hinge actually be somewhat rotated—which can happen if too much medial cortex is removed—then an internal/external rotation of the foot is an inevitable consequence. Simple geometry of closing-wedge osteotomy, for example, shows that if the correction angle is 10° but the osteotomy hinge is oriented at 30° to the frontal axis (which can happen if only 10 mm of extra medial bone is removed) then an additional 5° of internal rotation of the foot occurs. Internal rotation is associated with increased adduction moments and with poorer pain relief over time.[24] It is thus possible that the inability of two-dimensional planning to control for all of the angulation variables and poor selection of the patient as meeting the indications have contributed to the reputation of high tibial osteotomy as unpredictable.

An important clinical advantage of the computer-assisted technique is the placement of the medial hinge for closing-wedge osteotomy. With simple measurements it is relatively easy to control the thickness of the lateral portion of the wedge, but it is much more difficult to place the apex of the wedge within a millimeter or two of the medial tibial cortex. Jig systems can control the wedge angle, but again the placement of the apex is difficult to ensure even with fluoroscopic imaging. Apex placement is important because small lateral misplacement of the position of the wedge apex can produce a relatively large overcorrection—the small medial changes are propagated across the width of the tibia. If the wedge apex is placed too far medially then medial soft tissues can be disrupted, decreasing the stability of the osteotomy during healing.

The laboratory results show that the angle of the removed lateral wedge can be controlled to be at least as good as the best jig system. Because the location of the medial cortical hinge can also be controlled, it is expected that computer-enhanced osteotomy will provide better outcomes than the current course of treatment offers. Use of the computer-assisted HTO system has clarified the importance of incorporating all three dimensions in the planning and execution of this type of osteotomy. In particular, the laboratory tests have revealed some pitfalls that arose from neglecting three-dimensional aspects of osteotomy techniques, and shown that the standard deviation of angular error can be half that of the traditional technique. This is consistent with conclusions drawn by other groups who have used computer-enhanced systems for orthopaedic surgery. (For further work, see the Symposium section of *Clinical Orthopaedics and Related Research*, volume 354, such as Delp *et al.*,[25] Merloz *et al.*[26] and Nolte *et al.*[27].)

The clinical results are promising: to date, the maximum radiologically measured error is smaller than the standard deviation of the best jig systems. One difficulty with the early clinical technique was the implantation of markers into the tibia. The mathematically robust method[28] for registration is much preferred because the patients do not require the minimally invasive prior procedure. We will continue to recruit patients into our study, and also will follow the progress of the cohort to determine the quality of bone union and retainment of alignment that result from the computer-enhanced technique.

A shortcoming of the traditional and our computer-enhanced techniques is that neither adequately controls the flexion/extension correction or the internal/external rotation. Flexion/extension can be controlled by use of additional wires, or by determining an additional control point on each resection plane for the initial phase of the saw cut. The computer-assisted technique can also be modified to provide the surgeon with real-time feedback of the foot rotation, so that a desired overall limb alignment can be achieved. This is not trivial to do with a single mechanical arm for location sensing, but is relatively straightforward if optoelectronic position sensors are employed. It may also be possible to track the saw and/or an osteotome so that the surgeon can gain greater control of the osteotomy in the posterior aspect of the tibia, which is not readily seen from an anterolateral surgical approach.

This initial attempt at three-dimensional osteotomy planning concentrated on the development of a three-dimensional environment with geometric simulations. Future work could include biomechanical simulation accounting for the ligaments and for predicted medial/lateral displacement of the joint by normal walking forces. The high tibial osteotomy is a particular use of the closing-wedge osteotomy and the current system could be adapted for application in other anatomical regions. The closing-wedge osteotomy is only one of many corrective orthopedic procedures that could benefit from computer-assisted planning and image-guided surgical techniques.

Acknowledgements

This work was supported in part by the Natural Sciences and Engineering Research Council of Canada and the Information Technology Research Centre of Ontario. We are grateful to Gordon Goodchild for his careful programming of the guidance system and his assistance in performing the studies. Patricia McAllister and Cameron McLeod coordinated the clinical studies, and Ms. McAllister also performed the post-operative radiographic measurements. Dr. Paul Fenton performed the marker implantation.

References

1 Keene JS, Monson DK, Roberts JM, Dyreby JR, Jr. Evaluation of patients for high tibial osteotomy. *Clin Orthop Rel Res* 1989;243:157–65.

2 Rudan JF, Simurda MA. High tibial osteotomy—a prospective clinical and roentgenographic review. *Clin orthop Rel Res* 1990;255:251–6.

3 Hagstedt B, Norman O, Olsson TH, Tjornstrand B. Technical accuracy in high tibial osteotomy for gonarthrosis. *Acta Orthop Scand* 1980;51(6):963–70.

4 Hofmann AA, Wyatt RWB, Beck SW. High tibial osteotomy. Use of an osteotomy jig, rigid fixation, and early motion versus conventional surgical technique and cast immobilization. *Clin Orthop Rela Res* 1991;271:212–17.

5 Knight, JL. A precision guide-pin technique for wedge and rotatory osteotomy of the femur and tibia. *Clin Orthop Rel Res* 1991;262:248–55.

6 Koshino T, Morii T, Wada J, Saito H, Ozawa N, Noyori K. High tibial osteotomy with fixation by a blade plate for medial compartment osteoarthritis of the knee. *Orthop Clin N Am* 1989;20(2):227–43.

7 Myrnerts R. Clinical results with the SAAB jig in high tibial osteotomy for medial gonarthrosis. *Acta Orthop Scand* 1980;51(3):565–7.

8 Odenbring S, Egund N, Lindstrand A. A guide instrument for high tibial osteotomy. *Acta Orthop Scand* 1989;60(4):449–51.

9 Paley D, Herzenberg JE. New concepts in high tibial osteotomy for medial compartment osteoarthritis. *Orthop Clin N Am* 1994;25(3):483–98.

10 Rudan JF, Simurda MA. Valgus high tibial osteotomy—a long-term follow-up study. *Clin Orthop Rel Res* 1991;268:157–60.

11 Jakob RB, Murphy SB. Tibial osteotomy for varus gonarthrosis: indication, planning and operative technique. *Instruct Course Lect* 1992;41:87–93.

12 Tsumura H, Himeno S, Kawai T. The computer simulation on the correcting osteotomy of osteoarthritis of the knee. *J Jap Orthop Assoc* 1984;58:565–6.

13 Coventry MB. Upper tibial osteotomy for osteoarthritis. *J Bone Joint Surg Am* 1985;67(7):1136–40.

14 Insall JN, Joseph MD, Msika C. High tibial osteotomy for varus gonarthrosis: a long term follow-up study. *J Bone Joint Surg Am* 1984;66(7):1040–8.

15 Chao EYS, Sim FH. Computer-aided preoperative planning in knee osteotomy. *Iowa Orthop J* 1995;15:4–18.

16 Chao EYS, Lynch JD, Vanderploeg MJ. Simulation and animation of musculoskeletal joint system. *J Biomech Eng* 1993;115(4B):562–8.

17 Hanssen AD, Chao EYS. *High tibial osteotomy, volume 2 of Knee surgery*. Baltimore: Williams and Wilkins, 1994:1121–34.

18 Coventry MB. Osteotomy about the knee for degenerative and rheumatoid arthritis. *J Bone Joint Surg Am* 1973;55(1):23–48.

19 Hart JC, Francis GK, Kauffman LH. Visualizing quaternion rotation. *ACM Trans Graphics* 1994;13(3):256–76.

20 Shoemake K. Animating rotation with quaternion curves. *Comput Graphics* 1985;19(3):245–54.

21 Shoemake K. Arcball: a user interface for specifying three-dimensional orientation using a mouse. *Proc Graphics Interf* 1992;151–6.

22 Grood ES, Suntay WJ. A joint coordinate system for the clinical description of three-dimensional motions: application to the knee. *ASME J Biomech Eng* 1983;105:136–44.

23 Ellis RE, Toksvig-Larsen S, Marcacci M. Use of a biocompatible fiducial marker in evaluating the accuracy of computed tomography image registration. *Invest Radio* 1996;31(10):658–67.

24 Wang J.-W, Kuo KN, Andriacchi TP, Galante JO. The influence of walking mechanics and time on the results of proximal tibial osteotomy. *J Bone Joint Surg* 1990;72-A(6):905–9.

25 Delp SL, Stuhlberg D, Davies B, Picard F, Leitner F. Computer assisted knee replacement. *Clin Orthop Rel Res* 1998;354:49–56.

26 Merloz P, Tonetti J, Pittet L, Coulomb M, Lavallee S, Sautot P. Pedicle screw placement using image guided techniques. *Clin Orthop Rel Res* 1998;354:39–48.

27 Nolte LP, Zamorano L, Visarius H, Berlemann U, Langlotz F, Arm E, Schartzenbach O. Clinical evaluation of a system for precision enhancement of spine surgery. *Clin Biomech* 1995;10(6):293–303.

28 Ma B, Ellis RE. Robust registration for computer-intergrated orthopedic surgery: Laboratory validation and clinical experience. *Med Image Anal* 2003;7(3)237–50.

Chapter 18

ACL reconstruction—preoperative model system

F. Picard, James E. Moody, Anthony M. DiGioia III, Vladimir Martinek, Freddie H. Fu, Michael J. Rytel, Constantinos Nikou, Richard LaBarca, and Branislav Jaramaz

18.1 Clinical challenges

Outcome following anterior cruciate ligament (ACL) reconstruction is highly dependent on surgical technique, specifically tunnel placement in the tibial and femur. Important in positioning the ACL graft, proper tunnel placement along with proper graft tension results in improved long-term outcome after the surgical procedure.[1,2] It also minimizes complications such as graft failure and diminished range of knee motion.[3,4]

Unfortunately, proper placement of tunnels remains difficult with current arthroscopic techniques. This was evidenced in prior study by great variability in tunnel placement even when performed by surgeons experienced in ACL reconstruction.[5] Despite being a common procedure, the rate of misplaced tunnels in ACL reconstruction may be as high as 40%.[6,7]

The aim of a computer assisted ACL system is to improve accuracy and limit the range of surgical variability. The reliability of techniques to position ACL grafts are limited by the inaccuracy inherent in the instrumentation. The main obstacle encountered by mechanical alignment systems is the inconsistency in determining the anatomical frame of articulation, which are used to establish the references for the graft alignment actually, but X-ray and fluoroscopic control it is still difficult to correctly locate these articular frames either preoperatively or intra-operatively,[8] and this serves to further reduce the reliability of the mechanical instrumentation.

18.2 System description

18.2.1 Classification

Several image guided ACL navigation systems are now either under development or in clinical use. Image guided navigation for ACL reconstruction relies on identical principles and we describe below their common concepts. According to the classification, these systems are Surgical Navigation Systems (SNS). There are preoperative-model systems using patient-specific data.

18.2.2 Important concepts

Image Guided Navigation Technologies for ACL is based on concepts already described in the previous section for others surgeries such as TKR or osteotomies:

- the first is building a preoperative model on which the surgeon can simulate the surgery such as ACL sizing or placement and even simulated range of motion.

- the second is to intra-operatively navigate in order to implement the preoperative planning during the surgical procedure.

18.3 **Validation and accuracy**

We report a randomized study we conducted to compare tunnel placement between the traditional arthroscopic technique using standard guide-pin tools and an image based, computer assisted surgical navigation device. Accuracy, a measure of placing the tunnel at a predetermined position was assessed. We then described material, methods and surgical procedure.

18.3.1 **Equipment and material requirements**

The following list summarizes the main requirements for the experiment.

- Two surgeons experienced in ACL reconstruction, with no previous exposure to computer assisted surgical navigation systems.

- 21 foam knee bones (Sawbones Inc., USA) per surgeon. These were custom knee models complete with meniscus, collateral ligaments and PCL. All knees were fully enclosed in a simulated capsule of light-impervious elastic fabric (Fig. 18.1).

- A traditional ACL tools set (Paramax™ ACL guide system, Linvatec, USA).

- Computer assisted navigation system (KneeNav™, CASurgica Inc., Pittsburgh, PA, USA) including trackers to be attached to the femur, tibia, and the Paramax™ cruciate guide assembly (guide pin) (Fig. 18.2).

- Traditional tools included guide-pin guide and drill (Fig. 18.3).

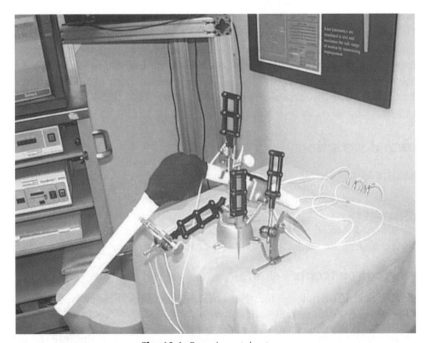

Fig. 18.1 Experimental set-up.

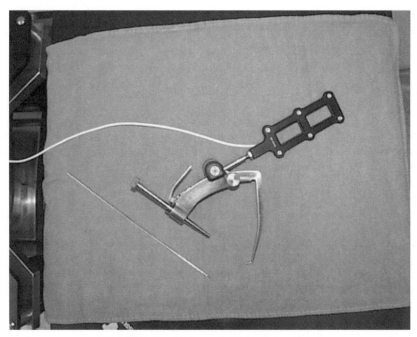

Fig. 18.2 Guide pin assembly with trackers.

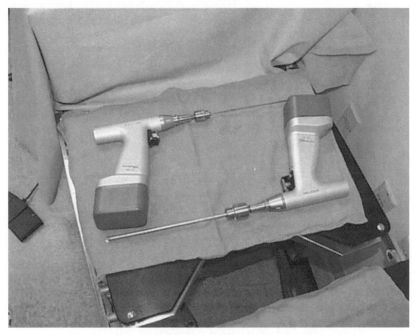

Fig. 18.3 Conventional drills.

- An arthroscopic station suitable for ACL reconstruction surgery included (1) a thirty degree arthroscope, (2) a camera, (3) central processing unit, (4) light cable, (5) monitor, and (6) a VCR to record all experimental data (Fig. 18.4).

18.3.2 Design and execution of the experiment

18.3.2.1 General

During the experiment, two surgeons independently prepared ACL tunnels on sets of sawbones knee models. Each surgeon used both traditional and computer-guided methods in attempting to place the femoral and tibial tunnels in a predetermined orientation and location. Post-operatively, the tunnel positions and orientations were measured via traditional planar radiographic and in three dimensions using computer measurement techniques.

Foam knee bones were used in the experiment since they were anatomically accurate, and (to within manufacturing tolerances) physically identical. Thus, meaningful results can be obtained by comparing follow-up measurements from all sawbones test specimens. Although not truly representative of an actual surgical environment, careful test site preparation and the use of sawbones knee models provided sufficiently realistic OR conditions for the purposes of this study.

18.3.2.2 Preparation

Several days before the experiment sessions, each surgeon was given a 'planning' sawbone knee model from which the simulated capsule was removed. On this model, the surgeon indicated the exact locations of the desired entry and exit holes for ACL tunnels. This reference knee then became, in

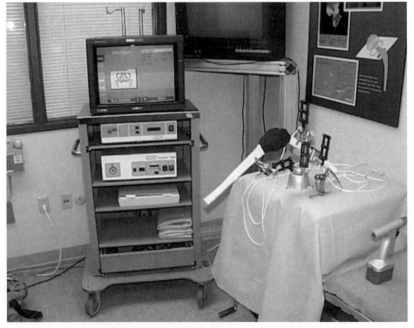

Fig. 18.4 Arthroscopic and computer stations.

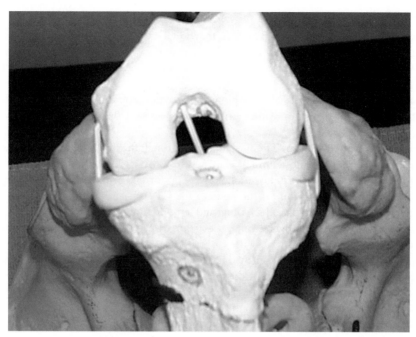

Fig. 18.5 Entry and exit holes for ACL tunnels.

effect, that surgeon's preoperative plan for the surgical experiment. The participating surgeons used their specific reference model throughout the experiment. This approach gave each surgeon the advantage of working within his personal reference.

Each 'planning' reference knee's tunnel locations were marked with radio-opaque fiducials (Fig. 18.5). The model was CT scanned using the following protocol: all slices were 1 mm thick; inter-slice density varies depending on the location in the model: 1 mm spacing was used in critical areas, e.g., areas used for registration and areas containing fiducials; 3 mm spacing was used in between high-density areas, and in other areas of anatomic interest; 10 mm spacing was used in all other areas (most proximal and most distal).

Three-dimensional surface models were generated from the CT images. These models were used intra-operatively to provide navigation as well as in the post-operative analysis for three-dimensional measurements of alignment accuracy.

18.3.2.3 Randomized procedure

The study was a randomized prospective parallel investigation comparing traditional and image guided navigation ACL reconstruction. Two groups of twenty identical knee models were selected. Each knee was numbered from 1 to 20 for the first surgeon and from 21 to 40 for the second surgeon. For each surgeon was given a set of 20 envelopes indicating whether the 'traditional technique' or 'navigation technique' was to be performed. The 20 envelopes for each surgeon were combined and thoroughly mixed, thus randomizing the subsequent selection order.

During the experimental sessions, the knee models were processed in numerical order. Once the model was set up, an envelope was selected and the indicated technique was used to perform the ACL tunnel placement on that model.

18.3.2.4 Surgical procedure

A single approach surgery was performed on each individual sawbone knee. Each model was placed in a natural posture and secured in a fixture designed to permit the surgeon to use their standard surgical approach. All the models have fully intact capsules so as to minimize any external visual cues for tunnel placement (Fig. 18.6).

In the traditional approach, the tibial guide pin was first arthroscopically positioned and drilled into the bone. Afterward, using a 10-mm reamer a tibia tunnel was over-drilled along the pin orientation (Fig. 18.7).

The second step consisted in fitting a femur guide-pin through the tibial tunnel. The pin was drilled through the femur in order to make a tunnel (Fig. 18.8).

For the navigation technique, the following steps were performed prior to the normal surgical flow: calibration of the guides, registration of the bone to the CT scan and verification. Then, using the calibrated guide-pin, the surgeon placed the tibial and femoral tunnels as above, with the assistance of the fully three-dimensional anatomy. Of note, the arthroscope was *not used* during the navigation assisted test (Fig. 18.9a).

Green dots were used on the three-dimensional images to mark the 'planned' ACL sites (surgical goal) and a red line was used to represent the guide-pin alignment (Fig. 18.9b, See Plate 4). Three different views of the knee were provided (tibial superior view, femoral inferior view and tibio-femoral sagittal view) and continuously displayed on the monitor. The surgeon could also select the view using a foot pedal control. The surgery then resumed in a traditional manner.

18.3.2.5 Evaluation protocol

Two assessment techniques were used for measuring the tunnel positions: a traditional radiographic method and a three-dimensional computer assistance measurement.

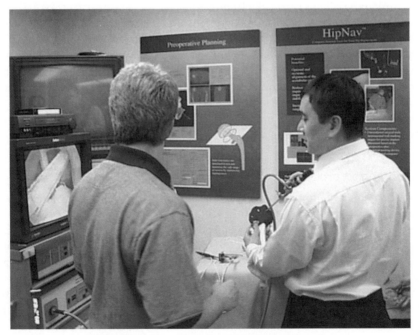

Fig. 18.6 Surgeon in action (Traditional surgery).

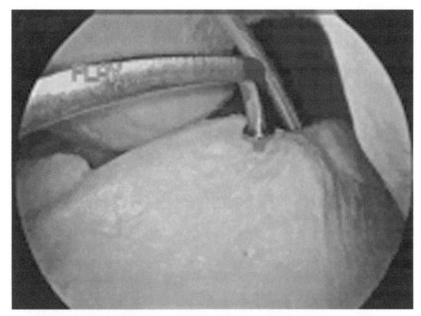

Fig. 18.7 Tibial guide pin orientation.

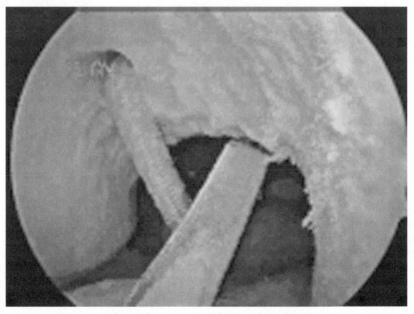

Fig. 18.8 Femoral guide pin orientation.

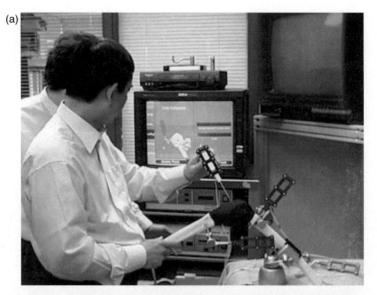

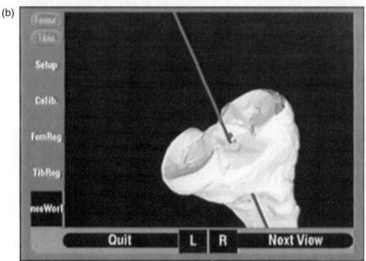

Fig. 18.9 (a) Surgeon in action (computer assisted). (b) Graphical interface.

18.3.2.5.1 X-ray assessment

The first assessment of alignment criterion was using the traditional radiological measurement of the femoral and tibial hole positioning. The following parameters were measured from X-rays for each of the foambone models: FSP = femoral hole sagittal positioning; FCP = femoral hole coronal positioning; TSP = tibial hole sagittal positioning; and TCP = tibial hole coronal positioning (Fig. 18.10).

Each model was filmed in the AP and lateral views (Figs 18.11, 18.12). Radiographic images were performed with Oralix 70 (Philips, Netherlands) using the following parameters: distance 36 inches (91.37 cm), 70 kV, 0.25 mA. Prior to radiography, the simulated soft tissue (including the whole capsule) was removed from the knee model in order to obtain separate tibia and femur images.

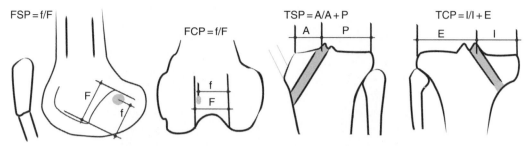

$FSP = f/F$ $FCP = f/F$ $TSP = A/A + P$ $TCP = I/I + E$

Fig. 18.10 Radiographic measurements.

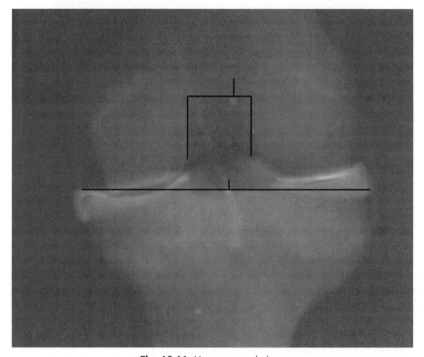

Fig. 18.11 X-ray coronal view.

A 10 mm tunnel obturator was placed in the tibial tunnels as a radiographic marker. This device enhanced contrast and facilitated the measurements of the tunnel positions. A single pin was secured in the femur at an isometric location. In order to standardize the X-ray measurements a casting was prepared to secure the identical sawbones models in exactly the same film orientation. The jig was composed of malleable urethane foam mounted to plywood (both essentially radiographically transparent). A reference sawbones tibia and femur were placed on the jig, positioned to perfect alignment, and pressed into the foam creating a unique 'footprint'. Subsequent test models were placed in the same footprint thereby providing identical alignment for all radiographs. Then, each bone was X-rayed in two planes (AP and lateral view).

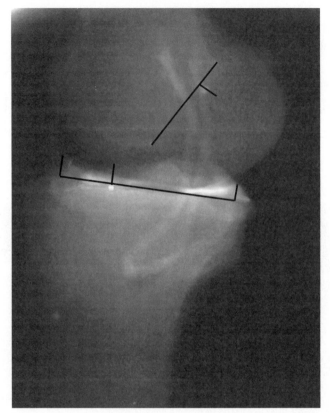

Fig. 18.12 X-ray sagittal view.

- *AP view.* the tibia and femur was placed in a flat position. The posterior femoral condyles and the posterior tibial condyles were in contact with undersurface and then aligned.
- *Lateral views.* The above technique was repeated to generate standardized lateral image of each model.

Two observers measured the X-rays.

18.3.2.5.2 Computer assisted assessment

In order to precisely measure the overall three-dimensional alignment of the tunnel each model was carefully reregistered and the final position of the femoral and tibial holes recorded. For the follow up measurements, the knee model was equipped with rigid bodies (one each for the tibia and femur) then registered in the normal fashion and registration was verified visually. A centering rod was inserted through the tibial tunnel so that each end of the rod could be easily accessed, as illustrated in Fig. 18.13. The ball probe tip was inserted into the distal detent, and the position was measured with respect to the tibia (Fig. 18.13a). The ball probe was moved to the proximal detent and a second measurement was recorded. For femoral alignment measurements, the ball probe was placed directly on each end of the femoral guide-pin tunnel (Fig. 18.13b). The points were collected with respect to the femoral tracker. The ball probe self-centered to the tunnel ends for most knee models. On models with oblique femoral

(a)　　　　　　　　　　　　　　　(b)

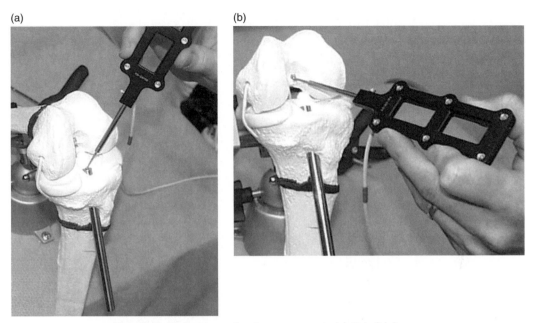

Fig. 18.13 Computer assisted measurements (a) tibia (b) femur.

tunnel care had to be taken to center the probe tip. Post processing software computed the intersection of the tunnel axes with the bone surface model.

18.3.3 **Results**

18.3.3.1 X-ray evaluation

There was no statistical differences between observer 1 and observer 2 for radiological measurements (Table 18.1).

But the sagittal tunnel alignment (TSP) for surgeon one, there was a trend that showed KneeNav™ to be more accurate than the traditional technique, no clear statistical differences were noticed between the two surgical techniques using planar radiographs as the basis for accuracy comparisons (Table 18.2).

18.3.3.2 Computer assisted measurement

Using the computer assisted system as a three-dimensional measurement tool, the 'surgical error' defined by the distance between the preoperatively marked ideal location and the surgically performed femoral and tibial holes. Surgical error was 3.1 mm (± 2.14 mm) for Group one (KneeNav™) and 4.6 mm (± 2.12 mm) for Group two (Scope) and was statistically different (Table 18.3) (Figs 18.14, 18.15).

The surgeons had no prior experience with KneeNav™ACL, yet after using it four times they reported being comfortable with it. Also, after this the tunnel placements tended to be more tightly clustered around the planned locations (Fig. 18.14).

Table 18.1 Comparison between the two observers

Tunnel position	Surgeon one				Surgeon two			
	Scope		KneeNav		Scope		KneeNav	
	Obs. 1	Obs. 2	Obs. 1	Obs. 2	Obs. 1	Obs. 2	Obs. 1	Obs. 2
FCP (%)	75.7 +/− 6.7	75.9 +/− 5.23	70.7 +/− 8.9	71.2 +/− 9.7	79.8 +/− 8.7	78.2 +/− 4.9	99.1 +/− 4.9	99.4 +/− 3.4
		p = 0.99		p = 0.52		p = 0.96		p = 0.90
FSP (%)	67.9 +/− 3.3	66.7 +/− 3.1	68 +/− 7.1	68.2 +/− 6.5	66.9 +/− 4.4	70.8 +/− 5.7	82.5 +/− 8.4	85.5 +/− 5.9
		p = 0.98		P = 0.98		p = 0.85		p = 0.91
TCP (%)	47.5 +/− 1.5	50 +/− 3.5	50.3 +/− 1.4	52.4 +/− 2.7	48 +/− 2	49 +/− 2.6	51.9 +/− 1.9	49.3 +/− 1.6
		p = 0.79		p = 0.74		p = 0.35		p = 0.84
TSP (%)	41.1 +/− 2	41.2 +/− 3.2	35.1 +/− 4.5	36.8 +/− 2	33.5 +/− 4.2	33.8 +/− 2.9	35.5 +/− 3	37.9 +/− 3.5
		p = 0.94		p = 0.64		p = 0.85		p = 0.91

FSP = Femoral hole sagittal position, FCP = Femoral hole frontal position, TSP = Tibial hole sagittal position, TCP = Tibial hole frontal position.

Table 18.2 Measurements of the bone tunnels positioning

Hole position	Surgeon #1		Surgeon #2	
	Scope	**KneeNav**	**Scope**	**KneeNav**
FCP (%)	75.7 +/− 6.7	70.7 +/− 8.9	79.8 +/− 8.7	99.1 +/− 4.9
	Goal = 70.1 (p = 0.08)		**Goal = 100** (p = 0.01)	
FSP (%)	67.9 +/− 3.3	68 +/− 7.1	66.9 +/− 4.4	82.5 +/− 8.4
	Goal = 72 (p = 0.94)		**Goal = 83.4** (p = 0.71)	
TCP (%)	47.5 +/− 1.5	50.3 +/− 1.4	48 +/− 2	51.9 +/− 1.9
	Goal = 52.2 (p = 0.98)		**Goal = 50.5** (p = 0.86)	
TSP (%)	41.1 +/− 2	35.1 +/− 4.5	33.5 +/− 4.2	35.5 +/− 3
	Goal = 39.1 (p = 0.02)		**Goal = 36** (p = 0.08)	

Table 18.3 Comparison between traditional and KneeNav techniques

Technique	Location	
	Femur	**Tibia**
Arthroscope		
Distances(mm)	4.2 +/− 1.8	4.9 +/− 2.3
TTest	p = 0.01	
KneeNav		
Distances(mm)	2.7 +/− 1.9	3.4 +/− 2.3
TTest	p = 0.04	

(a) 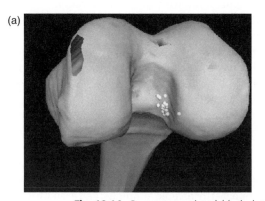 (b)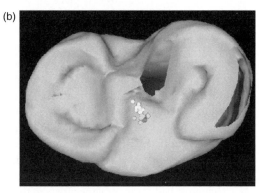

Fig. 18.14 Computer assisted (dark dots) vs Arthroscopic (light dots) surgeries.

18.4 **Discussion**

The computer assisted surgical navigation technique resulted in more accurate tunnel placements in the femur and tibia than the traditional arthroscopic technique. This surgical navigation system represents the second generation of computer-assisted surgical systems developed by the Center for Orthopaedic Research at UPMC Shadyside in collaboration with the Center for Medical Robotics and Computer Assisted Surgery (MRCAS) at Carnegie Mellon University. Building on principles and results obtained

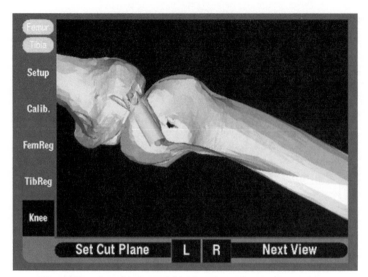

Fig. 18.15 Virtual ACL graft depicted on the monitor screen.

with the HipNav™ system [3], the KneeNav™ACL image guided system has been developed as a broad-based platform in order to improve many types of knee reconstruction surgery. The initial emphasis was on Anterior Cruciate Ligament Reconstruction (ACL-R).

This study demonstrated that traditional surgical tools could be easily adapted for use in with a computer assisted surgical navigation technique. It also demonstrated that image guided system enabled the surgeon to accurately place the tibial and femoral tunnels without visualization.

Each surgeon placed tunnels in accordance with a specific preoperative plan and they differed appreciably. The femur and tibial tunnel alignment targets were different between surgeon one and surgeon two. This occurred despite extensive prior study of proper tunnel placement for ACL reconstruction.[1,2] Prior study found similar variability in tunnel placement even when performed by surgeons experienced in ACL reconstruction.[5,9,10] This indicated the importance of allowing each surgeon to select individual, ideal tunnel placements and also suggested a requirement for any surgical navigation system to support customizable planning parameters.[8] Moreover, the surgeon must be given the option to verify and/or change his plan intra-operatively. Such capability is not currently available in robotic-based surgical systems.[11]

With radiographic assessment, there was not a undeniable statistically significant difference in tunnel placement between the two techniques. The initial conclusion might be that the KneeNav™ ACL technique had comparable accuracy to the traditional arthroscopic technique, and even worth for TSP parameter (surgeon one). But the computer navigation measurements demonstrated a difference in accuracy between the two techniques suggesting instead that the radiographic technique was inadequate in measurement of tunnel placement. This was also found in prior studies for ACL tunnel alignment assessment after ACL reconstruction as showed by Klos (Chapter 19), and also for total joint replacement.[12,13] A reason for this finding is that radiographic views are not able to establish the alignment in three dimensions.

It was also noted that the surgical system could provide navigation that could not be fully exploited due to limitations in the traditional instrumentation. For example, in our study the tracked tibial guide pin could be oriented such that the tibial tunnel, when over-reamed, would provide optimal access to the intercondylar notch for the subsequent femoral tunnel placement. However, this optimal orientation could not always be maintained during tibial guide pin drilling because the oblique angle between the ACL guide cannula and the tibia prevented a stable purchase of the guide. A lesser angle had to be used to ensure stable guide positioning during pin drilling. Thus, although traditional tools can easily be incorporated into computer assisted navigation systems, instrumentation may have to be redesigned before surgeons can take full advantage of a computer assisted system's capabilities. The second limitation of the computer assisted navigation system is the current image process. CT scan is certainly not the ideal medical imaging exam for ACL reconstruction because it is not routinely performed and, CTs provide poor cartilage and ligament visibility. Current work on 3D MRI reconstruction is expected to provide an accurate, safe, and traditional exam for CAS systems. A last limitation of the study was the use of foambone knees but identical bones were needed to provide a common baseline for follow-up comparison.

Studies using similar image guided technology (such Navitrack™, Sulzer) have been performed and will permit individual, ideal tunnel placements to be selected and trialed intra-operatively. Also a virtual ACL graft is created with a diameter that can be modified. Intra-operative determined cut planes would be defined so that the virtual ACL graft and anatomic structure such as the femoral notch can be depicted simultaneously. With passive range of knee motion the surgeon is able to change position of the virtual ACL graft if there is impingement or excessive graft lengthening (Figs 18.15, 18.16). Virtual ACL graft evaluation will be clinically evaluted in future experiments. No clinical report are available so far. This computer assisted procedure enables the surgeon to follow the traditional procedure using augmented assembly. A usual mechanical guide-pin equipped with a tracker enables the surgeon to visualize his own mark and the pin orientation. In KneeNav™ACL (CASurgica, Inc. Pittsburgh USA), four consecutive views can be displayed on the monitor screen by pressing the foot pedal control. Hence, the surgeon can verify interactively the tunnel orientations relative to the intra-operative planning before doing any drilling.

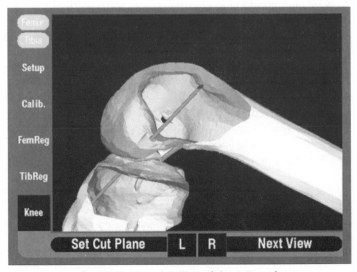

Fig. 18.16 Virtual drilling of the ACL graft.

In the described experiment, the surgeons were exposed to new technical concepts related to CAS systems. Tracking issues, tool calibration, model registration, and operation of the user-interface were quickly grasped and posed no problem in the execution of the experiment.[14] Computer assisted navigation systems will provide viable alternatives to current surgical tools. Regardless of the complexity of the underlying technology, a truly practical system must provide a simple and intuitive interface.

Acknowledgements

Chuck Cheetham from Linvatec Company, Bob Brown from Zimmer Randall Associate Inc. Company and Freddie Fu for additional support.

Patrick Mac Mahon (Department of Orthopaedic Surgery-University of Pittsburgh). The authors than his valuable assistance in the drafting of the document.

References

1 Frank CB, Jackson DW. The science of reconstruction of the anterior cruciate ligament. *J Bone Joint Surg* 1997;79-A:1556–76.

2 Fu FH, Bennett GH, Lattermann C, Benjamin C. Current trends in anterior ligament reconstruction: Part 1: biology and biomechanics of reconstruction. *Am. J. Sports Med.*, Nov-1999, 27:821–30.

3 Buzzi R, Zaccharotti G, Giron F, Aglietti P. The relationship between the intercondylar roof and the tibial plateau with the knee in extension: relevance for tibial tunnel placement in anterior cruciate ligament reconstruction. *Arthroscopy* 1999;15:625–31.

4 Yaru NC, Daniel DM, Penner D. The effect of tibial attachment site on graft impingement in an anterior cruciate ligament reconstruction. *Am J Sports Med* 1992;20:217–23.

5 Kohn D, Beusche T, Caris J. Drill hole position in endoscopic anterior cruciate ligament reconstruction. Results on an advanced arthroscopy course. *Knee Surg Sports Traumatol Arthrosc* 1998;6(Suppl. 1):S13–15.

6 Sati M, Bourquin Y, Stäubli H-U, Nolte L-P. Considering anatomic and funtional factors in ACL reconstruction: new technology. Pittsburgh, USA: CAOS, 2000:121–3, June 15–17.

7 Sati M, Staubli HU, Bourquin Y, *et al*. Clinical integration of computer-assisted technology for arthroscopic anterior cruciate ligament reconstruction. *Orthop Techn Orthop* 2000;10(1):40–9.

8 Klos TVS. Computer assisted anterior cruciate ligament reconstruction. Thesis Nijmegen, 2000. Cip Data Koninklijke Bibliotheek, 'S Gravenhage.

9 Dessenne V, Lavallee S, Julliard R, *et al*. Computer assisted knee anterior cruciate ligament reconstruction: first clinical tests. *J Image Guided Surg* 1995;1:59–64.

10 Julliard R, Lavallee S, Dessenne V. Computer assisted anterior cruciate ligament reconstruction of the anterior cruciate ligament. *Clin Orthop Relat Res* 1998;354:57–64.

11 Peterman J, Kober R, Heinze, *et al*. Computer assisted planning and robot assisted surgery in the reconstruction of the anterior cruciate ligament. *Orthop Techn Orthop* 2000;10(1):50–5.

12 Jiang CC, Insall JN. Effect of rotation on the axial alignment of the femur. *Clin Orthop Relat Res* 1989;248:50–6.

13 Stulberg SD, Picard F, Saragaglia D. Computer assisted total knee arthroplasty. *Orthop Techn Orthop* 2000;10(1):25–39.

14 Sati M, De Guise JA, Drouin G. Computer assisted knee surgery: diagnostics and planning of knee surgery. *Comput Aided Surg* 1997;2:108–23.

Chapter 19

Computer assistance in arthroscopic anterior cruciate ligament reconstruction

Tiburtius V.S. Klos, Raymon J.E. Habets, Anne Z. Banks, Scott A. Banks, Roger J.J. Devilee, and Frank F. Cook

19.1 Introduction

Anterior cruciate ligament reconstruction is the most frequently performed major orthopaedic procedure in the young adult population. Patients receiving a cruciate reconstruction at a mean age of 27 years will live an average of 50 to 60 more years. Thus, anterior cruciate ligament reconstruction should be considered a high precision procedure, requiring a durable reconstruction with excellent functional stability in an active and demanding population. Any improvements in the precision of graft placement will likely benefit patients.

Numerous different methods of graft placement are endorsed. Some authors[1-3] advocate isometric placement, as described by Sapega[4] on intra-operative isometry measurement. Recently, others have advocated more anatomic placement.[5-8] Anatomic reconstructions can be divided into two types: those based on the location of bony[9-11] or soft tissue[8] landmarks, and those based on measured parameters[12,13] derived from the intercondylar roof or soft tissue location. Most current anterior cruciate ligament instrumentation systems rely on intra-articular landmarks to guide tunnel placement.

The authors[14] reported studies characterizing parameters for graft placement using radiographic bony landmarks. The tibial attachment of the anterior cruciate ligament was found to have an average location of 46% ± 3% on a line extending from the anterior to posterior tibial cortices. For the femur, a consistent relationship was found between the intercondylar roof line (Blumensaat's line) and the nearly circular profile of the posterior and inferior contour of the lateral femoral condyle. In transepicondylar lateral radiographs, the center of this circular profile was located just beneath Blumensaat's line at 66% ± 5% of its anterior to posterior length, and the femoral insertion site was consistently found at 1/4 of the circle radius posterior to the center of the circle. These studies provide consistently identifiable radiographic features on the tibia and femur that can be used for fluoroscopic guidance of anterior cruciate ligament graft placement (Figs 19.1, 19.2).

The goal of the present study was to compare the variability of graft placement using conventional arthroscopic techniques with variability of graft placement in cruciate reconstructions performed with additional radiographic and computer graphic visualization. It was hypothesized that radiographic and computer guidance based on consistently identifiable radiographic landmarks could be used to improve the reproducibility of graft tunnel placement in arthroscopic anterior cruciate ligament reconstruction.

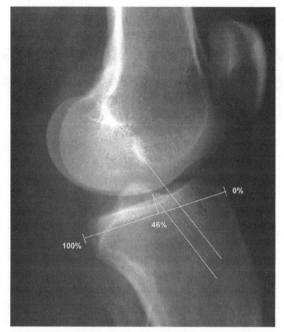

Fig. 19.1 Preoperative hyperextension lateral X-ray with radiographic parameters for graft positioning.

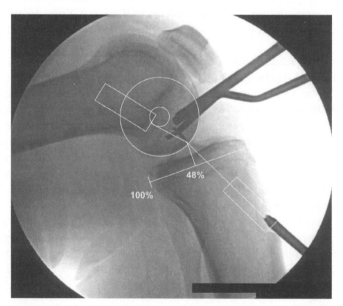

Fig. 19.2 Intra-operative overlay (computer) image with virtual graft placement and tibial guiding instrumentation.

19.2 **Materials and methods**

A consecutive series study was performed to evaluate anterior cruciate ligament graft placement variability with the use of contemporary arthroscopic instrumentation, arthroscopy with lateral fluoroscopic guidance, and arthroscopy with computer graphics enhanced lateral fluoroscopy (all using an endoscopic technique). One surgeon (TVSK) performed 29 cases of arthroscopic anterior cruciate ligament reconstruction between April 1994 and July 1995. Fifty-three patients were treated with arthroscopy and lateral fluoroscopy by the same surgeon between March 1995 and October 1996. Between October 1996 and September 1997, 50 patients were treated by two surgeons (TVSK and RJJD) with arthroscopy and computer enhanced fluoroscopy. Placement of tunnel guide wires was recorded with fluoroscopy in the last two groups and compared to graft placement in post-operative radiographs from the first group. Graft to tunnel placement was assessed using the methods of Staubli and Rausching[11] for the tibia and Harner *et al.*[15] for the femur.

During the procedure with computer assistance, fluoroscopic imaging is performed in the lateral plane. Optimal lateral positioning with overlapping condyles usually is acquired without any difficulty. The procedure is started with soft tissue removal, any required meniscal surgery, and harvesting of the patellar graft. A fluoroscopic image is taken after insertion of the tibial guiding instrumentation (Arthrex Inc., Naples, FL) to determine instrument and knee position. In this image, the tibial entry point and aiming position and the most anterior and posterior points on the tibial cortex are identified. The instrument and knee position are modeled with graphic overlays (Fig. 19.2) and can be tracked manually by the technician by moving the overlays with the mouse for each image.

Movements of the patient can be accommodated by repositioning the overlays with the mouse. Next, the system is calibrated using the size of the hook of the guide instrument. After the graft dimensions are entered into the program, the computer displays the position of the graft in relation to the

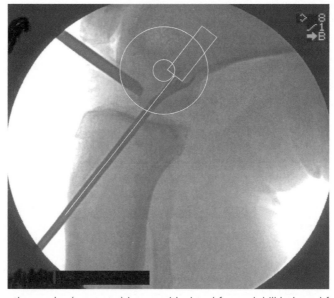

Fig. 19.3 Intra-operative overlay (computer) image with virtual femoral drill hole and femoral guiding instrumentation.

proposed entry point on the tibia (Fig. 19.2). When the tibial entry point is too shallow, the virtual placement will show the distal bone block to extrude from the tibia (graft to tunnel mismatch). By adequately adjusting the tibial entry point, graft to tunnel mismatch can be avoided.

The program predicts the placement of the femoral drill tunnel on a fluoroscopic image (Fig. 19.3) based on the position of the instrumentation. It is important to check the position of the tunnel and make certain no possible damage can occur to the posterior cortex. An intact posterior cortex is essential to provide sufficient tunnel strength for interference screw fixation. Finally, the graft is inserted and fixed with interference screws.

Software for this procedure was developed on a standard Intel Pentium computer (Intel Corporation, Santa Clara, CA) with Windows 95 (Microsoft Corporation, Redmond, WA) and a simple video capture board (Matrix Vision GmbH, Openweiler, Germany). The video capture board is used to acquire images directly from the video output of the fluoroscopic unit.

19.3 Results

Graft placement variability was significantly reduced when both fluoroscopy and computer assistance were used (Tables 19.1, 19.2). For the placement of the tibial portion of the graft, the standard deviation of the anterior/posterior graft location decreased from 6 to 4% with the use of fluoroscopy and to less than 3% with the addition of computer assistance.

Table 19.1 Radiographic measurement of drill hole placement tibia according to criteria by Staubli[11]

| | Tibia | | |
	A (%)	AF (%)	AFC (%)
Mean	45	46	46
Stand. Deviation	5.9	4.2	2.7
Minimum	37	38	38
Maximum	60	58	51
Range	23	20	13

A, arthroscopic (29 cases); AF, arthroscopic with fluoroscopy (53 cases); AFC, arthroscopic with fluoroscopy and computer assistance (50 cases).

Table 19.2 Radiographic measurement of drill hole placement femur according to criteria by Harner[15]

| | Femur | | |
	A (%)	AF (%)	AFC (%)
Mean	73	79	80
Stand. Deviation	9.0	5.1	2.8
Minimum	46	65	71
Maximum	90	89	86
Range	44	24	15

A, arthroscopic (29 cases); AF, arthroscopic with fluoroscopy (53 cases); AFC, arthroscopic with fluoroscopy and computer assistance (50 cases).

For the femoral graft placement, the standard deviation decreased from 9 to 5% with the introduction of fluoroscopy and to 3% with computer assistance. Statistical analysis (F-test) showed all differences between the three data sets to be significant ($p < 0.05$).

19.4 **Discussion**

Although many surgeons report satisfactory results with current anterior cruciate ligament reconstruction techniques, Kohn *et al.*[16] showed a high incidence of inaccurate graft placement in a group of 24 experienced anterior cruciate ligament specialists performing arthroscopic reconstruction on human anatomic specimen knees. Kohn *et al.* found inaccurate placement in 12 of 24 knees at the femoral site and in six of 24 knees at the tibial site. This provides convincing evidence that efforts should be made to reduce graft placement variability. The goal of this study was to evaluate the ability of enhanced intra-operative visualization to improve the repeatability of graft placement. Using proportional radiographic criteria for graft placement, it was found that both fluoroscopy and computer enhanced fluoroscopy significantly reduced graft placement variability.

Enhanced intra-operative visualization can reduce graft placement variability. However, the present study does not address the issue of optimal graft location. Many authors[1,3,5,6,8,11,15,17] have tried to define optimal points or areas for graft insertion, but there is currently no consensus. The computer system utilized for this study allows the surgeon (or technician) to input the desired graft position and allows the surgeon to use general radiographic, anatomical, or proportional criteria, or permits individual placement based on preoperative radiographs (Fig. 19.1). In this study, preoperative hyperextension radiographs were evaluated for the possibility of graft impingement. In all but two cases, no problems were recognized with the use of the our proportional parameters.

In addition to greater repeatability, the computer enhanced visualization permits accurate calculation of tunnel and graft lengths. In 42 out of 50 cases this permitted fixation of the tibial graft site with an interference screw, rather than a bone staple. Because painful staples often require removal, the use of intra-operative graft/tunnel length measurements (which permit intratibial attachment) may lower frequency of reinterventions.

The use of fluoroscopy has been a major concern to many surgeons. Some express concerns about radiation exposure; others fear the fluoroscopic equipment may obstruct the operation. Neither issue was problematic in this study. Goble[18] and Larson[19] have reported positively on the routine use of fluoroscopy and its limited radiation exposure, and an increasing number of training hospitals report using fluoroscopic feedback to monitor graft placement. Intra-operative images are superior for documenting graft location, eliminating the difficult task of identifying graft position from post-operative radiographs.[20] Increasing the accuracy of graft location assessment will facilitate outcome studies examining the relationships between graft location, function and longevity.[15,21]

The introduction of new technology to the operating room leads inevitably to concerns about higher costs and increased complexity. The radiographic equipment used for this study is readily available in most hospitals where arthroscopy is performed, and the computer system was based on inexpensive, off-the-shelf components. The visual nature of the task, and software designed for simplicity, make it easy for any operating room technician to learn (typical training time is less than 2 hours).

Arguments for increasing surgical repeatability and finding optimal graft locations intuitively are appealing and compelling. However, the scientific evidence does not yet support definitive relationships between outcomes and repeatability of positioning, or the superiority of one 'optimal' location versus another. Outcome studies which are already underway will certainly clarify these relationships. Regardless of these outcomes, however, the experience reported here clearly indicates that additional visualization techniques can significantly improve a surgeon's ability to place anterior cruciate ligament grafts in a desired location.

References

1 Hefzy MS, Grood ES, Noyes FR. Factors affecting the region of most isometric femoral attachments. Part II: the anterior cruciate ligament. *Am J Sports Med* 1989;17:208–16.

2 Hoogland T, Hillen B. Intra-articular reconstruction of the anterior cruciate ligament. An experimental study of length changes in different ligament reconstruction's. *Clin Orthop* 1984;185:197–202.

3 O'Brien WR. Isometric placement of anterior cruciate ligament substitutes. *Oper Techn Orthop* 1992; 2:49–54.

4 Sapega AA, Moyer RA, Schneck C, Komalahiranya N. Testing for isometry during reconstruction of the anterior cruciate ligament. *J Bone Joint Surg* 1990;72A:259–67.

5 Amis AA, Zavras TD. Isometricity and graft placement during anterior cruciate ligament reconstruction. *The Knee* 1995;2:5–17.

6 Barrett GR, Treacy SH. The effect of intraoperative isometric measurement on the outcome of anterior cruciate ligament reconstruction: a clinical analysis. *Arthroscopy* 1996;12:645–51.

7 Furia JP, Lintner DM, Saiz P, Kohl HW, Noble P. Isometry measurements in the knee with the anterior cruciate ligament intact, sectioned and reconstructed. *Am J Sports Med* 1997;25:346–52.

8 Morgan CD , Kalmam VR, Grawl DM. Isometry testing for anterior cruciate ligament for anterior cruciate ligament reconstruction revisited. *Arthroscopy* 1995;11:647–59.

9 Goble EM, Downey DJ, Wilcox TR. Positioning of the tibial tunnel for anterior cruciate ligament reconstruction. *Arthroscopy* 1995;11:688–95.

10 Miller MD, Olszewski AD. Posterior tibial tunnel placement to avoid anterior cruciate ligament graft impingement by the intercondylar roof. An in-vitro and in-vivo study. *Am J Sports Med* 1997;25:818–22.

11 Staubli HU, Rauschning W. Tibial attachment area of the anterior cruciate ligament in the extended knee position. *Knee Surg Sports Traumatol Arthrosc* 1994;2:138–46.

12 Howell SM, Barad SJ. Knee extension and its relationship to the slope of the intercondylar roof. Implications for positioning the tibial tunnel in anterior cruciate ligament reconstruction's. *Am J Sports Med* 1995;23:288–94.

13 Howell SM, Clark JA, Farley TE. A rationale for predicting anterior cruciate graft impingement by the intercondylar roof. A magnetic resonance imaging study. *Am J Sports Med* 1991;19:276–82.

14 Klos TVS, Barhs SA, Habets RJE, Cook FF. Sagittal plane imaging parameters for computer assisted fluoroscopic anterior cruciate ligament reconstruction. *Comp. Aided Surgery* 2000;5:28–34.

15 Harner CD, Marks PH, Fu FH, *et al*. Anterior cruciate ligament reconstruction: endoscopic versus two-incision technique. *Arthroscopy* 1994;10:502–12.

16 Kohn D, Busche T, Carls J. Drill hole position in endoscopic anterior cruciate reconstruction. Results of an advanced anthroscopy course. *Knee Surg Sports Traumatol Artheosc* 1998;6(Suppl. 1)S13–S15.

17 Fuss FK. Optimal replacement of the cruciate ligaments from the functional-anatomical point of view. *Acta Anat* 1991;140:260–8.

18 Goble EM. Fluoroarthroscopic allograft anterior cruciate reconstruction. *Tech Orthop* 1988;2:65–73.

19 Larson BJ, Egbert J, Goble EM. Radiation exposure during fluoroscopically assisted anterior cruciate ligament reconstruction. *Am J Sports Med* 1995;23:462–4.

20 Boden B, Migaud H, Gougeon F, Debroucker MJ, Duquennoy A. Effect of graft positioning on laxity after anterior cruciate ligament reconstruction. *Acta Orthop Belgica* 1996;62:2–7.

21 Khalfayan EE, Sharkey PF, Alexander AH, Bruckner JD. The relationship between tunnel placement and clinical results after anterior cruciate ligament reconstruction. *Am J Sports Med* 1996;24:335–41.

Chapter 20

CRA hip and knee reconstructive surgery: ligament reconstructions in the knee – intra-operative model system (non-image based)

Marwan Sati, Hans-U. Stäubli, Yvan Bourquin, Manvela Kunz, and Lutz-Peter Nolte

20.1 Introduction

Anterior Cruciate Ligament (ACL) rupture is a very common sports-related injury. Endoscopic or minimally invasive ACL reconstruction with an autogenous graft has become a standard due to the reduced trauma involved and the possibility to perform the procedure on an out-patient basis.

There was a recent consensus within the International Knee Society[1] that, according to state of the art knowledge on proper ACL placement, approximately 40% of ACL ligaments are currently being misplaced! An advanced arthroscopy course held by the society tested the misplacement rate of ligament placement in 24 cadaver knee following intensive instruction and practice on plastic model. When the knees were opened and evaluated according to the recent literature, only 4 of the 24 grafts were correctly placed, thus supporting the general misplacement rate finding. Through controlled cadaver studies we confirmed this large placement variation between surgeons using endoscopy alone.[2] These alarming findings expose a serious problem in the quality of a procedure that, if not performed correctly, can result in premature degeneration of knee structures that eventually requires total knee replacement.[3–6] This problem is particularly disturbing since ACL injury usually occurs in younger athletic individuals who would like to remain active.

Tunnel misplacements can partially be attributed to the restricted local endoscopic view that does not give the surgeon a global overview of ligament position with respect to the joint anatomy as seen in standard bi-planar X-rays. 30 degree endoscopes, lens distortions and the difficulty to judge depth from the two-dimensional (2D) view makes mental orientation of internal structures with respect to desired insertion even more challenging.

Surgeons often have the preoperative X-ray available on the light box during surgery to help make a mental picture for proper ligament placement, however no direct link exists to the intra-operative situation.

The limits of endoscopically identified landmarks for consistent ligament placement have lead some experienced surgeons to strongly advocate the use of fluoroscopy as a quantitative method to verify positioning intra-operatively.

In addition, there is no general consensus concerning the best graft choice and on the proper placement and tensioning of these grafts. As a result, there is a large variety of surgical techniques, graft types and fixation procedures.

To increase the challenge, many factors have been identified in the literature to be of importance for proper ligament placement:

(1) proper drill tunnel placement with respect to anatomical landmarks;[7–10]

(2) avoidance of impingement;[11]

(3) ensuring that elongation is not excessive;[12–17]

(4) proper graft tension and position to restore knee stability;[1,18]

(5) proper graft fixation in good-quality bone.[19,20]

20.1.1 State of the art in this field

There have been a few computer assisted surgery (CAS) systems proposed for ACL replacement over the past years to help solve some of the aforementioned problems. Previous work of the author involved the development of a noninvasive knee movement measurement system to help preoperatively plan prosthetic anterior cruciate ligament placement that minimizes bending and torsion loading.[21] Dessenne *et al.*[22] proposed the first intra-operative computer assisted ligament replacement system. They introduced the concept of a non-image-based system where the surgeon digitizes ligament attachment sites under endoscopic control. The system optoelectronically tracks and records movement of both femur and tibia in three-dimensional (3D) space and provides the surgeon ligament elongation data for different ligament insertions. Klos *et al.*[23] developed a system that creates a graphical template for planning of tunnel placement on preoperative X-ray images. During surgery an intra-operative fluoroscopic image is obtained and loaded to help plan ligament placement and bone block fixation. Clinical trials revealed that this technology statistically decreased variance in ligament placement.[23]

Anterior cruciate ligament replacement surgery is characterized by the large number of graft types, surgical techniques and philosophies. Present CAS systems are, however, each designed for specific surgical techniques and philosophies. We believe that there is a need for a computer-assisted knee ligament replacement system that can support both *functional* and *anatomical* placement criteria from the literature for a variety of graft types, surgical philosophies and surgical techniques and that does not require intra-operative imaging.

20.2 Proposed system

20.2.1 Factors to consider for proper ligament placement

The difficulties and limits of current endoscopic technology lead to common errors in the sagittal plane such as mistaking the characteristic ridge in the notch roof (residence ridge) to be the start of the posterior fossa resulting in far too anterior placement on the femur. Insertion too posterior on the femur due to the difficulty to judge this directly from endoscopy can result in the unfortunate situation of the tunnel exiting the posterior cortex which is termed *posterior wall blowout*. Another common error is too anterior placement on the tibia within the anterior aspect of the tibial footprint. Due to the oblique course of the ACL in the coronal and coronal oblique planes, correct medio-latera (M-L) ACL graft placement and orientation is of paramount importance.[24]

Besides anatomical considerations, there has been increased emphasis on functional considerations in ACL placement over the past few years.

Impingement can be difficult to avoid due to the restricted area available to the ACL graft: too anterior on the tibia hits the top of the intercondylar roof, too lateral on the tibia hits the side of the notch, too posterior on the tibia interferes with the PCL complex and insertion of the posterior horn of the lateral meniscus.[7,11] Variance between individual knee geometry can be very large. Intercondylar roof angle can vary for example from 22 to 64 degrees with an average of 38 degrees. ACL placement based on average knee geometry can easily lead to failure when geometric variations are extreme (notch hypoplasia, secondary notch stenosis).

Isometric ligament placement has been a controversial area.[12–17] The natural ligament is a complex structure in which a variety of fibers of varying elongation patterns can be identified.[25] At best, the graft can have only a few *isometric fibers* and one can only speak of an *area of minimal elongation*. Since planning is performed in an unstable knee, the use of abnormal kinematics for ligament placement is controversial. ACL-deficiency results in abnormal anterior subluxation of the tibia with respect to the femur, a factor that is not controllable under endoscopic visualization alone.

Considering these restrictions, placement must be a compromise that satisfies these criteria in the best possible manner according to the complex individual morphology.

20.3 Method

20.3.1 Preoperative planning with the CAS system

Standard preoperative X-rays are usually routine for ACL surgery since they warn of abnormalities in notch geometry such as steep notch roof, *guillotine osteophytes* or a particularly narrow notch. If preoperative X-rays are available, they can be prepared as *templates* for intra-operative guidance within the CAS system. X-rays should be taken in standard orientations, for example ML and AP (with the posterior condyles aligned), and contain a ruler with radio-opaque markings placed at the side of the knee. If available in numerical format, the X-ray is directly transferred to the computer, otherwise the radiographic film is scanned into the computer. The computer automatically detects radio-opaque ruler markings to determine image magnification. As in the system by Klos *et al.*,[23] desired ligament placement with respect to anatomical landmarks can be marked directly on this image through overlayed computer graphics.

Preoperative planning based on X-ray geometry is, however, limited since cartilage geometry is not visible in the radiographic and fluoroscopic image and plays a significant role in impingement.[24] Furthermore, notchplasty is often performed especially in knees having guillotine osteophytes or a particularly narrow notch. The preop plan is therefore only taken as a starting point and factors such as cartilage geometry and post-notchplasty geometry are considered within the intra-operative steps of the system.

20.3.2 Intra-operative use of CAS system

Tracking of both patient and surgical instruments is performed by an optoelectronic navigation system (Optotrak 3020, Northern Digital, CAN.) as in[22] that tracks an active infrared marker position with an accuracy of 0.1–0.3 mm. Two rigid shields that act as *dynamic reference bases* (Fig. 20.1), each containing four optoelectronic markers for tracking of the femur and tibia, are sterilized. During surgery they are attached to the femur and tibia with a specially-designed minimal-invasive two K-wire fixation device (Fig. 20.1, bottom). One is attached to the antero-lateral aspect of the femur through a mid-lateral approach, under the vastus lateralis. A small incision is made along the fibers of the ilio-tibial tract and the vastus lateralis mobilized from the intermuscular septum. Through this access, the K-wires are attached to the lateral femoral metaphysis as distal as possible without interfering with the femoral tunnel. The other reference base is attached onto the anterior aspect of the tibia, below the tibia tubercle (one hand distal to the joint line). Care must be taken so that it does not interfere with the tibial insertion tunnel or the drilling action and that the tracking shield is oriented such that it faces the tracking camera throughout knee flexion since these shields serve as reference bases to track the articulation's movement (six degrees of freedom).

Tools include a drill (or drill guide) tracked by a four-marker shield and a specially designed computer-integrated endoscopic palpation hook (Stille hook) equipped with 12 optoelectronic markers (Fig. 20.1). After sterilization, these devices are placed onto a calibration point to define the coordinates of their tip with respect to their tracking shields. Coordinates of the axis of the drill and palpation hook are *precalibrated* and assumed to remain constant. The large number of markers tracking the hook allows digitization of anatomic points for a variety of orientations. Like a previous CAS knee system,[3] potential ligament attachment sites can be directly digitized using this palpation hook in a minimally invasive fashion under direct visual endoscopic control. Unlike this previous technology, the proposed novel system allows surgeons to define freely and interactively the anatomical landmarks they require for proper ligament placement by using points, lines or surfaces to represent these reference structures. To digitize landmarks, the user selects the desired landmark from the menu and presses on a footswitch to register

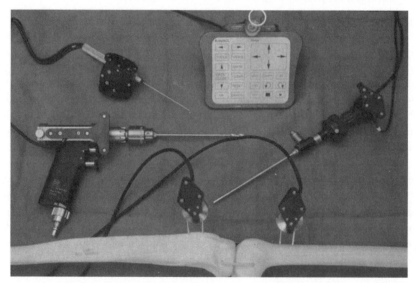

Fig. 20.1 Computer-guided tools for ACL surgery. Both tool and patient position are tracked by optoelectronic markers mounted on rigid shields that provide relative tool-bone positioning to the computer. From left to right, top to bottom: the palpation hook, the virtual keyboard, drill, endoscope, femoral and tibial dynamic reference bases. The reference shields are attached to the bone in a minimally invasive fashion with two K-wires each. The virtual keyboard is a sterile interface that is used to control the computer program using the palpation hook or drill tip.

points on that landmark. The digitizing point of the hook is at its very nose tip that should be placed directly on the desired landmarks. The hook can be use to digitize structures under direct visual endoscopic control or by palpation, when the tip is not in sight and the surgeon is sure to *feel* the right structure (for example the points within the posterior fossa of the knee).

20.3.3 Landmarks

One of the most important structures to consider for proper graft placement is the intercondylar notch on the femur because it determines the *available space* for both ACL and PCL. Particularly important is the roof of the notch and its lateral wall where *impingement* between ligament and notch is most likely to occur with the knee in extension. Impingement of the ligament with its surrounding structures limits the knee's range of motion and can cause premature ligament rupture. The position of the PCL defines the posterior limit of the graft placement. The central vertical part of the PCL and the anterior meniscofemoral ligament (Humphrey) are also important space constraining limits for the ACL-graft.

To digitize notch geometry, the user simply runs the tip of the tracked palpation hook over the notch surface under endoscopic control while pressing on the footswitch (Fig. 20.2a, b). The cloud of points generated from this action is organized into a surface via a custom made algorithm. Surgeons are free to define the area where they judge a potential impingement may take place (Figs 20.2b, 20.3). It is possible to depress and lift the footswitch to acquire points individually or to hold down the footswitch to rapidly digitize points in a *continuous acquisition* mode.

The roof of the intercondylar notch is a familiar sagittal X-ray landmark for ligament placement and is often referred to as the *Blumensaat line*. This landmark can be digitized intra-operatively under endoscopic control via a line that is drawn by pulling the Stille hook from the posterior fossa, up along the central top of the roof and finally over to the trochlear groove. This landmark is defined as the intercondylar roof (ICR) line (Fig. 20.2c).

Besides these suggested landmarks, the system allows surgeons to define any other landmarks they judge important for ligament placement. Some possible landmarks include the long axes of the femur and tibia to determine knee flexion angle more precisely. Some surgeons additionally digitize the posterior condyles and epicondylar axes of femur and tibia and the anterior tibia to gain a better spatial perception of joint geometry and orientation.

20.3.4 Anatomical surface generation from a cloud of points

Reconstruction of anatomical surfaces from intra-operatively digitized points required development of a specialized algorithm. Since the system was meant for general use, this technically required constructing an order surface from an arbitrarily distributed point cloud, which was a nontrivial problem.

The nature of this problem has its particularities compared to most surface reconstruction problems addressed in the literature. Previous work has mostly focused on determination of the surface of an object from a CT data set. The present problem is characterized by a small number of points and there are also no 'hints' to the location of the bone's interior, unlike with CT-based data where gray values give this additional information. Nonconvex surface generation gives strict speed constraints since the surgeon requires *real-time feedback* of the surface being digitized to know where subsequent points should be placed to form a meaningful structure. A surface is nonconvex if a line of the surface connecting two points in the cloud does not intersect with the rest of the surface.

Since the algorithm should not be dependent on *a priori* knowledge of the surface to be reconstructed, some preprocessing is performed using local information to organize the point cloud.

(a)

(b)

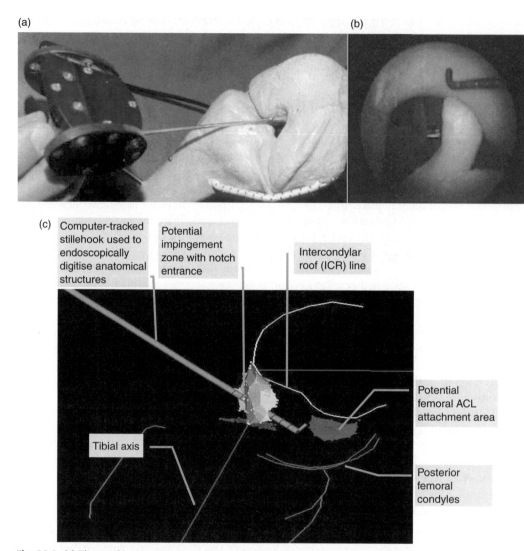

(c)

Computer-tracked stillehook used to endoscopically digitise anatomical structures

Potential impingement zone with notch entrance

Intercondylar roof (ICR) line

Potential femoral ACL attachment area

Tibial axis

Posterior femoral condyles

Fig. 20.2 (a) The tracking system records the relative position between the palpation hook and moving bones in real-time. (b) The surgeon can control the hook position under direct visual endoscopic control or by *feeling* with the hook when structures cannot be directly visualized. (c) The surgeon can define landmarks as color-coded points, lines or surfaces and can use these structures for digitizing potential ligament insertion sites for planning. The landmarks are shown from a lateral view. In this view one can see the ICR line that is equivalent to the familiar radiographic landmark called the Blumensaat line.

20.3.4.1 Local surface generation

Each point is first associated with a local tangent plane, defined by its surrounding points termed its *neighborhood*. We have empirically determined that best results are achieved when the number of points in each local neighborhood is approximately 6% of the total number of digitized points. The local surface is determined through linear regression.[26]

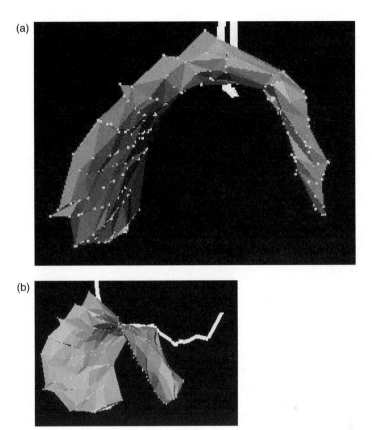

Fig. 20.3 (a) The digitized potential impingement surface of the intercondylar notch from a 'notch view' and (b) the intercondylar roof line (ICR) line (white) from an anterolateral view.

20.3.4.2 Surface orientation

The orientation of the local surfaces had to be processed to make them consistent (i.e. such that all adjacent planes were oriented in similar directions and not *flipped* with respect to one another), since the linear regression algorithm generated ambiguous plane orientation. This was done through a sequential *flipping* of the local surface normals until all adjacent normals were consistently oriented. The traversal path is important since propagation of this process through the data set can result in some vectors being flipped up then down, depending on the traversal path. Forming a so-called *Reimannian graph* ensures a proper propagation order.

Each digitized point is considered to be a node in the graph and nodes are connected to each of their neighborhood *nodes* (see definition above) by an edge. To each edge an associated *cost* is determined by

$$1 - |\mathbf{n}_j \cdot \mathbf{n}_i|$$

where $\mathbf{n}_j$ and $\mathbf{n}_i$ are the normal vectors of the tangent planes of each node point.

The cost of an edge is small if neighboring planes are nearly parallel. The starting point for the flipping sequence is taken arbitrarily as the point P_s having the smallest Z-coordinate. Starting at P_s, the neighboring node P_1 connected by the smallest cost edge is first considered. If the orientation between these two planes is different, then the plane is flipped to correspond to the orientation of the plane associated with P_s. The same process is repeated from node P_1 and so on throughout the whole point cloud. The graph traversal order is called the *minimal spanning tree*. This stage is the most time consuming of the whole surface reconstruction procedure.

20.3.4.3 Distance map

Consistent local normal orientation allows calculation of a distance map. For any point P in space, the distance map value of that point is calculated as the smallest distance to the nearest plane. The distance $d(P)$ from a point to each plane is calculated as:

$$d(P) = \mathbf{n} \cdot (\mathbf{P} - \mathbf{R}_1)$$

where $\mathbf{n}$ is the normal vector of the plane and $\mathbf{R}_1$ the center point of the plane.

20.3.4.4 Triangulation

Triangulation is performed using a modified *marching cubes* algorithm.[27] The traditional marching cubes algorithm forms the apex of a triangle if one cube corner lies on one side of the surface and another cube corner lies on the other side of the surface. Used directly on CT data, this algorithm uses the gray values of the cube corners to better determine the triangle's apex along each edge of the cube. Since no CT of the patient exists for *surgeon-defined anatomy*, we use the distance map to provide similar information. The distance map calculation gives information on whether a point of the cube is inside or outside of the surface plus the distance of that point to the nearest local surface. This distance information is used to help better determine the apex points of the each triangle. Note that the result of the marching cubes is an approximate surface that does not pass through the digitized points.

20.3.4.5 Surface point reduction

For surgery it is important that the surface is exact, i.e. that it passes through the digitized data points as much as possible. Since marching cubes typically generates a very large number of triangles, it is also desirable to reduce the number of triangles to increase rendering speed for real-time display.

Every marching cube triangulated triangle apex is merged with the nearest neighboring original data point. This has the effect of reducing the number of triangles and forcing the surface through the digitized data points.

For overall improvement of intra-operative use, the surface reconstruction algorithm is not called during continuous point acquisition (i.e. with the footswitch held down). This allows rapid acquisition of many points since there is no CPU overhead from the time consuming surface reconstruction. Once the footswitch is released, the algorithm recalculates the surface including the newly acquired points.

20.3.5 Template views

If a preoperative (preop) X-ray was available, it is used to create a personalized *template view* of the anatomy. In this view, the magnification of the landmarks is made to correspond to that of the preop

X-ray. The computer provides an approximate alignment of the digitized landmarks overlaid onto the preop X-ray (Fig. 20.4). The sterile interface can then be used to fine-tune the 2D/3D alignment through rotation and translation control. Once aligned, the surgeon navigates tool position on the preoperative X-ray template that can contain the preoperatively planned ligament placement. This template contains the preoperatively planned ligament placement based on radiographic landmarks representing bone morphology (Fig. 20.4).

20.3.6 Views

Standard views (ML, AP, notch) of the landmarks are set automatically by the system when the anatomical axes have been defined. Landmarks are often only of significance when seen from a standard viewpoint. For example, the intercondylar roof line (ICR) can be recognized as the familiar 'Blumensaat line' only in the medio-lateral view of the joint (Figs 20.2c, 20.4). Many surgeons use the extension of this line over the posterior cortex as an anatomical reference for ligament placement.

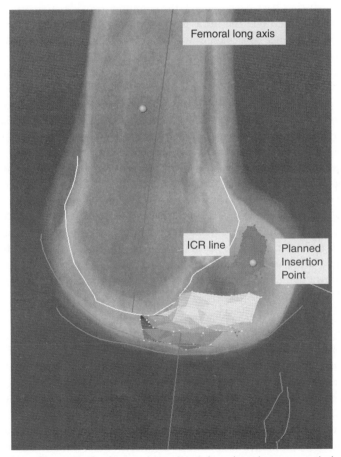

Fig. 20.4 Template view of knee. The background template is based on the preoperatively scanned standard X-ray. Digitized landmarks are aligned with their corresponding X-ray landmarks: the ICR and femoral axis.

20.3.7 **Interactive system use for ligament positioning**

Surgeons usually have a rough idea of intended graft attachment area that they can endoscopically identify. The system allows the surgeon to digitize an *area of potential attachment* under endoscopic control.[22] A surface is generated from this cloud of points using the same algorithm as for the notch entrance geometry. Unlike the notch representation, the coordinates of these points are recorded for later analysis of ligament elongation for different insertions. The potential attachment area on the tibia is also identified in the same manner.

The system then allows the surgeon to provide a first guess of the ligament attachment position. Ligament position can be defined by direct digitization of the internal attachment points within the knee allowing simulation of the intra-articular portion of the graft. These attachment points can be directly identified with the computer integrated palpation hook in a variety of ways: (1) directly under endoscopic control (Fig. 20.2b); (2) as preoperatively planned with respect to landmarks on X-ray template views (Fig. 20.4); or (3) on one of the *standard* views with respect to the digitized landmarks (Fig. 20.2c).

Once the attachment sites have been defined, the computer provides a virtual 3D representation of the planned ligament insertion. The intra-articular portion of the graft that spans the internal attachment points is represented as a cylinder with a variable length as determined by relative femur and tibia positions in space (Fig. 20.5a).

Drill tunnel orientation can be planned by directly digitizing an external point along the planned drill tunnel using the palpation hook. The femoral and tibial drill tunnels are each represented by a cylinder that has a different color than the intra-articular portion of the virtual graft. These virtual tunnels maintain a constant position with respect to their associated bone (Fig. 20.5a).

Impingement of the *planned* ligament placement can be predicted by the 3D location of the virtually planned ligament with respect to the digitized notch entrance surface geometry during knee flexion. Impingement can be best observed with the knee in extension from a femoral lateral view (Fig. 20.5b, left) or a view looking down the notch (Fig. 20.5b, right). Impingement is visualized by the graphical intersection of the virtually planned ligament with the intra-operatively-digitized notch surface as the knee is brought into full extension. The graphical overlap indicates that if the ligament were placed in this location, there would be impingement in extension, likely causing and extension deficit or premature graft wear. The diameter of the simulated ligament must be set to be equivalent to the harvested graft width during this analysis since ligament diameter has a significant effect on impingement. Ligament diameter is easily modified in the program during surgery after the graft has been prepared and its diameter known.

20.3.8 **Drilling**

Drilling of the planned tunnels can be performed using either a computer-tracked drill or computer-tracked drill guide. The computer-tracked drill or drill guide is represented by a graphical object with a line representing the axis, a cross at the drill tip and a circle at the tail of the drill. In the drilling mode, one can chose a view along either the planned femoral or planned tibial insertion tunnel.

Drill alignment with the planned *virtual* tunnels is performed in two steps: (a) the tip of the drill (cross) is first guided towards the center of the tunnel (in the tunnel view) and a small hole drilled in the bone to mark the entry point (Fig. 20.7a); (b) drill orientation is then adjusted until the tail of the drill (circle) is aligned over the tip (Fig. 20.7b). Because of some reluctance from the surgeons to use a drill directly, computer tracked Kirschner wire (K-wire) guides were developed.

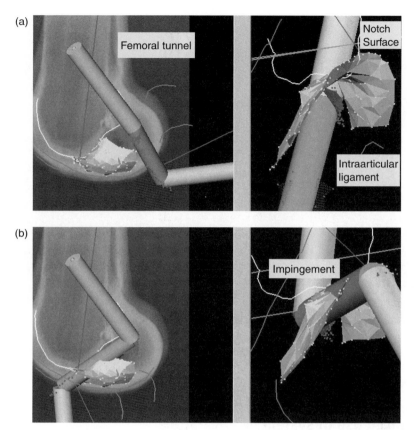

Fig. 20.5 Anatomical ligament position can be planned with respect to the digitized landmarks or the X-ray template. (a) Simulated 8 mm ligament with knee in flexion. X-ray overlay view (left) and view through the *notch* (right). (b) With knee in extension, impingement of the planned ligament with the notch roof can be seen graphically in the sagittal view (left) or even more clearly in the *notch view* (right) since the planned ligament graphically intersects with the digitized notch.

The system can also be used to assist in the placement of a graft using the one tunnel techniques as seen in Fig. 20.8. Computer tracked guides having an intra-articular targeting arm have been developed to place K-wires into the planned tunnel location. The target arm typically has a sharp point that can be computer-guided then fixed into position within the knee by pushing the tip into the remains of the ACL stump (this feature is similar to current mechanical K-wire guides). This point is registered by the computer to be the attachment point of the ligament and the resulting virtual ligament is represented for that position. With the internal point of the arm still in place, knee flexion can be performed to analyze ligament impingement and elongation change. If the internal point is chosen to be at an appropriate location, tunnel orientation can be modified while keeping the internal point in place. We have also developed and 'armless' K-wire guide that is computer-guided to the planned target point. A study on plastic and cadaver has been performed to determine the accuracy of this device.[28]

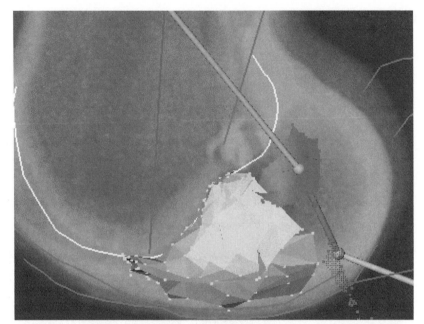

Fig. 20.6 The system can provide the surgeon with feedback on ligament elongation if a ***ligament attachment area*** has been defined. The ***red*** zone on the femoral attachment area indicates a region of insertion where elongation exceeds 3 mm. The meaning of these elongation values is, however, controversial. See Plate 4.

20.4 **Advanced use of system**

20.4.1 **Elongation analysis**

With the *virtual ligament* in place, the system can help to analyze graft elongation during a given knee flexion.[22] Ligament elongation is defined by the maximal length change of the middle most fiber of the virtual graft over a prescribed knee movement. This information is represented as a color map on the potential attachment areas of the femur and tibia (Fig. 20.6). For a given tibial attachment position and knee movement, the elongation for several femoral attachment points over the potential attachment area are calculated. Attachment points that would give elongation over 3 mm are colored red since grafts are known to undergo partial rupture when stretched more than 10% (total intra-articular graft length is usually approximately 30 mm). Attachment sites that would result in 2–3 mm elongation are colored yellow and elongation below 1 mm in green. This is particularly useful for those interested in finding *isometric* attachment location (see Figure 20.6).

The meaning of ligament elongation in the unstable knee is, however, controversial and unclear. It is for this reason that we do not recommend use of this functionality for the planning of ligament insertions.

20.4.2 **Planning in the unstable knee**

The ACL-deficient knee is often characterized by an anteriorly-displaced tibia with respect to the femur. For this reason, the surgeon may choose to plan ligament placement based on an X-ray image of the *contralateral knee.*

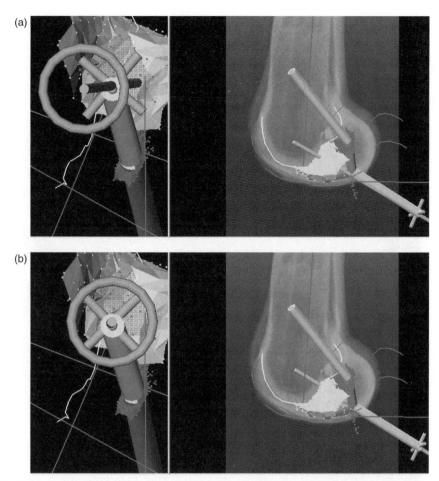

Fig. 20.7 The system provides the surgeon with real-time guidance of drill movement with respect to the *drill tunnel view* (left) which is a direct view down the selected drill tunnel axis and the *sagittal X-ray view* (right). The drill is represented by a graphical line for the drill axis, a cross at the drill tip, and a circle for the tail of the drill. (a) The first step in drill alignment is to align the center of the cross with the tunnel entry point and drill a small insertion indent. (b) Drill orientation is then adjusted until the circle is aligned directly over the cross tip in the *drill tunnel view* (left). An extended drill trajectory line gives additional information on possible femoral tunnel entry points for a one-tunnel technique.

Relative femoral and tibial posterior condyle position is very important for determining a reference *reduced position* for the planning of ligament placement since there is typically an anterior displacement of the tibia with respect to the femur in an ACL-ruptured knee. *Zero* anatomical compartment alignment is defined when tangents running parallel to the posterior cortex of the tibia and tangents to the subchondral contour of the posterior femoral condyles coincide.[29]

20.4.3 Tensioning

Since it has been shown that ligament tensioning is *tissue-dependant*,[30] the system is used to help evaluate this factor *in situ*. Although proper tibial positioning avoids knee extension limit, excessive ligament

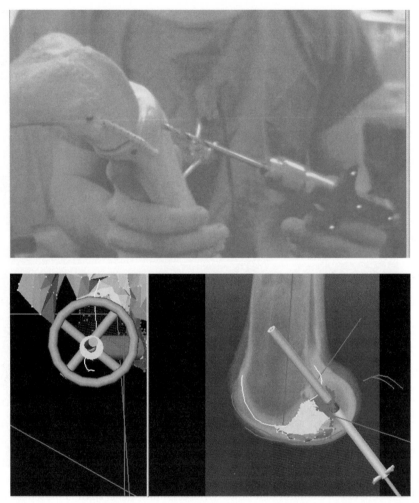

Fig. 20.8 Use of the system to help plan a one tunnel insertion is possible by manipulating both drill and knee joint until the virtual drill trajectory passes through the desired tibial and femoral insertion areas.

tensioning can result in an extension limit or flexion limit depending if the femoral attachment has been placed too posteriorly or too anteriorly respectively.[31] Too little tensioning will result in insufficient knee stability.[32] The computer can help support evaluation of proper tensioning by providing feedback on precise knee flexion angle and A-P laxity of the joint.

20.4.4 Custom views

Besides the standard views that are set automatically, the system also allows the surgeon to define custom viewpoints of the digitized landmarks. The view is aligned through interactive use of the palpation hook by physically aligning the long axis of the palpation hook in the desired view orientation with respect to the patient. The footswitch is depressed and the system provides real-time feedback of the current view. The footswitch is released when the desired view has been obtained.

To help the surgeon's orientation within the endoscopic view, a computer overlay of digitized land-marks onto the video image is optionally provided. The endoscope is equipped with an optoelectronic tracking shield and its projection parameters determined within this reference frame by a calibration procedure.[33] This provides a *one to one* correspondence between the endoscopic view and the computer view that helps the surgeon better locate structures and navigate even when soft tissue obstructs the direct sight of landmarks.

20.4.5 Bone block fixation

The system can help to decide the depth at which to fix the bone blocks into the tunnels. In the case of ligament replacement with a bone patellar bone graft, care must also be taken not to fix one of the blocks such that the other is no longer in the proper region of the tunnel. The total length of the graft and the location of the bone cortex determine the optimal tunnel fixation position. Since the system can give the intra-articular length of the graft, knowing total graft length allows calculation of the depth of the bone blocks.[23]

20.4.6 Documentation

The software has been designed to allow recording of (1) femoral and tibial landmarks, (2) ligament insertions, and (3) knee kinematics. Several knee movements can be recorded including pre- and post-graft insertion kinematics. After surgery, the system can play back the 3D animation of the knee motion with simulated virtual ligaments for post-operative analysis of knee kinematic restoration, ligament impingement and ligament elongation. This feature can be used to document the *quality* of the intervention, for example the proper placement of the ligament and the restoration of knee laxity. This feature was also used for experimental purposes, described below, to evaluate placement using endoscopy only versus placement with the CAS system.

20.5 Results

Various controlled tests in the laboratory and data sets obtained intra-operatively were used to fine-tune the parameters of the surface generation algorithm (6% of points for local tangent plane generation, etc.). Intra-operatively the algorithm proved quite robust and of sufficient rendering speed on an SGI O2 (SGI, Zurich, CH) and on a Sun Ultra 10 (SUN Microsystems Switzerland, Schwerzenbach, CH). There was a short learning curve for surgeons to obtain evenly spaced points and to properly coordinate footswitch and hand actions. When the surface was easily palpable, the continu-ous point acquisition mode allowed rapid digitization. For a large number of points (over 100), the algorithm took over 0.5 seconds to reconstruct the surface. The most time-consuming part of the process, the minimal spanning tree, is a nonlinear algorithm with calculation time increasing exponenti-ally with number of data set points. Suspension of the reconstruction algorithm during continuous point acquisition made addition of points to already large surfaces possible.

One problem with the reconstructed surfaces was that points at the very edge of some surfaces were not part of the final triangulation. Another problem was that in patients with a very narrow notch, more often the case in females or smaller individuals, the algorithm sometimes linked points between the medial and lateral sides of the notch forming a spider-web-like structure. In these cases, the surface had to be cleared and separate surfaces generated for the lateral and medial sides of the notch.

Digitization of lines was straightforward, although some of the optional landmarks were physically difficult to access, for example the posterior condyles. A study on the repeatability of the landmark digitization between surgeons will be published in a separate paper.

The incorporation of CAS into the various surgical steps inherent to ACL replacement involved a few days training on plastic bones, cadaver knees and a few operations before using the system routinely. The system has been presently used in approximately 50 surgeries within the first three trial clinics. The learning curve to generate the 'surgeon defined anatomy' was not too long since combined use of endoscope and palpation hook is a known skill for endoscopic surgeons. Various software and hardware improvements are constantly underway to facilitate operative use. Studies on inter-operator and intra-operator surgeon-defined anatomy digitization have shown excellent accuracy and repeatability and results will be published separately.

Preoperative X-rays were scanned into the computer and ligament placement was planned preoperatively using ratios with respect to radiological landmarks as an initial placement estimate. Intraoperatively, a notchplasty was performed immediately if judged necessary.

For the femoral insertion, ratios with respect to the intercondylar roof (Blumensaat's line), distal and posterior condyles, and the extension of the posterior cortex line were employed.[24] For the tibial insertion, ratios with respect to the AP limits of the knee were employed.[10]

The joint axes and the ICR-line where first marked allowing the alignment of the preop X-ray views that contained the planned position. Potential impingement areas of the notch entrance and potential ligament attachment sites were then identified. Care was taken to digitize cartilage structures that may impinge with the ligament. To ensure that the knee was in a reduced position during planning of ligament position, the position of the posterior femoral and tibial condyles was obtained. Ligament placement was then identified to satisfy landmark, impingement, elongation and posterior wall blowout criteria. To avoid impingement, the anterior limit of the ACL graft was placed to have a gap of 3 mm between the anterior border of the graft and the notch with the knee in extension. This allows play for when the action of quadriceps force and the weight of the subject on the posterior tilted tibia bring the tibia forward approximately 3 mm during active movements.

Drilling performed with a computer-guided K-wire guide with a target arm gave satisfactory results, although some bending of the K-wire was observed when going through hard cortical bone or when the drill was pushed too hard to the target. Separate tests with the 'armless' K-wire guide also gave satisfactory results on plastic and cadaver but no experience in a real surgery has been obtained yet. Several surgeons seemed hesitant to use a guide system that does not have a mechanical target point.

20.5.1 Flexibility of the technology for other techniques

Flexibility of the technology is best demonstrated by its use for different surgical techniques. For example, the system can be used in the following manner to help implement the most common *modified one-tunnel* technique.

The preoperative plan can be used to define a straight as possible tunnel through the tibia with the knee flexed at 120 degrees. An impingement-free tibial tunnel can be first guided, then a smaller drill bit can be guided through the tibial tunnel allowing a modified one-tunnel trajectory. The computer-generated trajectory ensures that the femoral tunnel was well anchored in the posterior cortex while avoiding posterior wall blowout. The graft was then fixed as in the standard procedure.

We have had some problems with guided drills that, although held by the surgeon in the planned direction, have sometimes been physically deflected from the hard cortical bone on the tibial plateau. Since at least a 4 mm drill bit must be used to ensure that there is no physical bending, a miss with such size of hole can be uncorrectable, especially when inserting a small graft of the order of 8 mm diameter.

The CAS system can also be used to simulate the unitunnel approach through the anteromedial arthroscopic portal with the knee flexed to 125 degrees.

20.5.1.1 General findings

Factors affecting impingement free ACL graft placement in the sagittal plane can be controlled using fluoroscopy and the radiographic quadrant method to define anatomic centers of guide pins prior to using cannulated reamers. With the endoscope in the standard anterolateral portal, correct ML placement according to the anatomic course of the ACL in the coronal oblique plane[24] is critical. Significant precision gain of correct ACL graft placement in the coronal (M-L) and coronal oblique planes was achieved by the CAS system. Furthermore, the digitization of the lateral part of the intercondylar roof of the intercondylar notch and its effect on potential ACL graft impingement zones could be demonstrated prior to using cannulated reamers to create the definitive tunnels.

20.6 **Discussion**

The estimated 40% ACL graft misplacement rate using standard clinical techniques can for the most part be explained by the limited local view provided by endoscopy that does not allow the surgeon to oversee tool position with respect to various landmarks. The situation is often further complicated by visual occlusion from soft tissue structures such as *Hoffa's fat pad* and restricted movements due to pivoting at the trochar entrance. The presented CAS technology combines locally identified landmarks in 3D to provide the surgeon with the desired overview.

Graft impingement is an all too common error that can lead to limited knee extension in the short term and to catastrophic failure through wear in the long term. Current endoscopic techniques do not allow proper evaluation of impingement until the tunnel has been surgically placed. The presented system allows simulation of virtual ligament placement, including customized graph sizing and functional analysis, before actual ligament drilling. The sagittal and notch views provide a powerful tool to modify ligament insertion as a function of the large variety of knee geometries encountered during surgery. Since notch shape and roof angle greatly vary between individuals, specialized mechanical guides cannot ensure optimal placement in all cases.

Knee ligament surgery is characterized by a variety of different graft types and surgical techniques and therefore warrants a versatile system. The versatility of the system has been shown through its described use for 'standard techniques', namely a variation of the single tunnel technique, and for more involved techniques that use the more advanced features of the system. The system can also be used to different degrees of complexity. Simplest use of the system would be to identify femoral and tibial graft attachment points endoscopically and verify elongation. Defining a notch entrance and ligament diameter allows impingement consideration in the plan. Defining attachment areas can help place a graft that minimizes elongation. Intra-operative digitization of anatomical structures and setting of views such as the ICR line and posterior condyles allows anatomical ligament placement. If preoperative X-rays can be obtained, ligament position can be planned with respect to radiological landmarks and reproduced through intra-operative X-ray templates.

The computer-integrated system also allows surgical views that are impossible using standard technology. For example it is possible to set a *through the notch view*. Using endoscopy, it is impossible to properly view directly inside the notch with the knee in full extension. The knee in extension is however the most critical orientation for studying ligament impingement.

The current system does not require nonstandard medical imaging since preoperative X-rays are routinely used for planning purposes to warn of a narrow notch or the presence of marginal notch osteophytes. The presented system represents the first link between these X-rays and intra-operative endoscopy. This plan can be transferred to the OR and subsequently refined.

Some groups have recently advocated the use of CT scan for computer assisted ACL replacement,[34] however there are several arguments against such an approach. First of all it exposes the patient to additional X-ray exposure and implies additional nonroutine costs. Secondly, a preoperative CT scan cannot reflect intra-operative changes to the notch geometry such as from a notchplasty, which is paramount importance in impingement analysis. Thirdly cartilage geometry does not appear on CT scan, and cartilage covering the distal end of the trochlear groove can be several millimeters thick, greatly effecting impingement analysis.

Direct digitization of cartilage structures, as currently presented, considers the true anatomical structures involved in impingement and combined with the tunnel view and realistic graft size representation provides a truly 3D analysis of this 3D problem. Direct digitization also eliminates the registration error and segmentation errors that occur when generating and *matching* the 3D geometry to the patient position.

The generation of local tangent planes using 6% of the total number of points assumes uniform density of points and a surface that does not contain holes. Other work in the literature has addressed the problem of nonuniform point distribution over a surface containing holes, however we found that this method could not satisfy the real-time requirements of the present application.

We believe that the erroneous triangulation at the edge of digitized surfaces comes from the point reduction process. The merging of marching cube triangulated vertexes with nearest original data points seems to be responsible for the omission of these external points. The present reduction algorithm has been chosen for simplicity and speed, however there is room for future improvement.

Drilling the graft insertion tunnels with a K-wire guide that is equipped with a mechanical target arm has the advantage that the virtual plan is never lost since the internal point is physically fixed within the knee. The K-wire guide without the internal arm has shown satisfactory results in cadaver tests and the accuracy of this device is currently being tested.[28] The general problem with K-wires is however that they can bend when crossing hard cortical bone, or if the surgeon pushes them too fast towards the target. Since these K-wires typically have about 2 to 2.5 mm diameter, small deflections can be corrected when overreaming to the desired tunnel size with a cannulated drill bit. Overreaming of a bent K-wire does however cause metallic debris that is undesirable.

The capacity to ensure good anchoring of the tunnel attachments into cortical bone is important since the ultimate strength of the construct is governed by the attachment strength.[19,20] The *registered* preoperative X-ray ensures good anchoring into cortical bone and computer-assisted support for tunnel length planning helps ensure that a more secure interference screw is used[19,20] rather than another means such as an endobutton.

Real-time tracking and recording allows 3D documentation never before possible in ligament surgery since ligament position cannot be properly seen on post-operative X-ray or CT scan without injection of a contrast medium. Current post-operative stability measurements remain unreliable.[16] The intra-operative reference base attachment and tracking allows an accurate measure of knee stability that immediately provides feedback on the benefit of the intervention.

The quantitative data supplied by this system should provide surgeons the ability to better fulfil their own surgical criteria and provide a strong basis for the objective comparison of these techniques. This study is restricted to the replacement of *single bundle* grafts that are fixed with one tunnel in the tibia and one tunnel in the femur. Work towards computer-assisted support for multi-bundle graft placement is described elsewhere.[35]

A controversial issue concerning the planning of ligament position based on kinematics is that the ACL-deficient knee is inherently unstable. Dessenne *et al.* compared passive kinematics for cadaver knees both with and without ACL and found no difference.[22] It is however clinically known that chronically ACL-deficient knees have large instabilities and anteriorly-subluxed tibial position.[31] Reuben *et al.*[36] compared pre- and post-ACL resected knees under simulated hamstring force and found differences in AP displacement, and ligament lengths during knee flexion. Isometric analysis for ligament placement therefore appears unjustified, especially in the chronically unstable knee. The appropriate role of elongation analysis in ACL planning remains yet to be determined and should be subject to ongoing research.

An alignment of the posterior condyles of both femur and tibia has been proven to be a reliable reference for the reduced position of the knee[29] and is used in this system as a reference position during impingement analysis. Since obtaining posterior condyle position is surgically challenging due to the restricted posterior access, a more practical method to obtain this data is currently under study.

We believe that the presented system represents an advance to satisfy various yet unanswered needs in ACL replacement surgery. Present CAS systems have been designed to satisfy specific surgical techniques and philosophies. The first[21] is restricted to minimal invasive planning of torsion and bending in the ligament. The second[22] principally measures knee movement to obtain a functional placement of the ligament that respects certain elongation (and impingement) criteria and the third[23] system seeks an anatomical placement of the ligament with respect to radiographic landmarks using intra-operative fluoroscopic guidance in the sagittal plane. The second system[22] presents the advantage of not requiring intra-operative fluoroscopy that surgeons tend to find inconvenient. The advantage of the third system[23] is that it allows two-dimensional (2D) X-ray anatomy-based preoperative planning of both ligament position and bone block length, but it does not provide a direct computer-assisted guidance of the planned tunnel insertion and a truly 3D analysis of ligament placement and elongation measurement. A fluoroscopy-based approach also cannot be used to consider cartilage geometry.

The presented system represents a new flexibly-combined anatomical and functional approach to ACL-planning compared to previous systems. This combined approach is advantageous since the surgeon can weigh their relative importance between anatomical placement and functional factors. In addition, the presented CAS system represents an objective teaching tool by allowing interactive analysis between knee anatomy and graft placement.

There is a relationship between anatomical and functional ligament placement. A good understanding of 3D anatomy of sites of attachment can help in accurate tunnel placement.[31] On the femur, anterior placement implies high strain in knee flexion and restricted knee flexion. Posterior placement can bring high strain in extension and cause and extension deficit. Tibial attachment was previously considered less important, however the need to avoid impingement has heavily refocused attention to this site.

20.7 Conclusions

This chapter has introduced a new combined anatomical and functional approach for ligament placement within the knee. Building on previous work in the literature,[22] the concept intra-operatively digitized points has been expanded to the concept of 'surgeon-defined' landmarks. The customized algorithm for surface generation from a cloud of points provides a general tool for reconstruction of structures such as the intercondylar notch that are important for ACL planning.

The system has been designed to be flexible which is shown by its use to support a variety of surgical techniques as well as its use as a simple or advanced planning tool. Landmarks and viewpoints of these landmarks can be defined by the surgeon according to the desired information, for example the 'notch view' which is not possible to see using standard techniques.

The novel incorporation of standard preoperative X-rays provides augmented information on bone geometry without exposing the patient or operating staff to additional radiation.

The 3D representation of the virtually planned ligament and dynamic interaction with digitized surgeon-defined landmarks allows detailed prediction of graft performance and placement correction before the actual drilling of the tunnels. This interactive playing with the virtual representation of the patient's particular knee geometry allows the surgeon to better evaluate the best insertion and feel confident about the chosen placement. This 'learning by playing' can be used as a valuable teaching tool to better understand the factors involved in proper graft placement.

The integration of this technology into the routine of several trial clinics has shown its usability in a realistic environment. Ongoing research and development includes better integration of the preoperative X-ray matching feature of the system, the study of the best computer-guided graft tunnel drilling method and fundamental study of how to plan ligament positioning in the unstable knee.

We hope that this technology will help us to understand and document the various factors involved in cruciate ligament graft replacement and help us to improve the high misplacement rate that occurs in clinics today.

Acknowledgements

The authors would like to thank the AO foundation for some financial support of parts of this project. The authors would also like to thank Chi Tso and Suzanne Larouche for their input in the early developments of the project.

References

1 Jakob RP, Amis AA. (*Workshop Summary*) *Proceedings of the Second ESSKA Scientific Workshop on Reconstruction of the Anterior Cruciate Ligament.* 1998; 6 (Suppl. 1):10.

2 Sati M, Stäubli H-U, Bourquin Y, Kunz M, Käsermann S, Nolte L-P. Clinical integration of new computer assisted technology for arthroscopic ACL replacement. *Oper Techn Orthop* 2000;10:40–9.

3 Hawkins RJ, Misamore GW, Merritt TR. Followup of the acute nonoperated isolated anterior cruciate ligament tear. *Am J Sports Med* 1986;14:205–10.

4 Hulth A, Lindberg H, Telhag H. Experimental osteoarthritis in rabbits. Preliminary report. *Acta Orthop Scand* 1970;41:522–30.

5 Kannus P, Jarvinen M. Conservatively treated tears of the anterior cruciate ligament. Long- term results. *J Bone Joint Surg Am* 1987;69:1007–12.

6 Noyes FR, Mooar PA, Matthews DS, Butler DL. The symptomatic anterior cruciate-deficient knee. Part I: the long-term functional disability in athletically active individuals. *J Bone Joint Surg Am* 1983;65:154–62.

7 Howell SM, Clark JA, Farley TE. Serial magnetic resonance study assessing the effects of impingement on the MR image of the patellar tendon graft. Arthroscopy. *J Arthrosc Rel Surg* 1992;8:350–8.

8 Jackson DW, Gasser SI. Tibial tunnel placement in ACL reconstruction. *Arthroscopy* 1994;10:124–31.

9 Peyrache MD, Djian P, Christel P, Witvoet J. Tibial tunnel enlargement after anterior cruciate ligament reconstruction by autogenous bone-patellar tendon-bone graft. *Knee Surg Sports Traumatol Arthrosc* 1996;4:2–8.

10 Staubli HU, Rauschning W. Tibial attachment area of the anterior cruciate ligament in the extended knee position. Anatomy and cryosections in vitro complemented by magnetic resonance arthrography in vivo. *Knee Surg Sports Traumatol Arthrosc* 1994;2:138–46.

11 Howell SM, Barad SJ. Knee extension and its relationship to the slope of the intercondylar roof. Implications for positioning the tibial tunnel in anterior cruciate ligament reconstructions. *Am J Sports Med* 1995;23:288–94.

12 Amis AA, Zavras TD. Isometricity and graft placement during anterior cruciate ligament reconstruction. *The Knee* 1995;2:5–17.

13 Feller JA, Glisson RR, Seaber AV, Feagin JAJ, Garrett WEJ. Graft isometricity in unitunnel anterior cruciate ligament reconstruction: analysis of influential factors using a radiographic model. *Knee Surg Sports Traumatol Arthrosc* 1993;1:136–42.

14 Fleming B, Beynnon BD, Johnson RJ, McLeod WD, Pope MH. Isometric versus tension measurements. A comparison for the reconstruction of the anterior cruciate ligament. *Am J Sports Med* 1993;21:82–8.

15 Fleming BC, Beynnon BD, Nichols CE, Renström PA, Johnson RJ, Pope MH. An in vivo comparison between intra-operative isometric measurement and local elongation of the graft after reconstruction of the anterior cruciate ligament. *J Bone Joint Surg* 1994;76-A:511–19.

16 Good L, Gillquist J. The value of intra-operative isometry measurements in anterior cruciate ligament reconstruction: an in vivo correlation between substitute tension and length change. Arthroscopy. *J Arthrosc Rel Surg* 1993;9:525–32.

17 Morgan CD, Kalmam VR, Grawl DM. Isometry testing for anterior cruciate ligament reconstruction revisited. *Arthroscopy* 1995;11:647–59.

18 Kohn D, Busche T, Carls J. Drill hole position in endoscopic anterior cruciate ligament reconstruction. Results of an advanced arthroscopy course. *Knee Surg Sports Traumatol Arthrosc* 1998;6(Suppl. 1):S13–15.

19 Kurosaka M, Yoshiya S, Andrish JT. A biomechanical comparison of different surgical techniques of graft fixation in anterior cruciate ligament reconstruction. *Am J Sports Med* 1987;15:225–9.

20 Robertson DB, Daniel DM, Biden E. Soft tissue fixation to bone. *Am J Sports Med* 1986;14:398–403.

21 Sati M, de Guise JA, Drouin G. Computer assisted knee surgery: diagnostics and planning of knee surgery. *Comput Aided Surg* 1997;2:108–23.

22 Dessenne V, Lavallee S, Julliard R, Orti R, Martelli S, Cinquin P. Computer-assisted knee anterior cruciate ligament reconstruction: first clinical tests. *J Image Guided Surg* 1995;1:59–64.

23 Klos TV, Habets RJ, Banks AZ, Banks SA, Devilee RJ, Cook FF. Computer assistance in arthroscopic anterior cruciate ligament reconstruction. *Clin Orthop* 1998;65–9.

24 Stäubli H-U, Adam O, Becker W, Rauschning W. Anterior cruciate ligament and femoral intercondylar notch in the coronal oblique plane. Cryosectional anatomy complemented by magnetic resonance imaging in cruciate ligament-intact knees. *Arthroscopy* 1999;15:349–59.

25 Mommersteeg TJ, Kooloos JG, Blankevoort L, Kauer JM, Huiskes R, Roeling FQ. The fibre bundle anatomy of human cruciate ligaments. *J Anat* 1995;187:461–71.

26 Eberly D. Least squares fitting of data. In: (Technical Report) Anonymous, eds. Department of Computer Science, University of North Carolina, 2000.

27 Lorensen WE, Cline HE. Marching cubes: a high resolution algorithm. *Comput Proc Graphics Proc SIGGRAPH* 1987;21:163–9.

28 Ménétrey J, Suva D, Poggi R, Sati M, Genoud P, Fritschy D. Validation of tunnel drill guide devices and free hand technique for anterior cruciate ligament reconstruction using the computer assisted orthopaedic surgery system. *5th International Symposium on CAOS*, 2000:64. Davos, Switzerland.

29 Staubli HU, Noesberger B, Jakob RP. Stressradiography of the knee. Cruciate ligament function studied in 138 patients. *Acta Orthop Scand* (1992); (Suppl. 249):1–27.

30 Burks RT, Leland R. Determination of graft tension before fixation in ACL reconstruction. *Arthroscopy* 1998;42:60–266.

31 Johnson RJ, Beynnon BD, Nichols CE, Renstrom PA. The treatment of injuries of the anterior cruciate ligament. *J Bone Joint Surg Am* 1992;74:140–51.

32 Hefzy MS, Grood ES, Noyes FR. Factors affecting the region of most isometric femoral attachments. Part II: the anterior cruciate ligament. *Am J Sports Med* 1989;17:208–16.

33 Sati M, Bourquin Y, Berlemann U, Nolte LP. Computer assisted technology for spinal cage delivery. *Oper Techn Orthop* 2000;10:69–76.

34 Petermann J, Kober R, Heinze R, Froelich JJ, Heeckt PF, Gotzen L. Computer-assisted planning and robot-assisted surgery in anterior cruciate ligament reconstruction. *Oper Techn Orthop* 2000;10:50–5.

36 Reuben JD, Rovick JS, Schrager RJ, Walker PS, Boland AL. Three-dimensional dynamic motion analysis of the anterior cruciate ligament deficient knee joint. *Am J Sports Med* 1989;17:463–71.

Chapter 21

Ligament reconstruction in the knee: the use of the CASPAR system

Joerg Petermann, Alirezah Pashmineh Azar, and Leo Gotzen

21.1 Clinical challenges

21.1.1 Traditional ACL reconstruction

ACL rupture is the most common acute ligamentous lesion of the knee joint. As the ACL controls the whole range of motion and has an important role in proprioception, the loss of ACL function is a serious injury, both morphologically and functionally. The incidence of secondary meniscus tears in ACL insufficient knee joints is about 70% and posterolateral instabilities also often occur. The result is post-traumatic osteoarthritis.[1–3] The indications for ACL replacement in physically active patients are therefore, no longer controversial.

Traditional techniques in ACL reconstruction have one procedure in common: at least one tunnel is drilled into the bone on the femoral and tibal side, and the ACL substitute is fixed in the tunnels. The correct localization of the tunnels is the most important parameter.[3,4] Brown[5] showed that in 15–25% of reconstructed knee joints, a revision had to be performed as a reinstability could be detected. In about 85% non-isometric positioning of the tunnels was the main cause.[5,6] The choice of transplantat, the method of graft fixation, pretensioning, twisting, mini-open or endoscopic techniques are all significantly less important. The discrepancy between the theoretical consensus on the correct points of insertion and the large number of revisions show that positioning of the tunnels remains the main problem.

21.1.2 Computer assisted orthopedic surgery (CAOS) applications in ACL reconstruction

As most surgeons perform isometric functional placement in the conventional hand-held fashion; only a few have experience of computer assisted methods. The first reconstruction techniques with computer-assisted tools were procedures using navigation systems.[7,8,9,10] The navigation techniques based on CT or fluoroscopy (see Chapters 18, 19, and 20) are used in a few centers. Most of the systems are at an experimental stage, and large number of patients have not been operated on. When looking at the accuracy of COAS it was shown that there was a range of up to 2.5 mm, i.e. 25% of the used drill tunnel diameter of 10 mm. The length of operation is such that this kind of reconstruction cannot be performed routinely.[7] The other major issue is that the navigation techniques, including the intra-operative planning and simulation of the graft, are performed on the unstable knee joint. That means that the correct relation of the femur to the tibia in the knee joint, as expressed when planning with the stable contralateral knee, is not taken into consideration. These methods in ACL reconstruction (using navigation systems) should be discussed critically and a careful follow-up has to be performed. In ACL reconstruction the CASPAR system (U.R.S.-ortho GmbH & Co., Rastatt, Germany) is the only active system.

21.2 Systems

In traditional ACL reconstruction the most common mistake is to use the former points of insertion of the torn ACL as the reference point, although the skeletal structures should be used to define the correct positioning of the graft.[4,11] As there is a pathological hyperextension and increased external rotation capacity combined with a translation of the biomechanical center to the medial compartment,[4,12,13] the planning of the correct tibial tunnel position should be performed on the stable contralateral knee joint using the lateral side view x-ray in hyperextension.[11] Only by performing this planning procedure can the correct relation between the osseous partners of the knee joint be determined. The anterior edge of the tibial tunnel is defined by the cross point of Blumensaat's and tibia plateau line.[4,11,14,15]

When analysing our results (we started with this two dimensional preoperative planning procedure in 1992) we were surprised to find that about 40% of patients still had an impingement grade 1 according to Howell and Taylor's classification.[16,17] Because of these results we began to use a computer-assisted three-dimensional preoperative planning system based on CT scans. The best accuracy was achieved by using a robot assisted system to drill the tunnels, and we decided to develop this procedure with the CASPAR system.

21.2.1 Placement of fidicual markers

After the anamnesis, clinical and radiological investigations, and a measurement of stability the indication for ACL reconstruction is checked. On the day of operation, and the fidicuals are placed in the operating room.

The fidicuals (self-cutting screws) are set while the patient is under a local anaesthetic. The screws are placed bicortically to keep them in a stable position. The tibial pin is positioned about 6 cm below the medial joint line at the level of the tibial tuberosity, midway between the anterior and posterior surface of the tibia (Fig. 21.1). The positioning of the drill channel therefore coincides with the stab incision for the tibial reference pin. The femoral reference pin is placed about 8 cm above the lateral joint line and in the middle of lateral aspect of the distal femur. Then registration crosses are fixed on the screws. These plastic crosses have four metal pearls at the ends of the cross (Fig. 21.2a) During the CT scans no artefacts will occur and the 3-D position of the fidicual in relation to the tibia and femur is defined. During the operation these crosses are changed into metal crosses with holes in the corresponding diameters there by allowing registration.

21.2.2 CT scanning and preoperative planning

For the helical CT the legs of the patient are fixed in a special frame to achieve a standardized postioning with hyperextension of the knee joints (Fig. 21.2b). To detect movement of the patient's leg a calibration rod is added. The CT is then performed and the data transferred online to our planning room. Here the surgeon calls up the patient's data for identification and storing.

On the screen the surgeon can see three planning slices of the knee joint: an ap, a lateral, and a coronar view. These scan levels are always marked with colour frames. Red is the ap view, green the lateral

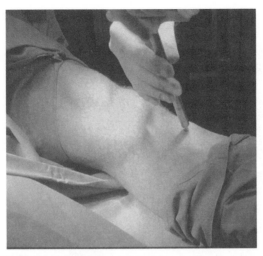

Fig. 21.1 Positioning the tibial fidicual through a stab incision.

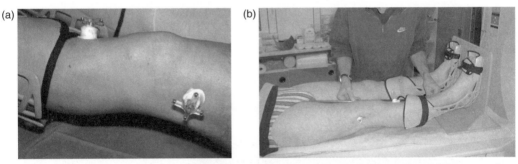

Fig. 21.2 (a) The plastic registration crosses are screwed on the fiducials; (b) the patient's legs are put in a special frame in hyperextension and a calibration rod for movement detection is fixed.

side view and blue the coronar scan. In all scans the planning is performed at the same height as the, cutting level. The surgeon is able to scroll up and down at each scan level. If you click on the right frame on the right-hand corner of the picture, the image gets the only scan on the screen. The surgeon can then zoom up or down with the magnification. The level of each planning step is shown by pearls on the right side of the screen, marked by a blue arrow. Special functions such as the chosen diameter of the cutting miller or the length of the tunnel are demonstrated. Distances and angles necessary or useful for preoperative planning are indicated. If the planning step is finished, the yellow padlock is clicked. Then this level is closed and the next step can be performed (see Fig. 21.3).

The first step in the preoperative planning process is to identify the fidicual markers on the CT scans (Fig. 21.4): first the pin at the distal femur, then at the proximal tibia.

After the tibial and femoral pin registration, the segmentation of the CT scans is controlled (Fig. 21.5). Using this means that mistakes caused by the patient's movement during the CT can be avoided.

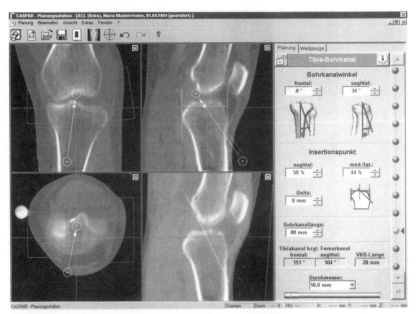

Fig. 21.3 Blumensaat's line of the stable and unstable knee joint (blue and yellow), the planned tibial drill tunnel (yellow) with the chosen diameter (10 mm), and the areas which must not be crossed in order to avoid impingement syndromes are marked. See Plate 5.

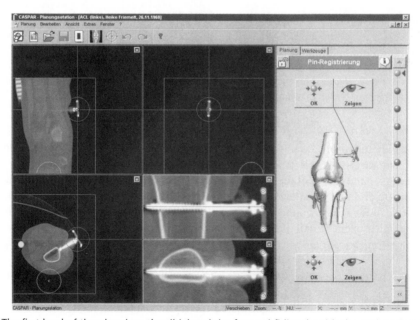

Fig. 21.4 The first level of the planning: the tibial and the femoral fiducials with the registration crosses are shown.

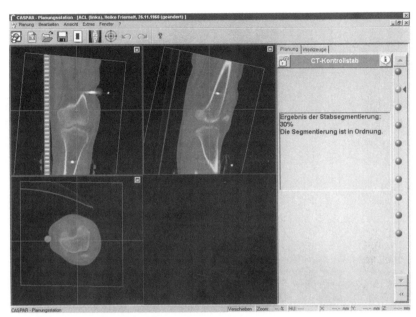

Fig. 21.5 The segmentation with 33% is exact, there was only a few movements during the CT scan and the planning can continue.

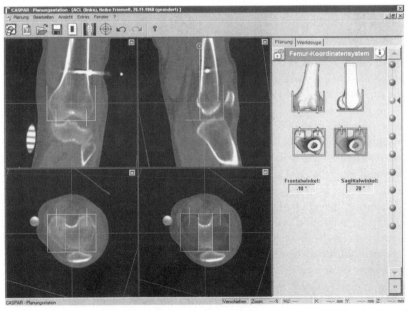

Fig. 21.6 During the femoral calibration process the femur shaft axis, the width, the depth and the middle of the condyles are marked. This allows the femur to be shown in a 3D data set.

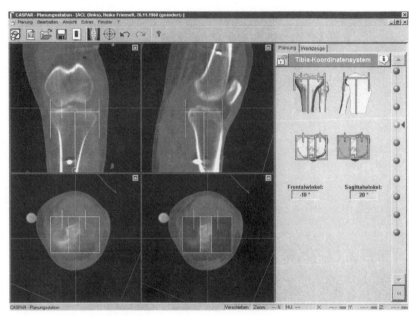

Fig. 21.7 Normalization of the proximal tibia. The tibial axis and the width and depth of the tibia head plateau are marked, and the dimensions of the femoral condyles are the red areas. In this region no tunnel has to be planned to avoid graft impingement syndromes. See Plate 6.

The next step is to define the anatomical structure of the distal femur known as normalization or calibration (Fig. 21.6) A right angle is put around the distal femur at the height of the distal epicondylus, the region with the most expended diameter. Additional special lines mark the internal sides of the medial and lateral femur condyl, used to avoid wall impingements of the ACL graft. These areas are marked with red fields during the following planning stages. The axis of the femur is defined by the dorsal femur corticalis.

Now the position of the proximal tibia in the 3D data set is determined (Fig. 21.7), also by putting around a right angle at the region with the most width. The axis of the tibia is marked. Performing these two last procedures now gives a clear definition of the position of the knee joint.

The next step is the matching of the femur (Fig. 21.8). The injured unstable side is marked yellow and the contralateral knee joint blue. With the mouse, the surgeon puts the yellow above the blue knee joint and all the planning data can now be matched from one knee joint to the other. The shapes of the femur look identical after the closing of the matching process (Fig. 21.9). This management can be performed as there is now symmetry of the osseous structures.[18]

After the matching of the femur, the matching process for the tibia follows (Fig. 21.10). Comparing the lines (blue for the stable and yellow for the injured side) at the intercondylar roof the different range of hyperextension is demonstrated and measured. Additionally, the different range of rotation is shown on the screen. The importance of the preoperative planning procedure on the stable contralateral knee joint is now demonstrated and the value of the interactive matching process (to define the correct insertion points) is underlined.

After normalization and matching, the correct positioning of the insertion points is the next step, first on the femur, then on the tibia. The Blumensaat's line is put exactly parallel to the roof of the intercondylar notch. The basis of the right angle is defined by the anterior end and the posterior

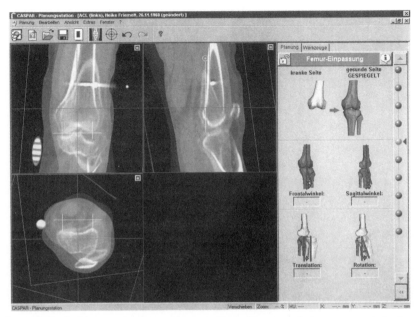

Fig. 21.8 The pathological hyperextension and external rotation are well demonstrated. As there is also a lateral instability, an opening of the joint line of the injured knee joint can be seen.

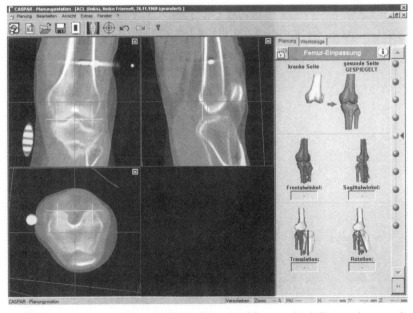

Fig. 21.9 After finishing the interactive matching of the distal femura, both lie exactly on each other.

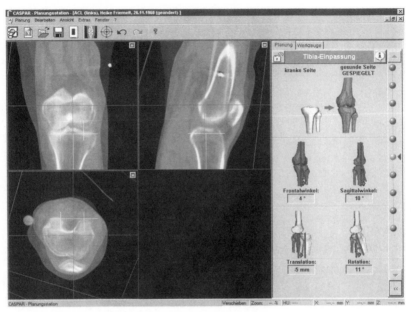

Fig. 21.10 After the matching of the tibia, the different positions are measured and shown on the screen. Now the all planning data can be transferred from the stable to unstable knee joint.

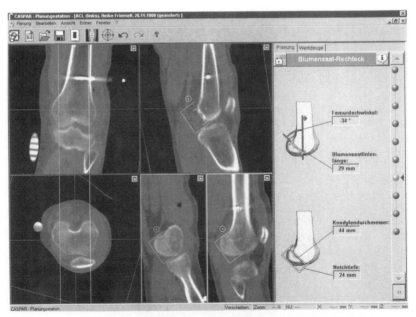

Fig. 21.11 To measure the dimensions of the medial side of the lateral condyle a right angle is adapted to the posterior, the anterior border, and tangential to the distal curve with the basis of Blumensaat's line.

margin of the middle of the lateral conydyle (Fig. 21.11). The intercondylar roof angle is measured and the pathological angle can be detected.[19]

The surgeon now has two options. He can use templates according to the different planning procedures described by for example Aglietti, Amis, or Harner.[3,4,14,20] These are easily adapted by using the data sets. The other option is to use free navigation, so that the dorsal distance of the posterior border of the femoral tunnel is 2–3 mm to the dorsal cortical edge. This latter procedure is the most common technique in ACL reconstruction using drill guidances.[3,4] Then the proximal end of the femoral drill tunnel is lead to the end point by using the mouse. The surgeon can plan blind sacks or the point of tunnel outcome using a two tunnel two incision technique (Fig. 21.12). We plan the proximal end of femoral tunnel in such a manner that the incision necessary for the graft fixation is the same as the incision necessary for the pin fixation.

After the femoral, the tibial tunnel is planned. The position depends on the Blumensaat line of the femur in hyperextension on the healthy side and thus on the position of the tibia relative to the femur (Fig. 21.13). After the normalization and matching procedures, malpositioning of the insertion point and the tunnel can be avoided as the planning is performed on a correctly positioned knee joint. Parallel to Blumensaat's line in the stable knee joint the drill tunnel is planned in the lateral side view. In the ap and coronar plane the orientation is adapted to the anterior eminence. The marked areals of the femoral condyles avoid wall impingement. The distal point of entrance of the drill tunnels is planned in such a manner that the incision for the tibial fidicual is used and irritation of the pes anserinus is avoided.

After the planning of both tunnels, it should be checked again at every level and scrolled through on the screen. Then the data have to be stored and the planning map is printed for the patient's documents. During the storing process a control of plausibility is performed. If there are any mistakes it is

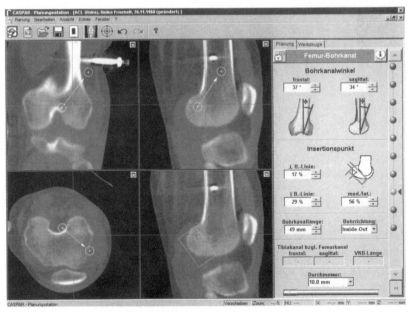

Fig. 21.12 The femoral tunnel is positioned and by scrolling through the 3D data set the correct position is controlled.

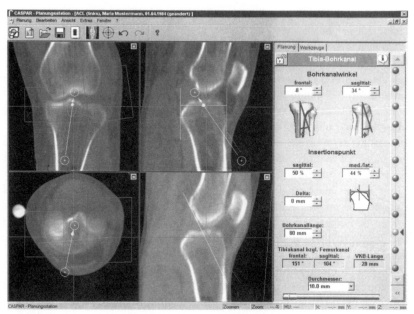

Fig. 21.13 The tibial drill tunnel is positioned, notch and wall impingements are avoided, and the tunnel is planned in correct relation to the femur and tibia according to the postion in the stable contralateral knee joint.

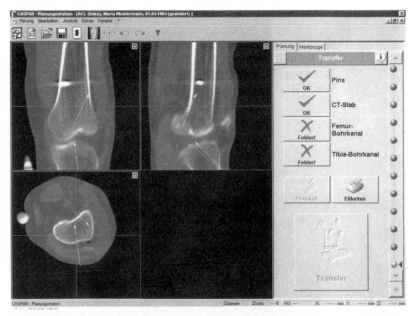

Fig. 21.14 In this example, mistakes in the planning were made in the positioning of the tibial and the femoral tunnel placement. The storing of the data onto the pc card and transferring the data to the CASPAR robot is impossible.

shown on the screen (Fig. 21.14). After detecting the level on which the mistake happened the surgeon goes back to this position and performs the necessary corrections. After the correction the planning is stored on a pc card and this is used to transport the data to the CASPAR robot.

21.2.3 **Surgical technique**

After storing the data onto the pc card, it is brought to the robot in the operating room. The time of reconstruction should be as close as possible to the setting of the fiducials. The preoperative preparations consist of sterile draping of the robot, calibration of the tools, and transfer of the planning data. Additionally we perform a lateral side-view x-ray of the hyperextended contralateral knee joint in case of complications with the computer assisted technique, so that we could continue with conventional reconstruction methods. Immediately before surgery, the leg is postioned by using a foot plate and a special boot for those steps of surgery that are performed without the robot. The knee instability is measured preoperatively and postoperatively with the sterile KT 1000 S (MEDmetric Corp, San Diego, CA). Then the knee is scoped, and additional damage such as meniscal lesions are treated. Then two different options are possible: to harvest the graft first or to perform the drilling process of the tunnels with the robot. All types of grafts can be used—we normally used the 10 mm central third of the patellar tendon as a bone-tendon-bone graft, protected by a 3 mm telos ligament (telos GmbH, Marburg, Germany). The drilling process is normally done first in our own procedure.

For the CASPAR assisted ACL reconstruction the femur and the tibia are temporarily immobilized in special a frame flexed to 115° (Fig. 21.15). The fixation device is connected by two arms to the robot. To control the movement of the knee joint, a mechanical sensor is attached to the fixation frame or an optical system (a modified navigation system, orthopilot, aesculap AG, Tuttlingen, Germany) works as a detector. The drilling process is stopped in case of movement of the knee joint.

After fixing the knee joint in the frame, the first step is the tibial registration procedure. The detector is lead by hand to the metal registration cross fixed on the tibial fidicual. All four holes on the cross are detected with the sensor and the computer performs the registration.

Having identified the position of the tibia the registration stab is changed into the diamond-plated cutting miller and the water cooling system is adapted. The registration pin is removed and the drilling process started (Fig 21.16a). After finishing drilling the planned tunnel the robot stops and the

(a)

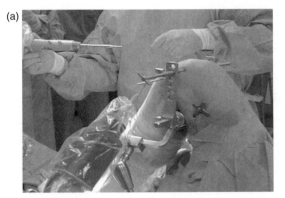

(b)

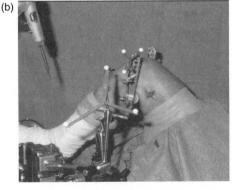

Fig. 21.15 The knee joint is fixed in the frame and the sensors for movement (a) mechanical, (b) optical— are adapted. To start the tibial registration process the registration stab is fixed on the CASPAR robot and lead by hand to the fidicual with the registration cross.

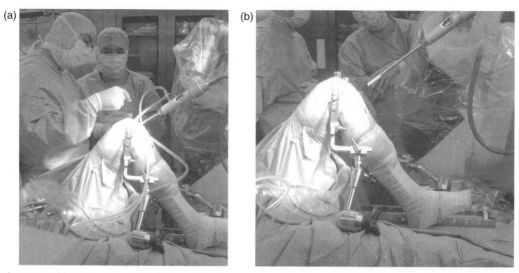

Fig. 21.16 (a) Starting the tibial drilling with the water-cooled diamond-plated cutting miller and; (b) after its removal with the osseous cylinder of the tunnel.

surgeon can control the tibial tunnel. If the tunnel should be longer, the surgeon can define the grade of lengthening individually. The water cooling system is stopped and the cutting miller is moved out of the knee joint by the robot, normally with the osseous cylinder. Then the same procedure is performed for the femoral tunnel (Fig. 21.16b). If you do a mini open procedure, you need no more skin incision, if the technique is performed endoscopically a new incision has to be performed.

After the successful drilling processes the frame and the robot are removed and the ACL reconstruction is completed. Postoperatively, we document the correct position of the graft with an x-ray of the reconstructed knee joint in lateral side view and hyperextension (with the patient still under general anaesthetic). After the ACL reconstruction an accelerated rehabilitation program is performed.

21.2.4 Validation

Because the fiducials are measured both on the CT scan and by the robot, and the position of the tunnels relative to the pins is known from the planning, the robot is able to drill the tunnels with great precision. An error simulation has shown maximum deviations of less than 0.8 mm.[21] Analysing the first knee joints with a CASPAR assisted ACL reconstruction the deviation analysis can be confirmed.[22]

21.3 Comparison with traditional techniques

The traditional and navigated techniques for ACL reconstruction do not mind the pathological hyperextension and malrotation of the injured knee joint during the planning process or during the positioning of the tunnels.[3,4,7,9,10] This is the main reason why in about 20% of ACL reconstructed knees a revision has to be performed, because of incorrect tunnel placement.[6] As the robot only drills the tunnel in the position, length, width and angle, as was planned, the reconstruction technique every surgeon is used to, can be performed. The traditional technique will also be improved by the correct placement of the insertion points. To achieve this, CT scans are necessary. The number of CT scans can be reduced and is now about 370 scans for both knee joints. Comparing the CASPAR assisted reconstruction method with traditional techniques the CASPAR method takes longer, but the operation is significantly quicker than using navigation techniques. Initially we needed more than 30 minutes longer, but after having performed 20 operations with the CASPAR assisted procedure the time of operation decreased to about 10 minutes. Time needed for pin placement and for the preoperative planning must be added. For the patient the positioning of the fiducials must be seen as a second invasive procedure. The clinical outcome in patients with our new procedure cannot be compared to the traditional technique follow-up results yet, as the follow-up time is different. Comparing the tunnel positions we could find no graft impingement on the postoperative x-rays in lateral side view and hyperextension or on the MRIs performed two years after reconstruction and removal of the augmentation band.

21.4 Clinical trials

After our first cadaver studies, the first CASPAR assisted ACL reconstruction was performed in March 1999. We have now operated on 94 patients. In the first year we followed-up patients with an acute isolated ACL instability (27 patients). The mean age was 29 (range 18–52) years; and about one third were female. Fourteen knee joints were injured at the left side. The length of the tibial drill cylinders was 50 (40–55) mm of the femoral tunnel 66 (52–80) mm. The mean tibial registration error was 0.3 mm and femoral 0.6 mm. In the post op x-rays at lateral side view no signs of graft impingement were found. One patient had a superfical thrombosis. We had one complete break off caused by a hardware defect. In 3 cases we had slight collisions with the lower patella pole or with the medial condyle during the drilling process, but after rewriting the software no more collisions were noted. No lesions of the synovia of the PCL were noted. There were no problems associated with the diamond plated cutting miller. One patient with an empyema was excluded from follow-up. Two who had a traumatic rerupture followed by a second reconstruction were excluded too. In one patient we found a reinstability without a reasonable cause, but this had been reconstructed at the date of the follow-up examination and could therefore be included. The IKDC ranging is shown in Table 21.1.

After a sports injury we had to reathroscopy one patient 7 months after the ACL reconstruction. We found a type I ACL transplant according to our classification[17] and no signs of graft impingement in the lateral side view x-ray under anaesthesia. In the MRI a well-structured substitute was seen without any signs of tunnel enlargement and with a good bony ingrowth (Fig. 21.17).

Table 21.1 One year follow-up results of patients with an acute isolate ACL reconstruction (IKDC scoring)

			A	B	C	D
Group 1:	Pat. subj. assessment	Knee function	11	14	2	0
		Affect on activity level	11	14	2	0
Group 2:	Symptoms	No pain on activity	17	8	2	0
		No swelling	18	7	2	0
		No giving way	25	2	0	0
Group 3:	Range of motion	Extension deficit	24	3	0	0
		Flexion deficit	21	6	0	0
Group 4:	Stability	Lachman (KT 1000 mmd)	10	13	3	1
Group 8:	One-leg-hop	% side-to-side difference	10	12	5	0
Overall ranging			10	13	3	1

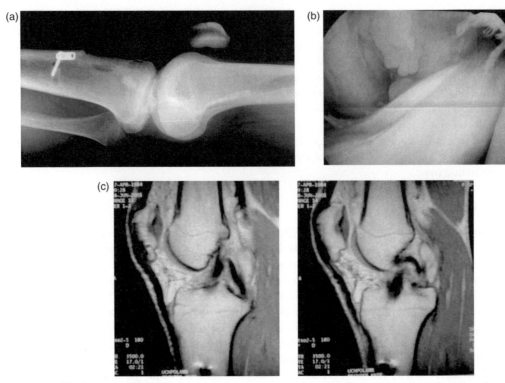

Fig. 21.17 (a) The postoperative X-ray in hyperextension and lateral side view shows no sign of graft impingement; (b) the ACL substitue (type I) 7 months after arthroscopic reconstruction; (c) MRI scan one week after the removal of the augmentation band and the fixation devices, good bony ingrowth, no graft impingement, and well structured.

21.5 **Discussion**

Our 2 years of using the CASPAR system showed it to be safe, effective, and efficient for the accurate placement of tibial and femoral canals in ACL surgery. The degree of accuracy achievable with it is in the range of 0.5–0.8 mm, which cannot be met by any manual or navigation technique.[21,22] The positions of the insertion points are planned preoperatively at the stable contralateral knee joint and thus, the correct relation between femur and tibia for the joint position is defined. Problems caused by increased external rotation or hyperextension, which can occur in the conventional or computer assisted planning procedures in the navigation techniques are avoided.

The use of fidicuals should be viewed critically, the manufacturers are working on software developement for a surface detection system. Principally the problem is solved, but the accuracy of this pinless procedure is not yet as accurate we would like.

The following steps must be standard when planning the preoperative process in the 3D data set. Free navigation in the planning procedure of the insertion points and drill tunnels has to be changed in defined positions. Therefore, anatomic markers must be found which allow a reproducible positioning of the x-, y- and z axis of the femur and tibia. Then the described different insertion points have to be controlled with cadaver knee studies to measure the isometric behavior. This procedure of standardization is necessary so that, we can drill the tunnels exactly in the ideal isometric position, and, if you compare the published data to the so-called correct insertion points, a great variation can be found.[23] Furthermore, an intraoperative simulation of the graft behavior in the planned positions should be possible, including the ability to measure the length and graft tensioning.

After solving these problems, a double blinded randomized study should be performed to compare the outcome between traditional and computer assisted techniques, including an analysis of the costs, the rate of graft malpositioning, and revisions.

In the future we think that planning procedures for ACL reconstruction and associated ligamentous lesions should be developed. A combination between intraoperative surface detection procedures used by the navigation techniques and the computer assisted preoperative planning should help to solve the problems with the fidicual markers.

21.6 Summary

Our initial clinical experience with the CASPAR system in ACL reconstruction showed it to be safe, effective, and efficient for the accurate placement of the drill tunnels. The degree of accuracy achievable with this technique cannot be met by manual techniques or navigated procedures in a reliable and repetitive manner. Current disadvantages, such additional surgery for the placement of the fidicual markers, and slightly longer time for surgical treatment, have to be weighed against obvious benefits for the patient. Additionally, the documentation of the planning and surgical procedure is an important part of quality control in orthopedic surgery.

References

1 Friederich NF, O'Brien WR. Gonarthrose nach Verletzung des vorderen Kreuzbandes. *Z Unfallchirurgie Versicherungsmedzin* 1993;86:357–68.

2 Lobenhoffer P. Kniebandverletzungen I. Anatomie, Biomechanik, Diagnostik, Indikationsstellung. *Chrirg* 1999;70:219–30.

3 Lobenhoffer P. Kniebandverletzungen II. Operative Therapie bei vorderer und hintere Knieinstabilität. *Chirurg* 1999;70:326–38.

4 Fu FH, Bennett CH, Ma CB, *et al.* Current trends in anterior cruciate ligament reconstruction. *Am J Sports Med* 2000;28:124–30.

5 Brown CH, Carson EW. Revision anterior cruciate ligament surgery. *Clin Sports Med* 1999; 18(1):109–71.

6 Wetzler MJ, Getelman MH, Friedman MJ, *et al.* Revision anterior cruciate ligament surgery: etiology of failure. *Operat Tech Sports Med* 1998;6:64–70.

7 Ellermann A, Buelow J, Siebeold R. Computer Guided ACL—Reconstruction 9th ESSKA Congress, 2000; 16–20th September, London.

8 Klos TVS, Habets RJE, Banks AZ, *et al.* Computer assisted fluorscopic arthroscopic anterior cruciate ligament reconstruction. *Clin Orthop* 1998;354:77.

9 Sati M, de Guise JA, Drouin G. Computer assisted knee surgery: diagnostics and planning of knee surgery. *Comput Aided Surg* 1997;2:108.

10 Staeubli HU, Bekic J, Käsermann S, *et al.* Surface anatomy based real time navigation for ACL— reconstruction. Abstract book, *4th North American Program on Computer Assisted Orthpaedic Surgery,* CAOS 2000:121–4.

11 Gotzen L, Petermann J. Die Ruptur des vorderen Kreuzbandes beim Sportler. *Chirurg* 1994;65:910–9.

12 Luites JWH, Wymenga AB, Blankevoort L, *et al.* Double—bundle anatomic ACL—reconstruction with computer assisted surgery part II: an in-vitro study of the anterior laxity in knees with anatomic

double—bundle versus isometric single bundle reconstructions. Abstract book, *4th North American Program on Computer Assisted Orthopaedic Surgery*, CAOS 2000:132–4.

13 Vergis A, Gillquist J. Persistence of altered knee motion in ACL deficient subjects after ligament reconstruction. Wiesbaden: European Orthopedic Research Society; 2000, October 15th.

14 Aglietti P, Zaccherotti G, Simeone G, *et al*. Patellar tendon versus doubled semitendinosus and gracilis tendons for anterior cruciate ligament reconstruction. *Am J Sports Med* 1994;22:211–18.

15 Howell SM. Principles for placing the tibial tunnel and avoiding roof impingement during reconstruction of a torn anterior cruciate ligament. *Knee Surg Sports Traumatol Arthrosc* 1998;6:2–12.

16 Howell SM, Taylor MA. Failure of reconstruction of the anterior cruciate ligament due to impingement by the intercondylar roof. *J Bone Joint Surg* 1993;75A:1044.

17 Ziring E, Ishaque BA, Petermann J, Gotzen. Arthroskopische und klinische Evaluierung nach isoliertem, augmentierten VKB—Ersatz. *Unfallchirurg* 2000;104:158–66.

18 Teitz CC, Lind BK, Sacks BM. Symmetry of the femoral notch width index. *Am J Sports Med* 1997;25:687–90.

19 Petermann J, Reinecke J, Ishaque BA, *et al*. Praxisorientierte Klassifikation der Fossa intercondylaris des Kniegelenkes. *Unfallchirurgie* 1999;25:215–23.

20 Amis A, Jakob RP. Anterior cruciate ligament graft positioning, tensioning and twisting. *Knee Surg Sports Traumatol Arthrosc* 1998;6(Suppl. 1):2–12.

21 Petermann J, Kober R, Heinze R, *et al*. Computer—assisted planning and robot—assisted surgery in anterior cruciate ligament reconstruction. *Operat Tech Orthop* 2000;10:50–5.

22 Petermann J, Schierl M, Niess C, *et al*. Computer assistierte Planung und Roboter assistierte Ersatzplastik des vorderen Kreuzbandes mit dem CASPAR—System. *Arthroskopie* 2000;13:270–9.

23 Gotzen L, Pashmineh Azar R, Petermann J. Experimentelle und klinische Grundlagen für den Einsatz des CASPAR—Systems beim VKB—Ersatz, CAS 2000, Pro und Contra, 17 November, Berlin.

Chapter 22

Pelvic trauma

David M. Kahler

22.1 Introduction

Orthopaedic trauma surgeons are experienced in minimally invasive techniques using two-dimensional video output during either arthroscopy or C-arm fluoroscopy. Standard C-arm fluoroscopy is sometimes sufficient for percutaneous placement of screws in various trajectories about the pelvis and acetabulum. The biggest limitation of this technique is that imaging is generally available in only one plane at a time. The surgeon must position the implant in one view, and then obtain additional images in other planes for 'trial and error' placement of guide wires or screws. The complex anatomy of the pelvis houses a large number of vital structures; when relying on only one planar image at a time for guidance, an erroneous first pass of the guide wire can potentially have disastrous consequences.

Significant operating room time is expended while the fluoroscopy technician positions the C-arm to supply views in multiple planes, both during and after implant placement. Although most orthopaedic surgeons are comfortable with this technique for hip fractures and intramedullary nailing, these procedures expose both the patient and surgeon to significant radiation doses. This radiation exposure and operative time is greatly increased when working around the pelvis, due to the increased soft tissue mantle, as well as the precise oblique projections necessary for adequate pelvic imaging. For all of these reasons, it became clear that we had to search for a new technology that would allow more versatile screw trajectories with less radiation exposure and greater first pass accuracy. The advent of Computer Assisted Orthopaedic Surgery (CAOS) provided this technology.

In 1998, a jointly-sponsored NIH/AAOS workgroup convened to define CAOS and identify potential applications that warranted research support. CAOS, or *Image Guided Surgery*, was defined as the use of either a 3D data set or multiple stored 2D images to define and execute a surgical plan using real-time surgical navigation. Orthopaedic trauma (pelvis and acetabulum), spine surgery, and total joint arthroplasty were identified as the key potential impact areas for this new technology.

CAOS provides access to either a three-dimensional data set (*3D-CT guidance*) or multiple simultaneously displayed stored fluoroscopic images (*virtual fluoroscopy*). For both techniques, most current image-guided surgery systems use an optical tracking system (digital camera array and digitizer) to follow both the position of the patient and special surgical instruments during the course of the procedure. The predicted position of the surgical instruments is then displayed on a computer monitor relative to the position of the stored images. This process is known as *surgical navigation*. In the author's experience, optimal accuracy is provided by tracking the drill guide used to place guide wires for cannulated screws, rather than by tracking the drill itself. The two basic types of computer guided surgery systems (3D-CT vs. virtual fluoroscopy) each have unique advantages and disadvantages when applied to orthopaedic trauma.

Surgeons are often quick to note several obvious drawbacks in choosing CAOS over standard technique. Those wishing to use this technology must invest some time in learning to use the interfaces and software. The surgeon, scrub nurse, and assistants must also learn to operate without obstructing the digital camera's view of the operative field. The operating room must be large enough to accommodate the computer system and camera, as well as the C-arm unit. Cables connecting the two units may interfere with mobility of personnel and equipment in the operating suite. There is inevitably some setup time involved in interfacing the system with the C-arm and placing a reference array on the patient prior to obtaining images. In the author's experience, this process adds ten to fifteen minutes at the start of the surgical procedure. Although this time is essentially always recouped during the procedure by gaining increased first pass accuracy, many surgeons still find the setup time objectionable.

In general, orthopaedic surgeons in the United States have been relatively slow to embrace computer assisted technology. This appears to be due primarily to concerns about cost and complexity of the systems. Many surgeons remain unaware of the fact that these systems and software packages are now commercially available, and several hundred such systems have been installed in hospitals in the United States. The European orthopaedic community appears to be adopting the use of these systems more quickly than surgeons in the United States.

22.1.1 Pelvic and acetabular fracture applications

Percutaneous fixation of the posterior pelvic ring disruption (crescent fracture, sacral fracture, or sacroiliac joint disruption) has gained favor in the orthopaedic trauma community. This approach is much less invasive than traditional open anterior or posterior exposure of the posterior pelvis. When combined with appropriate anterior ring fixation, a single iliosacral screw placed into the S1 body is often sufficient for stabilization of the unstable posterior ring.

Formal internal fixation of acetabular fractures has traditionally required large surgical exposures. These exposures can be associated with significant complications, including infection, wound healing problems, major blood vessel or nerve injury, denervation or devascularization of the abductors, and heterotopic ossification. For the most part, these complications are related to the surgical exposure itself, rather than to the initial traumatic injury. It therefore seems reasonable to consider percutaneous stabilization of selected acetabular fractures in order to avoid exposing the trauma patient to the morbidity of an extensive surgical exposure.

The following groups of acetabular fractures may be amenable to minimally invasive surgical fixation:

1. Nondisplaced (1–3 mm) but potentially unstable fractures involving the weight bearing dome. Transtectal transverse fractures with roof arcs measuring less than 45 degrees may fall into this category.[1] Tornetta has recently provided a technique for stressing nondisplaced fractures under fluoroscopic guidance that helps to confirm potential instability in slightly displaced fractures.[2] Percutaneous stabilization of these fractures may prevent late fracture displacement and allow beneficial early mobilization of the trauma patient.

2. Slightly displaced fractures (3–5 mm) with gap displacement that may be reduced with percutaneously placed lag screws. In the absence of translational displacement, certain anterior column, transverse, anterior column/posterior hemitransverse, and posterior column fractures can be adequately fixed with large diameter lag screws placed perpendicular to the fracture lines.

3. Displaced fractures (>5 mm) that fall into one of the above two categories following a closed reduction maneuver. Occasionally, transverse and column fractures with subluxation or dislocation

of the femoral head may assume acceptable position following a maneuver to reduce the femoral head beneath the weight bearing dome. The surgeon may also apply preoperative or intra-operative traction to improve the reduction. More recently, a distraction frame that applies lateral traction through both greater trochanters has been used to reduce hip subluxation prior to fixation in transverse and posterior column fractures. The surgeon may also potentially reduce selected anterior column fractures with Schanz pin joysticks placed in both iliac wings, and hold the reduction with a temporary external fixator during percutaneous fixation.

4. Displaced both column fractures with good secondary congruity. In the both column fracture that has medialized with gap displacement but good secondary congruity, the fracture can be stabilized *in situ* with two cannulated screws placed into the anterior and posterior columns. This can prevent further fracture displacement, and eliminates the need for prolonged traction or restricted mobilization of the patient. Reduction can sometimes be improved with the bilateral distraction frame. Percutaneous stabilization allows the elderly patient with the typical geriatric both column fracture to be mobilized immediately; the hip may later be reconstructed, if necessary, by elective total hip arthroplasty after the patient's medical status is optimized.

5. Displaced acetabular fractures in morbidly obese patients. In this situation, the trauma surgeon may be willing to accept somewhat greater final fracture displacement than usual, as the perceived risk of surgical complications related to a formal surgical exposure is increased. Precise percutaneous lag screw placement may provide some reduction and stabilize the fracture adequately to allow mobilization, while minimizing risks related to an extensile surgical exposure. It may be more prudent to accept 3 mm of articular displacement in a very large patient rather than to strive for an anatomic reduction through an extensive open exposure.

Fractures of the posterior wall of the acetabulum are rarely amenable to percutaneous reduction and fixation. Given the anatomy of the sciatic nerve in close proximity to the fracture fragment, it is difficult to safely place percutaneous screws across posterior wall fractures without risking nerve injury. Open reduction is also usually necessary to adequately debride the hip joint and reduce marginal impaction. The unstable posterior wall fracture/dislocation remains an indication for formal open reduction and internal fixation using a buttress plate, with or without supplemental lag screw or spring plate fixation.

The surgeon contemplating percutaneous fixation of any acetabular fracture must be mindful that these techniques have not yet been validated in randomized clinical trials. The early clinical results of percutaneous fixation have been extremely encouraging, both in decreasing hospital stay and morbidity in longitudinal studies, and in case reports for selected fractures.[3–7] Although patients will generally opt for less invasive surgical techniques when given a choice, they should be informed that this technique is currently viewed as an experimental procedure. These techniques should be performed only by experienced acetabular fracture surgeons, in the event that a change in surgical plan and conversion to an open procedure is necessary. A thorough knowledge of the nuances of pelvic osseous and soft tissue anatomy is necessary to plan trajectories and safely place percutaneous screws; advanced appreciation of radiographic anatomy is essential when relying on nonstandard fluoroscopic projections to provide guidance. The surgeon must always be prepared to revert to a formal open approach in the event of inadequate imaging or inadequate reduction for percutaneous technique. It is unlikely that an inadequately reduced fracture treated with percutaneous technique will ever have better outcome than a well-reduced fracture treated with standard open technique, in the absence of complications related to the approach.

22.2 **3D (CT based) vs. 2D (fluoroscopy based) surgical navigation for pelvic and acetabular fractures**

A 3D-CT CAOS system became available for spine surgery in the early 1990s (Stealth Station, Sofamor-Danek, Memphis, TN). With minor software and instrument modifications, this system was first adapted for pelvic and acetabular fracture fixation in 1996. Approval for clinical use was granted in 1997 following accuracy validation in a cadaver study.[8,9]

The 3D-CT based CAOS technology proved to be very versatile in planning novel screw trajectories for pelvic fracture fixation, and also proved to provide exceptional accuracy during execution of the preoperative plan. Surgical plans could be defined and stored preoperatively by identifying precise entry and target points for screws on the virtual 3D model. The preoperative planning software helped to define safe pathways for screw placement in many applications about the pelvis. Early work showed that this technology provided sufficient accuracy to place both iliosacral screws and percutaneous screws for fixation of the acetabular columns.[8,10] Optimal accuracy was obtained by attaching an external fixator with spherical aluminum fiducials to the patient prior to obtaining the CT. When coupled with an external fixator for registration, the 3D-CT technique provided exceptional accuracy (Fig. 22.1). In actual clinical use for posterior pelvic ring fixation, both operative time and fluoroscopic time were significantly reduced when compared to standard fluoroscopic technique, and there were no screw malpositions noted.[10]

Although 3D-CT guidance remains a powerful clinical tool, the applications of this technology in fracture care were relatively limited, as a three-dimensional model had to be 'built' using CT data obtained prior to surgical fracture reduction. The model could not be easily updated to provide guidance for fixation following fracture reduction. In general, fractures could be stabilized using 3D-CT guidance only if they were minimally displaced, or if a closed reduction could be obtained and maintained with an external fixator prior to obtaining the preoperative CT scan. Surgeons were concerned about performing a separate surgical procedure for attachment of the fiducial array prior to obtaining the CT. As such, this technology found only limited utility in selected applications about the pelvis and

(a) 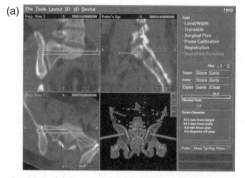   (b)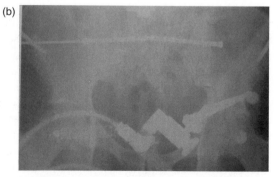

Fig. 22.1 (a) Screen output with stored surgical plans for placement of bilateral iliosacral screws for stabilization of bilateral sacroiliac joint disruptions, following closed reduction with an external fixator. The 3D-CT model is visible at lower right, and the navigation views show the planned path of screw placement in two orthogonal planes. A third plane is perpendicular to the path of the screw. The 3D-CT technique provided exceptional accuracy; (b) tip-to-tip accuracy in screw placement intra-operatively. This patient also had percutaneous stabilization of a transverse acetabular fracture with lag screws.

acetabulum.[7–10] It could not be easily adapted to long bone applications, or to any application where bone fragments would be manipulated after the CT scan was performed. Nonetheless, the experience gained in performing percutaneous fixation of selected acetabular fractures proved invaluable in later adapting the newer virtual fluoroscopy systems to percutaneous fixation. The screw pathways defined in clinical cases from 1997 to 1999 are still used in the newer virtual fluoroscopy applications.

Virtual fluoroscopy (fluoroscopic navigation) was refined and approved for clinical use in 1999. Before this time, the distortion inherent in analog C-arm images prevented their use in surgical navigation. Software algorithms were developed for powerful computer workstations that allowed them to rapidly warp the C-arm images to make them optically correct and allow their use for guidance. The surgeon uses a standard C-arm unit to harvest multiple two-dimensional images in the operating room. A camera tracks the position of the C-arm unit during image acquisition and the images are warped, stored, and displayed on a workstation. Up to four individual stored images may be displayed at any one time. The camera can then track special instruments (such as a drill guide) and display their position relative to each of the stored images. The need for the time consuming 'registration' step is eliminated in this newer technology. In addition, the virtual model could be easily updated at any point during the procedure by simply obtaining new images. The surgeon may be well away from the surgical field during image acquisition, and there is no radiation exposure to patient or surgeon during surgical navigation. The arrival of virtual fluoroscopy greatly broadens the potential applications of CAOS in orthopaedic trauma. Computer assisted technique may now be applied to essentially any orthopaedic procedure that traditionally relies on intra-operative fluoroscopy for guidance.

The development of virtual fluoroscopy has expanded the applications of CAOS to essentially all procedures that have traditionally required intra-operative fluoroscopy for fracture reduction or positioning of implants. For the first time, CAOS techniques could be applied to routine long bone fracture management, and are no longer limited to the spine and pelvis.[11] Newer angle/distance features in the software packages facilitate planning and execution of osteotomies for joint realignment and correction of deformity. The systems have proven to be well suited to a variety of pelvic and acetabular fracture applications, including minimally invasive techniques that were first made possible by the 3D-CT technology. The newest systems are entirely surgeon driven, using a touch screen interface that eliminates the need for an unscrubbed assistant or technical support staff (Fig. 22.2). Replacement of the previous mouse driven (or so called 'shout and click') interface has led to improved acceptance of

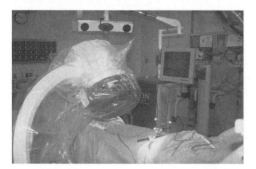 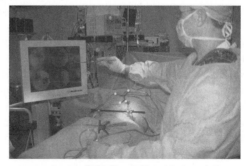

Fig. 22.2 The figures depict a modern virtual fluoroscopy system in use (iON-FluoroNav, Medtronic/ Smith + Nephew, Memphis, TN). A reference frame has been attached to an anterior pelvic fixator, and the C-arm has been retrofitted with a calibration target that allows the camera to track the C-arm. The touch screen interface is more surgeon-friendly than the previous mouse-driven interface. The surgeon is manipulating navigation images using a sterile stylet.

this technology in the operating room, both on the part of surgeons and nursing staff. In the author's practice, the newer virtual fluoroscopic navigation has now essentially replaced the 3D-CT technology.

When using virtual fluoroscopy for surgical navigation during implant placement, it is essential that the surgeon take the time to harvest adequate images. The surgeon must be very familiar with radiographic anatomy in a variety of customized oblique imaging planes, particularly when working around the pelvis and the columns of the acetabulum. Image quality in pelvic applications is sometimes compromised by patient obesity, bowel gas, or retained intra-abdominal contrast. In many applications, it is difficult logistically to obtain the two ideal orthogonal images perpendicular to the path of intended drilling and fixation, leading to increased reliance on nonstandard oblique radiographic projections. In all applications, the surgeon must have the diligence to ensure that the images are adequate to safely proceed. In the event that adequate fluoroscopic images cannot be obtained, the surgeon must have the discipline to abandon the surgical navigation and use an alternative method. The surgeon then has the responsibility to either proceed with formal open reduction, or consider 3D-CT technique at a separate operative sitting.

CAOS equipment and instruments are costly, and financial considerations will likely hinder widespread acceptance in the short term. Nonetheless, the technology offers substantial potential benefits, including improved accuracy, decreased operative time, and decreased invasiveness. The greatest benefit, however, may lie in decreasing the orthopaedic surgeon's reliance on intra-operative ionizing radiation for guidance during surgery. Radiation exposure to the surgeon's body and hands is essentially eliminated using CAOS techniques.

22.3 Iliosacral screws (posterior pelvic ring disruption: SI joint, sacral, or crescent fracture)

This application is particularly well suited for virtual fluoroscopy. The surgeon initially reduces the pelvic ring using closed methods (traction, external fixator, or Schanz pin joystick), and confirms adequate reduction with C-arm images. It is helpful to maintain the reduction with either a temporary external fixator or a 2.8 mm wire passed from the ilium into the sacral ala. Multiple images are then harvested and stored on the computer workstation. Up to four images are used; the author prefers to use AP, inlet, outlet, and oblique lateral views for intra-operative guidance. The oblique lateral view is oriented such that it is parallel to the path of intended screw fixation. The trajectory feature is used to identify the optimal starting point on the skin, and the drill guide is passed bluntly down to the ilium. The ideal trajectory into the center of the S1 body is chosen in all four views, and a guide wire is drilled to the appropriate depth using the trajectory length feature. Confirmatory images are obtained, and the cannulated screw is then passed over the guide wire. In the author's experience, fluoroscopic time is reduced by over 50%, total surgical time (including setup) is decreased, and the first pass of the guide wire has been acceptable in nearly every case. Rare instances of intraosseous pin deflection have been observed, and mandate that confirmatory images be obtained prior to actually passing the screw over the guide wire. There have been no complications or screw malpositions noted in over 30 individual screw placements using virtual fluoroscopic technique.[12]

22.4 Pelvic ring disruption

Bony disruption of the pelvic ring may often be managed using percutaneous technique, provided that an acceptable reduction can be obtained and maintained during imaging. It has not yet proven possible to safely stabilize a pure symphyseal disruption percutaneously. Nonetheless, it has often been possible to stabilize many osseous anterior and posterior ring injuries using large diameter cannulated screws. This is usually done in the supine position using a retrograde anterior column screw for the anterior ring, and an 'LCII screw' for the posterior ring.

The retrograde screw starts just inferior and lateral to the ipsilateral pubic tubercle, and courses through the superior pubic ramus across the fracture and just anterior/superior to the hip joint. A 7.3 mm screw can usually be used in male patients; safe passage of this screw is sometimes impossible in female patients, and the surgeon must be prepared to perform an open reduction in such cases. Obturator/outlet and iliac/inlet views are helpful, although standard Judet views may be adequate for navigation. A true AP is always used to provide initial orientation in almost all applications.

The LCII screw starts at the anterior inferior iliac spine, passing through the broad column of bone just above the acetabulum, coursing above the sciatic notch, and terminating near the posterior iliac spine adjacent to the sacroiliac joint. Standard Judet and inlet views are used for this screw, although an image should optimally be obtained in line with the planned trajectory of the screw as well.

22.5 Screw trajectories for specific acetabular fracture patterns

In general, anterior column, posterior column, transverse, and anterior column/posterior hemitransverse fractures are best suited for percutaneous technique, provided an acceptable closed reduction or lag screw reduction can be performed. Both column fractures with good secondary congruity can also be stabilized *in situ*, particularly in elderly patients. It has not yet been possible to safely reduce and stabilize posterior wall fractures with percutaneous technique. Excluding posterior wall fractures, almost 50% of acetabular fractures at the author's home institution are now treated percutaneously, and clinical outcomes are being monitored.

22.5.1.1 The high anterior column acetabular fracture

These coronal plane fractures traverse the superior weight bearing dome of the acetabulum, exiting through the iliac wing. Abdominal and gluteal muscle forces frequently cause significant displacement. The anterior fracture fragment, including a variable portion of the weight-bearing dome, is typically displaced cephalad, but may be reduced by application of longitudinal traction. The fragment is usually externally rotated and sometimes medialized as well. Schanz pin joysticks are used to manipulate the fracture, and reduction is maintained by application of a temporary external fixator. Reduction is assessed using Judet iliac and obturator oblique views. In the event of an unsuccessful closed reduction with an external fixator, a limited lateral window ilioinguinal exposure provides sufficient access for improvement of reduction.

For virtual fluoroscopic navigation, four individual radiographic projections are stored on the image guided surgery workstation. Anteroposterior, inlet and Judet views provide sufficient information for safe screw placement; the obturator oblique Judet view may be angled cephalad or caudad so that the C-arm is oriented in line with the intended path of screw placement. A true lateral of the pelvis is often helpful as well, but is difficult to obtain in the obese patient. The fracture is stabilized using two 7.3 mm cannulated screws passed over 2.8 mm guide wires placed just inferior to the anterior superior iliac spine. The first screw is similar to the LCII screw, and the second starts at the anterior inferior iliac spine and is angled toward the ischial spine (Fig. 22.3). During the past ten years, the author has stabilized over 20 high anterior column fractures using this technique. There has been no case of loss of reduction or development of arthrosis to date. The average HHS hip score at two year follow up is 91.[13] The average post-surgical hospital stay for patients with isolated injuries treated percutaneously has been two days. Percutaneous technique may prove to be the treatment of choice for this particular fracture pattern.

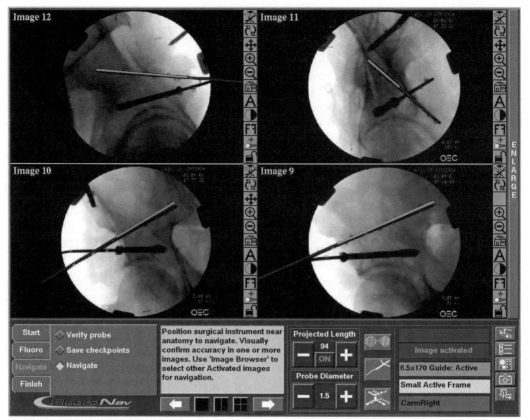

Fig. 22.3 A high anterior column acetabular fracture is reduced intra-operatively with a temporary external fixator. Two screws placed in standard trajectories are then used to stabilize the fracture. In the navigation views for virtual fluoroscopy, the drill guide is represented as a red line, and the predicted trajectory in green is superimposed on the actual position following guide wire placement. (See Plate 7.)

22.5.1.2 Transverse acetabular fractures

Nondisplaced fractures with worrisome roof arcs, and displaced fractures reducible with lateral traction are amenable to percutaneous internal fixation. A lateral traction (distraction) external fixator may be applied using Schanz pins placed in both greater trochanters. Residual gap displacement is often reducible using a lag screw placed perpendicular to the fracture line. True AP and true lateral views are usually sufficient for lag screw placement. Additional screws may be placed into the anterior column using antegrade or retrograde technique, and into the posterior column using retrograde technique through the ischial tuberosity (Fig. 22.4). The ideal radiographic views for surgical navigation are still evolving, but in general the surgeon should strive to obtain two orthogonal views perpendicular to the intended path of fixation. Anterior column/posterior hemitransverse fractures are stabilized with a lag screw and an LCII screw.

22.5.1.3 Posterior column fractures

Fractures of the posterior column are usually associated with subluxation or dislocation of the femoral head. Occasionally, an acceptable closed reduction can be obtained by simply reducing the

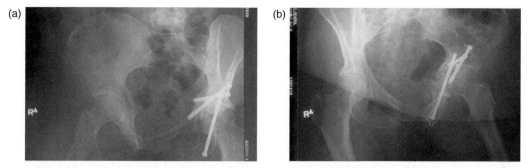

Fig. 22.4 Judet views (a and b) of a transverse acetabular fracture nonunion stabilized with a lag screw, an antegrade anterior column screw, and a retrograde posterior column screw.

hip dislocation, or by applying a distraction frame. The fracture may be stabilized by placing a long cannulated screw from just inferior to the ASIS, passing posterior to the hip joint to engage the dense cortical bone in the region of the ischial spine.

22.6 Reduction of radiation exposure to patient and surgeon

Ionizing radiation exposure is probably an underappreciated risk for both trauma surgeons and trauma patients. Reduction of radiation exposure to patient and surgeon is a tangible advantage of using computer assisted technique, rather than standard fluoroscopy, for placement of fixation screws. One minute of intra-operative fluoroscopy about the pelvis is equivalent to about 40 mSv (4 Rads, 4,000 mRem) of radiation, or approximately equivalent to 250 chest X-rays or a CT scan of the pelvis.[14] The careful surgeon absorbs very little direct radiation during fluoroscopic imaging, but is still subject to scatter from the patient's anatomy; the patient absorbs most of the radiation dose. In actual practice, surgeons frequently place their hands in the radiation beam, especially during fracture reduction and freehand locking of intramedullary nails. The Occupational Safety and Health Administration's guidelines recommend no more than 50 rem per year of hand exposure, and this corresponds to only 12 minutes of fluoroscopy time per year.[15] It is quite possible for an orthopaedic surgeon to exceed this threshold.

Measurable health effects can occur at much lower doses of radiation. For example, air travel above 30,000 feet results in a slight increase in background radiation exposure, due to reduced atmospheric absorption of gamma and X-irradiation. Career high-altitude airline pilots receive about 3–6 mSv of radiation over environmental background (0.6–2.0 mSv) per year, or about twice the dose received by the general population. This small additional radiation dose would be equivalent to about 10–15 seconds of fluoroscopy about the pelvis or hip. It is distressing to note that pilots have a fivefold increase in myeloid malignancies and a threefold increase in skin cancers when compared to the population at large.[15] Although the skin cancer risk may be related to increased sun exposure, increased background radiation exposure is felt to be responsible for the hematopoietic malignancies.

22.7 Conclusion

Virtual fluoroscopy, a new development in the field of CAOS, has numerous potential applications in the field of orthopaedic trauma. Using this technique, cannulated screws may be precisely placed within the pelvis using only a few individual fluoroscopic images. This versatile technology has supplanted 3D-CT technique in the author's practice. Despite the need for specialized equipment and instruments, this technology has the potential to greatly decrease the orthopaedic surgeon's reliance on intra-operative ionizing radiation during the performance of minimally invasive surgery. With improved acceptance by the orthopaedic community, virtual fluoroscopy may eventually replace real-time C-arm fluoroscopy in orthopaedic practice. The decreased invasiveness and improved accuracy of CAOS holds the potential to improve outcomes in pelvic fracture management when compared to standard operative technique.

References

1 Olson SA, Matta JM. The computerized tomography subchondral arc: a new method of assessing acetabular continuity after fracture (a preliminary report). *J Orthop Trauma* 1993;7:402–13.

2 Tornetta P III. Nonoperative management of acetabular fractures: the use of dynamic stress views. *J Bone Joint Surg Br* 1999;81-B:67–70.

3 Gay SB, Sistrom C, Wang G-J, Kahler DM, Boman T, Goitz HT, McHugh N. Percutaneous screw fixation of acetabular fractures with CT guidance: preliminary results of a new technique. *Am J Radiol* 1992;158:819–22.

4 Kahler DM, DeGrange D, Wang G-J. Percutaneous fixation of selected acetabular fractures using computed tomographic (CT) guidance. *Presented at American Academy of Orthopaedic Surgery Annual Meeting*, 1996, February 24. Atlanta, GA.

5 Parker PJ, Copeland C. Percutaneous fluoroscopic screw fixation of acetabular fractures. *Injury* 1997;28:597–600.

6 Starr AJ, Reinert CM, Jones AL. Percutaneous fixation of the columns of the acetabulum: a new technique. *J Orthop Trauma* 1998;12(1):51–8.

7 Zura RD, Kahler DM. Case report: a transverse acetabular nonunion successfully treated with computer assisted percutaneous internal fixation. *J Bone Joint Surg* 2000;82-A:219–24.

8 Kahler DM, Zura R. Evaluation of a computer-assisted surgical technique for percutaneous internal fixation in a transverse acetabular fracture model. *Lect Notes Comp Sci* 1997;1205:565–72, Springer.

9 Kahler DM. Computer assisted fixation of acetabular fractures and pelvic ring disruptions. *Techn Orthop* 2000;10(1):20–4.

10 Kahler DM, Mallik K. Computer assisted iliosacral screw placement compared to standard fluoroscopic technique. *Comput Aided Surg* 1999;4(6):348.

11 Kahler DM. Virtual fluoroscopy: a tool for decreasing radiation exposure during femoral intramedullary nailing. *Poster Presentation. American Academy of Orthopaedic Surgery Annual Meeting*, March 2001. San Francisco, CA.

12 Kahler DM, Mallik K, Tadje J. Computer-guided percutaneous iliosacral screw fixation of posterior pelvic ring disruption compared to conventional technique. *Presented at 5th North American Program on Computer Assisted Orthopaedic Surgery*, July 7, 2001. Pittsburgh.

13 Johanson NA, Charlson ME, Szatrowski TP, Ranawat CS. A self-administered hip-rating questionnaire for the assessment of outcome after total hip replacement. *J Bone Joint Surg Am* 1992;74:587–97.

14 Agarwal SK. Ionizing radiation exposure during orthopaedic and radiologic procedures at the University of Virginia. Unpublished data, 1998.

15 Mehlman CT, DiPasquale TG. Radiation exposure to the orthopaedic surgical team during fluoroscopy: 'How far away is far enough?' *J Orthop Trauma* 1997;11(6):392–8.

Chapter 23

Hip trauma

Roger Phillips, Amr M. Mohsen, Warren Viant, and
Kevin Sherman

23.1 Clinical challenges

23.1.1 Fixation devices in hip trauma surgery

Fractures of the proximal femur, hip and pelvis are among the most frequent dealt with by orthopaedic surgeons. This chapter focuses on the proximal femur where the fracture sites may be classified as shown in Fig. 23.1. Extracapsular fractures may be treated by *compression hip screw* internal fixation. Undisplaced intracapsular fractures may be treated by *cannulated screw* or by compression hip screw internal fixation. Displaced intracapsular fractures are often treated by hemiarthroplasty for the elderly, but for young patients cannulated screw fixation is preferred in order to preserve the femoral head. A common denominator of compression hip screw and cannulated screw devices is that both pass through the neck and head of the femur at a predetermined angle. A primary functional aim of Computer Assisted Orthopaedic Surgery (CAOS) is the accurate and effective placement of these fixation devices.

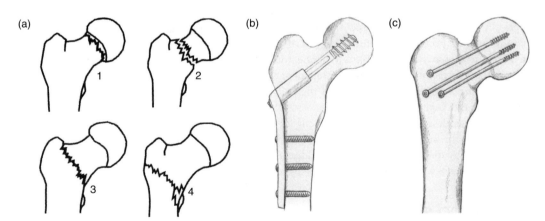

Fig. 23.1 (a) Classification of proximal femur fracture sites: (1) subcapital-intracapsular, (2) transcervical-intracapsular, (3) intertrochanteric-extracapsular along base of neck, (4) petrochanteric-extracapsular. (b) Internal fixation with compression hip screw. (c) Internal fixation with three cannulated screws.

23.1.2 **Shortfalls of hip trauma surgery**

The incidence of hip fractures is increasing as the life expectancy of the population is increasing. Melton *et al.*[1] reports that the lifetime risk of a hip fracture is 17.5% and 6% of white women and men, respectively. It is also estimated that in the United States there over 200,000 intertrochantic fractures a year and hip fractures account for 30% of all hospitalized patients.[2] For these reasons many have called hip fractures an orthopaedic epidemic.

The traditional surgical approach for hip trauma surgery has many shortfalls. Positioning a guide wire or screw is a trial and error approach; this is undesirable as it prolongs operation time, increases tissue damage and it relies on surgical expertise. As each try involves fluoroscopic imaging, both the patient and the surgical team are exposed to additional, but potentially unnecessary, radiation. Non-optimal placement of the fixation device may also affect the mechanical stability of the femur.[3] Furthermore Flores *et al.*[4] report that failure of fixation is a significant complication of the treatment of unstable intertrochanteric fractures.

It is clearly desirable to improve surgical techniques to avoid these shortfalls as complications contribute to the high morbity and mortality rate of hip fracture patients where between 15% and 20% die as a result of these fractures.[2] CAOS techniques offer the opportunity to address shortfalls of existing hip trauma surgery and thus improve healthcare delivery.

23.1.3 **Review of CAOS approaches to proximal femur fractures**

This chapter describes a computer assisted system for hip trauma surgery known as CAOSS (Computer Assisted Orthopaedics Surgical System). A recent alternative CAOS approach for hip trauma surgery that is starting to gain acceptance is known as Virtual Fluoroscopy (VF).[5] Fluoroscopic imaging with a C-arm image intensifier is used extensively in traditional proximal femur trauma surgery. VF extends the capability of image intensification by producing virtual images of the patient and surgical tools without radiation. Current VF systems include Medtronic Sofamor Danek's Fluoronav™ and Medivision's SurgiGATE.

In VF systems a number of images of the operation site are taken using a C-arm image intensifier; the C-arm may then be removed from the operation site. The position of a surgeon's tool is tracked optically through attached reference frames. This allows the computer to overlay a real time projection of the tool on previously captured images. By attaching an optically tracked frame (known as a dynamic reference frame—DRF) to the bone, tools can be overlaid onto images even when the bone moves. In VF systems the normal arrangement is that the C-arm is tracked optically by attaching IREDs to the X-ray receptor housing of the C-arm. An image calibration plate is also permanently attached to the X-ray receptor.

This chapter describes next the components of CAOSS and explains how CAOSS is used to implant compression hip screw and cannulated hip screws. It then reports on the status of clinical studies. It concludes by discussing how CAOSS addresses the surgical shortfalls of hip trauma surgery and compares CAOSS with VF systems.

23.2 **System description**

23.2.1 **Classification of CAOSS**

CAOS systems may be classified in terms of diagnosis, surgery planning, registration of plan with patient and implementation of surgical plan. CAOSS is classified below under these categories.

Hip fractures are diagnosed with plain radiographs, and where the diagnosis is inconclusive other imaging modalities (e.g. MRI, CT, etc.) may be used. Surgical planning for CAOSS uses intra-operative fluoroscopic images. CAOSS creates a 3D surgical plan by reconstructing information from a pair of fluoroscopic images. The surgical plan space for CAOSS is in the coordinate space of an optical tracking system. The patient is registered with this surgical space by mapping the fluoroscopic image space onto the surgical planning space. The key step in implementing the surgical plan is drilling a hole into the proximal femur. CAOSS uses a passive lockable approach for this. The surgeon, under computer guidance, positions an optically tracked guiding cannula that is locked in position with a passive arm whilst the surgeon drills.

23.2.2 Important surgical concepts

23.2.2.1 Basic orthopaedic principle

A basic principle of orthopaedic surgery relevant to hip trauma is the 'placement of an object (guide wire, screw, tube or scope) at a specific site within a region, via a trajectory which is planned from X-ray based 2D images and governed by 3D anatomical constraints'.[6]

The current traditional method for implementation of this *basic orthopaedic principle* is a scientific trial and error—best guess with expertise acquired on a long learning curve. The accuracy and safety of the procedures depends on a surgeon's judgement, experience, ability to integrate images, utilization of intra-operative vision systems, knowledge of anatomical and biomechanical constraints and dexterity. Hence the implementation of the basic orthopaedic principle is technically demanding, time consuming and operator dependent.

23.2.2.2 Compression hip screw

The compression hip screw is a cannulated screw and plate combination (Fig. 23.1b). The screw must be positioned accurately so that it passes through the neck into the femoral head and terminates in subchondral bone close to, but a safe distance from, the hip joint surface.

In traditional surgery, the fracture is first reduced. Anteroposterior (AP) and lateral fluoroscopic images are taken with a C-arm image intensifier to confirm appropriate reduction of the fracture. A lateral incision exposes the bone and the surgeon partly inserts a guide wire through a hand-held jig at the predetermined appropriate position. Correctness of position is checked by further fluoroscopic images and additional attempts are made to insert a guide wire correctly. Each extra attempt weakens the bone structure, exposes both patient and surgeon to additional radiation and prolongs the operation. Once the guide wire is positioned, it is overdrilled and the cannulated screw is slid over the guide wire and screwed into the femur neck and head. The screw support plate is then fitted to the screw and fastened to the femoral shaft.

23.2.2.3 Cannulated hip screws

It is common practice to use three cannulated screws for the fixation of an intracapsular neck of femur fracture. The three cannulated screws should be placed along parallel trajectories through the lateral femoral cortex, the femoral neck and into the femoral head (Fig. 23.1c). A good spread of the screws within the bony structure is bio-mechanically desirable to provide stability to the fracture.

The traditional surgical approach involves reducing the intracapsular fracture using both AP and lateral fluoroscopic images. The first guide wire is inserted and its position confirmed by fluoroscopic imaging. The position of the guide wire is adjusted and reinserted. This process is repeated for the other two guide wires. A cannulated drill is passed over each of the guide wires to enlarge the hole and the cannulated screws are inserted. The procedure can be performed either as an open or percutaneous technique. Most surgeons require multiple attempts to achieve a favorable position, and often the position is not optimal.

23.2.3 Patient positioning and surgical exposure

For both hip trauma operations under consideration, the patient is positioned in the conventional manner with the leg firmly held in a boot. Reduction of the fracture and exposure of the operation site follows the traditional approach.

23.2.4 Positioning of the CAOSS equipment in the operating theatre

The CAOSS equipment comprises a CAOSS trolley, an optical tracking system, an optically tracked end-effector attached to a lockable passive arm, a registration phantom and various guiding cannulas. The CAOSS trolley (Fig. 23.2) houses the main PC-based computer system, the computer system for the optical tracker, a monitor, an isolated power supply and a frame grabber which has a video feed from the C-arm image intensifier. CAOSS is designed to work with any modern image intensifier.

The optical tracking system uses a two camera array that tracks the position of InfraRed Emitting Diodes (IREDs) in 3D space. The camera array is mounted on the theater laminar flow enclosure next to the pole used for draping and out of the sterile field. The camera is between 60 and 100 cm above the operation site.

The end-effector and passive arm are rigidly mounted to the side bar of the operating table using a standard Maquet clamp (Fig. 23.3). This assembly is on the sterile side of the drape. The passive arm is proprietary equipment and its two ball and hinge joints are lockable via a single twist handle. The position of this end-effector is tracked by an arrangement of seven IREDs attached to the end-effector.

The end-effector is used by the surgeon to position the registration phantom and to position the guiding cannulas. It is manufactured from PEEK (polyetheretherketone), thus it is autoclavable, largely radiolucent, and lightweight.

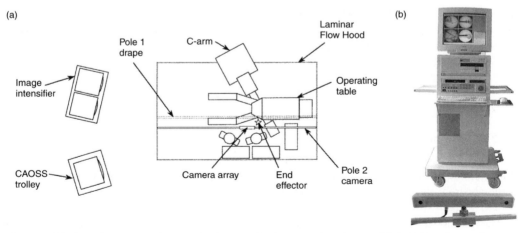

Fig. 23.2 (a) Plan of CAOSS equipment deployment in the operating theater. (b) CAOSS trolley and camera array.

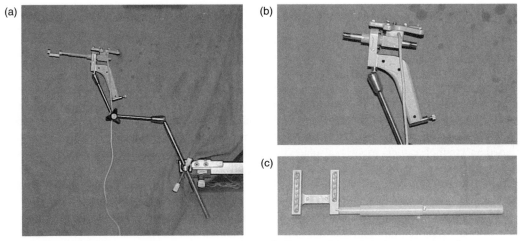

Fig. 23.3 (a) CAOSS equipment set-up showing the end-effector with registration phantom; the end-effector is held by a lockable passive arm which is attached to the operating table using a Maquet clamp. (b) The end-effector with guiding cannula. (c) The registration phantom.

The guiding cannula has a sharp serrated end and this allows good purchase on soft tissue and bone during drilling. To drill into bone, a secondary (inner) cannula is inserted inside the outer cannula.

23.2.5 Calibration and registration

The image guidance principle of CAOSS is to extract 2D anatomical features from fluoroscopic images and reconstruct them to produce a surgical plan in 3D. This plan is created in the coordinate space of an optical tracking system. To achieve this requires, firstly, accurate 2D calibration of fluoroscopic images and, secondly, accurate registration of the fluoroscopic image space with the coordinate space of the tracking system.

23.2.5.1 2D Calibration of X-ray images

Fluoroscopic images suffer from a number of distortion effects, such as pincushion, S shaped distortion, etc.[7,8]. The amount of image distortion is dynamic both in time and with the position of the C-arm. A major factor of this dynamic variation of distortion is the strength and orientation of the magnetic fields surrounding the C-arm. Sufficient image accuracy for trajectory planning is obtained by calibrating in just two positions, i.e. with the C-arm axis vertical and horizontal.

Calibration involves preoperative imaging of an X-ray translucent grid containing an evenly spaced grid of 64 × 64 balls. This calibration plate is placed on the X-ray receptor cover of the C-arm and an image taken. Software automatically detects the grid and calculates a distortion-undistortion map that is filed. Intra-operatively, CAOSS removes the distortion from each fluoroscopic image before using it for planning and before displaying it to the surgeon. This calibration need only be performed monthly.

23.2.5.2 Registration of fluoroscopic image space

This registration involves accurate determination of the position (in the coordinate space of the optical tracking system) of the X-ray source and the virtual image plane (i.e. the grid plane of the calibration plate) of the C-arm. This registration occurs for each fluoroscopic image taken of the patient.

Registration is achieved by placing a small registration phantom (Fig. 23.3c) in the image space of the C-arm and as close as possible to the patient. For an AP image the phantom is placed between the X-ray receptor and the patient. For a lateral image the phantom is placed between the X-ray source and the patient. To assist positioning of the phantom for lateral images, a laser cross showing the center of the image beam is projected onto the patient.

The phantom consists of an H arrangement of 21 metal balls whose projection appear in a fluoroscopic image. The phantom is held in an end-effector whose position is tracked optically. When a patient is imaged, software undistorts the image and then automatically detects the position of the phantom in the image. Then knowing the optical position of the phantom, a registration algorithm (based on a pinhole camera model) calculates the position of the C-arm in the coordinate space of the optical tracking system. Significant obscuration of the phantom frequently occurs in the image due to shadow of muscles, bone edges, retractors, etc., but the phantom extraction software is resilient to such obscuration.

The registration technique compensates for C-arm flex and the linear elements of dynamic distortion. A C-arm span can typically flex between 1 and 5 mm and this results in a change of orientation between the X-ray source and the X-ray receptor.

23.2.6 Intra-operative surgical planning and simulation

The same anatomical features are used for planning the position of both compression hip screws and cannulated screws. Computer-based planning uses an AP and a lateral fluoroscopic image of the fracture site taken after fracture reduction. The anatomical features used are the shaft axis of the proximal femur and the femoral neck and head.

An assistant in theater identifies these three anatomical features on the two images with a mouse. The femur shaft is identified by six points on the lateral side and one point on the medial side; each side of the neck is identified by three points; and the head is identified by six points. The 2D projection of the femur shaft axis and the femoral neck and head centers is then determined. These 2D projections are then reconstructed to create a 3D surgical plan.

23.2.6.1 Surgical planning of compression hip screw

The computer plans a trajectory for the guide wire of the compression hip screw by constructing a 3D line from a way point in the femoral head that intersects with the femoral shaft axis at the same angle as the hip screw and plate (typically 115° to 135°). The way point is taken to be one quarter distant along the 3D line joining the center of the head with the center of the neck. This trajectory is then overlaid on both AP and lateral images (Fig. 23.4). The depth of the drill hole is also calculated as part of the surgical plan. The surgeon reviews the suggested guide wire trajectory and, if necessary, modifies it using three controls. The entry point of the guide wire on the femur shaft may be moved anteriorly/posteriorially, and the way point in the femoral head may be moved anteriorly/posteriorially and laterally/medially.

23.2.6.2 Surgical planning of cannulated screws

The computer plans parallel trajectories for the three cannulated screws by first constructing a common direction for all the trajectories.[9] This direction is calculated to maximize the amount of bone mass the three screws penetrate. Based on this direction, the computer then plans the three parallel trajectories for maximum separation, whilst ensuring both adequate bone clearance and clinical validity. The computer achieves adequate bone clearance by matching the partial anatomical data from two fluoroscopic images with a generic anatomical model of the femoral neck region. The surgeon can

(a)   (b)

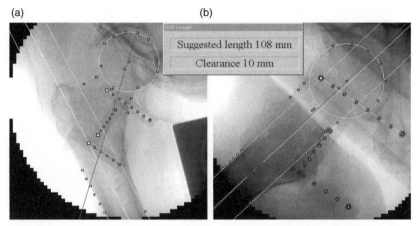

Suggested length 108 mm

Clearance 10 mm

Fig. 23.4 (a) AP and (b) lateral fluoroscopic image for compression hip screw planning. Both figures show: identification points for the femoral shaft, neck and head, the planned trajectory for the guide wire, the projection and detection of the registration phantom (note that in the lateral image 5 of the 21 markers of the registration phantom are obscured). The figure also shows the suggested length of the guide wire.

review and adjust the clinical parameters and observe the resulting trajectory plans overlaid onto the fluoroscopic images of the femoral neck region.

23.2.7 Surgical implementation of the intra-operative plan

CAOSS uses a passive approach to implement the intra-operative surgical plan for both operations. To insert a guide wire the surgeon positions a guiding cannula using guidance displayed by the computer. This guiding cannula is mounted in the end-effector that is optically tracked and held by a passive arm. When the surgeon achieves the desired position for the cannula, the arm is locked and this holds the end-effector and cannula rigidly in place. The surgeon then uses a standard orthopaedic drill to implant the guide wire along the planned trajectory (Fig. 23.5a). Progress on insertion of the guide wire may be checked by fluoroscopic imaging.

To position the cannula the surgeon first moves the cannula's tip across the cortex of the bone until the required entry point is reached. The cannula is then pivoted about this entry point to achieve the desired angular approach. The computer guides (Fig. 23.5b) the surgeon by a quantitative and a graphical indication of the movements required.

Minimizing drill whip and drift is essential to achieve accurate and reproducible results when using CAOSS. A toothed cannula is used that grips the bone and this reduces drill whip and drift.

23.2.8 Ergonomics

The ergonomics of the CAOSS approach are good. Additional equipment is introduced into the operating theater at a readily acceptable level. At the operation site a conveniently placed optical camera tracks surgical tools and a passive arm helps the surgeon position tools. Currently, a separate trolley houses the two computer systems and a monitor, but increasing miniaturization and integration of image guidance functionality into the fluoroscope equipment would improve considerably floor space

(a)

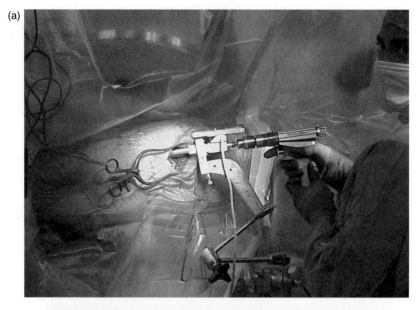

(b)

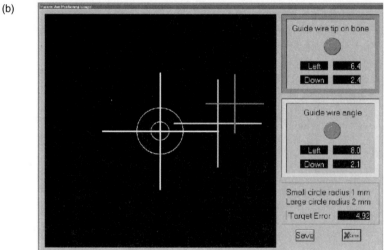

Fig. 23.5 (a) Implementation of guide wire according to surgical plan; the guiding cannula is held in place by the end-effector and locked passive arm. (b) The computer display that guides the surgeon in positioning the guiding cannula prior to drilling; once in position the passive arms is locked.

ergonomics. There is scope to reduce surgeon-computer interaction and to improve reproducibility of outcome by automatic detection of anatomical features in fluoroscopic images.

23.2.9 Safety

CAOSS was designed specifically for clinical use; thus the end-effector, passive arm, registration phantom and cannula are all sterilizable to requisite EC standards. Also all electrical and electronic components have been designed and satisfactorily tested to meet all the requisite EC electrical and electromagnetic radiation standards for medical equipment.

As CAOSS is a passive system the surgeon is always in full control of the equipment. The surgeon can take fluoroscopic images at key stages to confirm that image guided implementation is proceeding correctly.

23.2.10 Validation and accuracy

There has been extensive validation and evaluation of CAOSS. It has included software simulation, performance evaluation of system components, extensive laboratory trials (in excess of 200 trials) on plastic sawbones and laboratory trials on butcher's specimens.

The design of the registration phantom was developed using extensive computer simulation that modelled the fluoroscopic image intensifier and the propagation of errors. The design simulation was used to determine the best trade-off between optimizing reconstruction performance and the clinical requirements of being as unobtrusive in fluoroscopic images and as small as possible.

In terms of CAOSS components, tests have shown that an image has a maximum calibration error of 0.5 mm. It has also been shown that using the passive arm and guidance system that the entry point on the bone is typically positioned with an error of less than 0.7 mm whilst the angle position of error on the bone is less than 0.2°. This positioning is typically achieved within 30 seconds.

The CAOSS system has been validated with a number of plastic bone and butchers' specimen trials. In a trial of 10 plastic bones the accuracy of guide wire placement in the femoral head had a worst case error of 2.6 mm and a mean error of under 0.5 mm. This error represents total system error and it includes drill drift and whip. The results were measured with a coordinate measurement machine (accuracy better 0.02 mm).

23.3 Comparison of CAOSS with other approaches to hip trauma surgery

23.3.1 Traditional surgery

CAOSS provides a right first time approach to insert a guide wire whereas traditional surgery uses a trial and error approach. Also the placement of a guide wire using CAOSS is less dependent on surgical expertise.

The pair of fluoroscopic images used for surgical planning in both traditional and CAOSS approaches are not true AP and lateral views. In traditional surgery this increases variability of guide wire placement. CAOSS is less effected as the actual 3D positions of views are parameters in the surgical plan calculation.

23.3.2 Early CAOS approaches

CAOSS differs from typical CAOS systems for hip trauma of the early to mid 1990s in the following ways.

1 CAOSS software produces a surgical plan based on anatomical features whereas the surgical plan in earlier systems was simply drawn on images by the surgeon.

2 In CAOSS (and other recent CAOS systems) there have been improvements in calibration, registration and position tracking techniques that have led to improved overall accuracy of fluoroscopic image guided surgery.

3   CAOSS uses a passive arm to help the surgeon maintain the tool / guide wire on the surgical plan; this considerably reduces the fiddle-factor of the hand-held tool approach of many early CAOS systems.

Consequently surgical performance using CAOSS is more reproducible and easier to assess. This improved reproducibility is important for prospective outcome analysis.

23.3.3 Virtual fluoroscopy systems

The VF systems have a permanently mounted grid attached to the camera for image calibration and registration of the image space with the optical tracking system. This leads to the following differences with CAOSS.

1   The optically tracked volume for CAOSS is close to the operation site and it interferes very little with the set-up in operating theaters. For VF systems the tracked volume is very much larger as the X-ray receptor has to be tracked through a 90° vertical rotation of the C-arm and it is more likely to interfere with theater set-up, for example interference with vertical sterile drapes. CAOSS also suffers less from losing line of sight for tracking, as the tracked volume is very much smaller.

2   For CAOSS there is significantly less image obscuration. In CAOSS just 21 opaque markers of the registration phantom appear in just one portion of the image whereas in VF the whole image is splattered by markers. However, in some VF systems many of the markers in the image are replaced by their surrounding background; this is undesirable.

3   In CAOSS the registration phantom has to be manually placed in the image space. This is an extra step compared to VF and occasionally multiple images are required to achieve correct placement.

Typically in VF the implementation of a surgical plan is by hand-held tools. The CAOSS approach of a lockable passive arm is preferable as it removes the fiddle-factor and improves surgical reproducibility.

In the hip trauma operations considered by CAOSS there is minimal movement of bones at the operation site. Thus a dynamic reference frame (DRF) is not required to track bone movement as is the case for VF systems. However, if bone movement is detected then replanning of the guide wire may be required.

Another difference concerns the approach to image calibration. In CAOSS, images are calibrated in two positions preoperatively. In VF systems the image is calibrated intra-operatively with every image of the patient. Compared to VF systems, CAOSS's calibration is more precise (due to a denser calibration grid), interferes less with surgical intervention but some affects of dynamic distortion remain. These effects are minimal as the rotation and translation aspects of dynamic distortion are taken account of by CAOSS's registration technique. Others have calibrated preoperatively the C-arm image intensifiers in a large number of positions.[10,11] For each intra-operative image the calibration parameters of the closest preoperative calibrated position is used. This approach has drawbacks of being cumbersome, time consuming and it does not handle fully the temporal aspects of dynamic distortion.

23.4 Clinical trials

23.4.1 Pilot clinical studies

CAOSS has been developed collaboratively between the University of Hull and the East Yorkshire Hospitals Trust.[12,13] In 1999, CAOSS received Medical Device Agency approval for a single-centered clinical trial in the United Kingdom. A complete CAOSS is installed in an operating theater at the Hull Royal Infirmary. A Philips BV 29 image intensifier is being used for the clinical trials of CAOSS.

Clinical trials have been approved to evaluate the effectiveness of CAOSS for insertion of compression hip screws and insertion of cannulated hip screws. For each a double blind trial is planned involving 70 patients in each trial. The outcomes of the CAOSS approach will be evaluated by analysis of measures of implant position, operation time, X-ray dosage, blood loss, post-operative complications, hospital stay, etc. Post-operative evaluation will be by clinical and radiograph assessment at 6, 12 and 26 weeks.

CAOSS was first used in the operating theater in May 2000. CAOSS has been used so far in 15 operations. Data from these sessions has been closely analyzed and minor adjustments made to CAOSS concerning image processing, surgical planning, computer guidance for positioning, etc. It is too early in the pilot study to quantify benefits.

23.5 Discussion

23.5.1 Acceptance of CAOS for hip trauma surgery

The aim of CAOS systems for hip trauma surgery is to improve healthcare in the broadest sense. Potential benefits of computer assisted systems to orthopaedic surgery are well established.[14,15] CAOS for hip trauma surgery is important because of the following potential benefits:

(1) improved patient outcome (e.g. more accurate fixator placement, less implant failures, less revision surgery, and less morbidity);

(2) improved treatment (less radiation to patient and surgeon, less blood loss, reduced operating times and hospital stay, less tissue damage);

(3) improved surgical procedures (reduced invasiveness);

(4) enables development of new fixation devices which take advantage of CAOS's ability to position implants accurately;

(5) reduces the skill level (e.g. dexterity, mental 3D reconstruction, etc.) required for surgery; this should reduce training costs and improve outcomes.

These benefits address the shortfalls identified at the start of the chapter.

Some CAOS systems such as CAOSS calculate a surgical plan using 2D projection of anatomical features from 2D images to form a 3D surgical plan. The surgical plan is thus dependent on the anatomical variation of patients and the pose of the patient in the image. These dependencies need further study.

A barrier to the acceptance of CAOS in hip trauma surgery is cost justification. The cost of hip trauma is relatively low and patient outcomes are generally considered acceptable even though there are numerous shortfalls. The introduction of CAOS would probably increase direct costs of operations. However, the long term healthcare benefits of using CAOS, the very large volume of hip trauma surgery and the wide applicability of image guided fluoroscopy will probably overcome the cost justification barrier.

23.5.2 Challenges for the future

Achieving clinical efficacy for CAOS systems is challenging due to the hostile environment of the operating theater (e.g. sterilisation, ergonomics, cost, safety), the multitude of skills required to develop them, and the novel and technically complex nature of CAOS systems. Developments in technology and innovative ways of integrating technologies are, slowly but surely, providing clinically acceptable image guidance systems that are able to produce real benefits for patients and healthcare providers.

Future developments of CAOSS and VF systems for hip trauma surgery include: image processing to reduce unnecessary surgeon/system interaction, more ergonomic and accurate position tracking (ideally without line of sight constraint between tracked object and sensor) and improved ways of drilling.

The introduction of digital C-arm fluoroscopes will improve CAOS for hip trauma. These have flat X-ray digital receptor plates instead of image intensification tubes. These plates improve image resolution and reduce image distortion. C-arms need to be better designed to reduce the imaging effects caused by flex. C-arms also need to be designed from the outset for more effective and less obtrusive position tracking.

A further challenge is closer integration and standardization between fluoroscopic imaging and image guidance. For example a C-arm image intensifier could provide all the computing facilities for fluoroscopic image guidance with image guidance software being loaded from CDROM or over the Internet.

Whereas CAOS provides better ways of treating hip trauma injury, a major orthopaedic challenge is to reduce the incidence of hip trauma by preventive treatments such as bisphosphonate treatment for osteoporosis.

23.6 **Summary**

C-arm image intensifiers are extensively used in traditional hip trauma surgery. They were designed to provide qualitative images during surgery. Through image calibration and registration of image space, they are able to provide a quantitative imaging capability. This has led to a number CAOS systems based on fluoroscopic image guidance being developed and used clinically for hip trauma surgery. These systems typically support intra-operative surgical planning and guidance to implement this plan. These systems are in their infancy and future developments will undoubtedly lead to improved patient care and improved implants.

References

1 Melton LJ, III Chinchville EA, Cooper C, *et al*. How many women have osteoporosis? *J Bone Min Res* 1992;7:1005–10.

2 Crenshaw AH, ed. *Campbell's operative orthopaedics*, 8th edn. St Louis, Mosby Year Book; 1992.

3 Wu CC, Shih CH. Biomechanical analysis of the dynamic hip screw in the treatment of intertrochanteric fractures. *Arch Orthop Trauma Surg* 1991;110:307–10.

4 Flores LA, Harrington IJ, Heller M. The stability of intertrochanteric fractures treated with a sliding screw—plate. *J Bone Joint Surg Br* 1991;72:37–40.

5 Hofstetter R, Slomyczykowski M, Sati M, Nolte L-P. Fluoroscopy as an imaging means for computer-assisted surgical intervention. *Comput Aided Surg* 1999;4:65–76.

6 Mohsen AMMA, Sherman KP, Cain TJ, *et al*. End user issues for a surgical computer—robotic assisted systems. *Trans Institut Measure Contr* 1995;17:265–71.

7 Boone JM, Seibert JA, Blood W. Analysis and correction of imperfections in the image intensifier TV-digitiser imaging chain. *Med Phys* 1991;18:236–42.

8 Pietka E, Huang HK. Correction of aberration in image intensifier systems. *Comput Med Imag Graphics* 1992;16:253–8.

9 Viant WJ, Phillips R, Mohsen A. Computer assisted positioning of cannulated hip screw. In: Lemke HU, Vannier MW, Inamura K, Farman AG, eds. *CARS'99 Computer assisted radiology and surgery*. Amsterdam: Elsevier, 1996;751–5.

10 Brack C, Burgkart R, Czopf A, *et al*. Accurate X-ray-based navigation in computer-assisted orthopaedic surgery. In: Lemke HU, Vannier MW, Inamura K, Farman AG, eds. *CAR'98 Computer assisted radiology and surgery*. Amsterdam: Elsevier, 1998;716–22.

11 Fahrig R, Moreau M, Holdsworth DW. Three-dimensional computer tomographic reconstruction using a C-arm mounted XRII: correction of image intensifier distortion. *Med Phys* 1997;24:1097–106.

12 Mohsen AMMA, Cain TJ, Sherman KP, *et al*. The CAOS projects. *First International Symposium on Medical Robotics and Computer Assisted Surgery*, 1994:49–56. Pittsburgh.

13 Phillips R, Viant WJ, Mohsen AMMA, *et al*. Image guided orthopaedic surgery—design and analysis. *Trans Institut Measure Contr* 1995;17:251–64.

14 Taylor RH, Lavallee S, Burdea GC, Mosges R, eds. Orthopaedics. In: *Computer-integrated surgery technology and clinical applications*. Cambridge: MIT Press, 1996:371–2.

15 Mohsen AMMA (1995). A non invasive intelligent orthopaedic guide: concepts, issues and efficacy assessment. PhD Thesis, University of Hull, Hull, UK.

Chapter 24

Long bone trauma

Norbert Suhm

24.1 Clinical challenges

24.1.1 Intra-operative guidance with the C-arm fluoroscope

There is a trend towards less invasive, percutaneous techniques in the operative treatment of long bone fractures. The concept includes closed fracture reduction with correct alignment of axes, rotation and correct reconstruction of bone length without open surgical exposition of the fracture site. The former concept of open fracture reduction and plate fixation accepted large skin incisions and dissection of muscles to allow the surgeon direct view on the fracture site. As percutaneous osteosynthesis techniques respect the important role of soft tissues in fracture healing, these techniques suggest improved outcome from both the aesthetic and the functional point of view.[1]

Since the view through small skin incisions are limited, percutaneous osteosynthesis techniques increase the demand for intra-operative fluoroscopy to determine the position of anatomy, surgical tools and implants relative to one another; to monitor the advance of guide wires and drills; and to make corrections if necessary.[2]

Intra-operative C-arm fluoroscopy fails to provide direct visual feeback because fluoroscopic images are static two-dimensional (2D) projections. Reconstruction the spatiotemporal intra-operative situation based on such projections may be difficult for the surgeon. The need to rotate the fluoroscope to visualize different planes makes fluoroscopy a burdensome tool that prolongs the operation times. The simultaneous use of two C-arm fluoroscopes would disable the surgeon`s access to the patient. Long fluoroscopy times are responsible for relevant exposure of the surgeon and the patient to radiation.[3] Moreover X-rays fail to visualize soft tissues and cartilage.

Operative technique and requirements to the C-arm fluoroscope have changed a lot from former open fracture reduction and plate fixation to percutaneous, image guided osteosynthesis techniques. However the C-arm fluoroscope has not yet been adapted to these needs. Some of the problems mentioned above can be solved by applying surgical navigation techniques to orthopaedic surgery.

24.1.2 Computer-assisted osteosynthesis of long bone fractures

Surgical navigation systems, as currently used in various surgical disciplines, make use of three-dimensional preoperative tomographic image data sets for visualization. Their application in orthopedic surgery was therefore limited to spine surgery and pelvic ring surgery, where preoperative CT data are commonly acquired.[4,5] Development of systems for fluoroscopy based image-interactive navigation made it possible to apply surgical navigation technology to the treatment of long bone fractures.[6]

Virtual fluoroscopy makes the fluoroscope a tool which allows surgeons to manipulate the bony structures and implants as if they were getting multi-planar continuous fluoroscopic feedback. Use of stored intra-operative fluoroscopic views for visualization saves fluoroscopy time and therefore limits radiation exposure. Continuous multiplanar intra-operative guidance may increase the accuracy of the surgical procedure. As the C-arm fluoroscope can be removed from the patient after the initial image acquisition, it no longer obstructs the operating room for the remainder of the procedure.

Virtual fluoroscopy therefore adapts the C-arm fluoroscope to provide intra-operative guidance during image guided osteosynthesis techniques.

24.2 **Virtual fluoroscopy**

24.2.1 **Definition**

Virtual fluoroscopy refers to a surgical navigation technique that is based on intra-operative fluoroscopic images. The images are used to continuously visualize the spatial relationship between referenced major bone fragments or the referenced implant and referenced surgical tools in multiple views. The clinical demand is approximation of multiplanar life fluoroscopy by continuous repositioning the surgical tool's projection within multiple stored fluoroscopic views.

24.2.2 **Important concepts**

The application of virtual fluoroscopy requires computer equipment, a C-arm fluoroscope, and tracking equipment. Software performs the mathematical transformation underlying virtual fluoroscopy: a projection from three-dimensional intra-operative space into stored plane fluoroscopic images. Input data required are fluoroscopic image data, the C-arm fluoroscope's imaging geometry, position data from tracking and geometric data from the surgical tools.

A standard C-arm is used to obtain fluoroscopic images as input image data. Nonlinear image distortion is corrected. The imaging geometry of the C-arm fluoroscope is calibrated by introducing a calibration kit into the X-ray beam. Since both geometry and position of the kit are predetermined, the representation of any spatial point within the imaged volume in the plane fluoroscopic image is available for the navigation system. This procedure replaces the registration procedure required by other types of surgical navigation system.

The fluoroscope, anatomical structures, implants and surgical tools need to be equipped with position sensors to allow for position definition by the system's tracking unit. Most surgical navigation systems use optoelectronic position sensors for tracking.

Geometric data from the surgical instruments are established during instrument calibration and are stored in the system. These data are needed for correct simulation of the tool geometry, e.g. the position of the drill's tip. Any change of tool geometry after instrument calibration requires recalibration to achieve a correct simulation.

For intra-operative application the fluoroscope is prepared in the usual manner and may be draped for sterile use. During image acquisition both the reference of the object to navigate on and the reference attached to the C-arm fluoroscope need to be visible for the tracking unit. This allows definition of the spatial relationship between the imaged object and the projection plane. Any relative movement between the object's reference base and the object itself after image acquisition would destroy this essential relationship and would require to repeat image acquisition.

Referenced surgical tools are applied to the patient during the procedure. Both the objects DRB and the surgical tool's DRB need to be visible for the tracking unit. The system calculates the tool's projection within the stored fluoroscopic images. As all calculations are based on relative position data there are no limitations for relative movements between the tracking unit and the objects with attached DRBs.

Virtual fluoroscopy is adapted to clinical needs as it is very close to the current clinical procedure. Application of the technique requires minimal preoperative preparations. Equipment requirements are moderate because most of the surgical instruments can be used without change but only need to be referenced. As the system does not need a preoperative CT-study, a registration procedure does not have to be performed and the surgeon does not depend on the cooperations, e.g. with the radiology department to apply virtual fluoroscopy.

24.2.3 Surgical technique

We used the SurgiGATE system with the C-arm Navigator Module (Medivision, Oberdorf, Switzerland) for intra-operative guidance during percutaneous osteosynthesis such as intramedullary nailing or screw fixation. In all applications the system was used to guide the implants to the ideal position.

All computation processes run on a SUN ULTRA 1 workstation (Sun Microsystems, Inc.). A standard Philips BV 29 C-arm fluoroscope (Philips Medical Systems, Best, The Netherlands) was prepared for use with virtual fluoroscopy by attaching a reference shield to the image intensifier component. The calibration procedure to acquire the C-arm's imaging geometry is performed once prior to the first use of the SurgiGATE system and the data are stored within the system. Other systems for virtual fluoroscopy repeat acquisition of data on the imaging geometry with every fluoroscopic shot. This concept requires the calibration kit to be included within the X-ray beam. The distance in between X-ray source and image intensifier where the patient is placed during image generation is therefore reduced.

The SurgiGATE system applies an optoelectronic position sensor (Optotrack 3020, Northern Digital, Waterloo, Ontario Canada) for tracking. Position reference units are equipped with infrared light emitting diodes (LEDs). Optoelectronic tracking technology demands a line of sight between the DRB and the tracking unit. The LEDs are triggered from the navigation system via a cable connection (:= active marker technology). Passive marker technology does not require cable connection between the DRB and the navigation system which improves intra-operative handling.

The SurgiGATE's user interface is adapted to the hands occupied—eyes occupied situation in modern image guided orthopaedic surgery. A virtual keyboard gives the surgeon complete control of the C-arm navigator via a sterile interface. Up to four projections can be used simultaneously to control the position of the active surgical tool.

24.2.3.1 Intra-operative guidance by virtual fluoroscopy for distal interlocking

In one clinical application we applied intra-operative guidance by virtual fluoroscopy for drilling the distal locking holes during intramedullary nailing osteosynthesis.

Though locked nailing is a standard surgical technique in the operative treatment of diaphyseal fractures, insertion of distal interlocking bolts remains technically demanding. Mechanical or fluoroscopic guidance are commonly applied to pass the drill through the interlocking hole. For mechanical guidance methods, the precision of bolt placement is typically problematic; for fluoroscopic guidance methods, the fluoroscopic time is the issue. Applying virtual fluoroscopy to drill the holes for distal locking suggests improvements in these two points.[7]

The intra-operative setup as position of the computer cart, tracking device, C-arm fluoroscope and nail reference base varied with the fracture to be treated and with the type of implant used. Principally the computer cart should be placed opposite to the surgeon in order to guarantee direct view of the computer screen. The tracking unit should be positioned behind the surgeon to secure visibility of all reference bases during image acquisition and drilling the interlocking holes. Guidance is required in a single plane for distal interlocking and the nail is the object to target at.

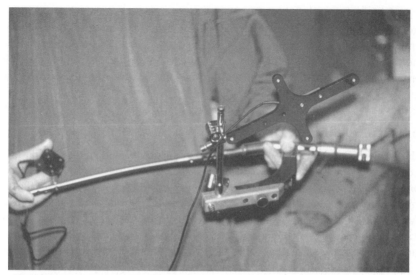

Fig. 24.1 Collecting procedure during computer assisted distal locking. The nail DRB (cross shaped) is rigidly attached to the insertion handle. The referenced nail pointer is inserted in the distal locking holes and the configuration is presented towards the tracking unit (not visible).

Computer assisted distal locking of intramedullary implants was performed in two steps:

First, computer controlled precision alignment of the fluoroscope. Proper alignment of the fluoroscope prior to image acquisition is an essential prerequisite for successful distal locking: after implantation into the medullary canal of the long bone the implant's locking holes must be imaged as perfect circles. To perform computer controlled precision alignment of the fluoroscope, the nail reference base was rigidly connected with the nail insertion handle prior to implantation. The position of the interlocking holes and the orientation of their longitudinal axis relative to the nail reference base were tracked and transferred to the workstation: the referenced nail pointer tool was inserted into the locking holes and this configuration was tracked by the digitizer (see Fig. 24.1). These positional data were visualized in a computer animation to guide the radiology technician during positioning the fluoroscope after nail insertion into the medullary canal prior to image acquisition. A single fluoroscopic shot was transferred to the SurgiGATE system.

Second, drilling interlocking holes with online visual control (see Fig. 24.2). The drill-bit was calibrated for the actual position within the referenced driver. When the referenced driver approached the interlocking holes, its actual position is projected into the fluoroscopic image that was displayed on the workstation screen.

The position of the interlocking holes is defined at the skin level and a 1.5 cm stab wound is made. The drill bit was moved along the surface of the bone until the simulated drill tip was projected into the center of the distal interlocking hole. The entrance point was fixed by pushing the drill's tip into the bone. Next, the longitudinal axis of the drill was aligned parallel to the axis of the interlocking hole and the length measuring algorithm was initiated. After penetration the bone's second cortex, the length measuring algorithm was stopped and the distance passed by the drill was displayed. Thus the correct length of the interlocking bolt could be determined.

Clinical evaluation included recording precision of the interlocking procedure, fluoroscopy time and procedure time needed for computer assisted distal locking. Problems with technical equipment during the procedure were reported.

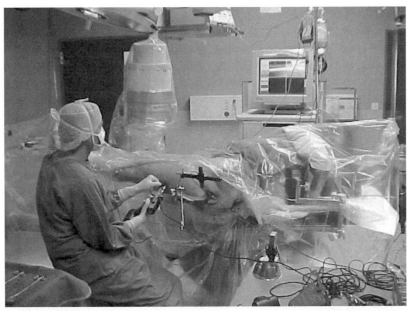

Fig. 24.2 Computer assisted distal locking of a PFN^R implant. The cross-shaped nail DRB is attached to the insertion handle. The referenced drill is moved along the bone surface. The actual drill's position is projected into the stored fluoroscopic images on the computer screen in front of the surgeon. The C-arm fluoroscope is removed from the patient.

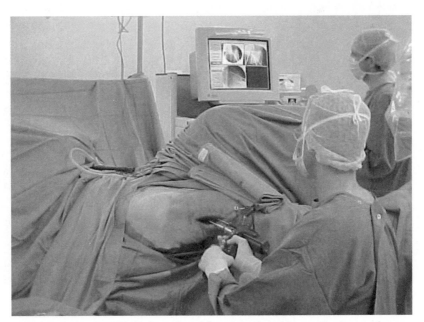

Fig. 24.3 Guidewire placement with biplane virtual fluoroscopic guidance. The bone reference and the referenced driver are visible for the tracking unit (not visible). The C-arm fluoroscope is removed from the patient.

24.2.3.2 Virtual fluoroscopy for guidewire placement

In a second application, intra-operative guidance by virtual fluoroscopy was applied to place guidewires during DHS implantation to stabilize pertrochanteric femoral fractures and during screw fixation of femoral neck fractures. In these applications simultaneous guidance in multiple views is required and the proximal femoral bone is the referenced object to target at.

The principle is to perform fracture reduction and temporary fracture fixation with Kirschner wires. Next, the DRB is fixed to a Schanz screw that is inserted into the proximal femoral bone through a stab wound. Anterior-posterior and axial fluoroscopic shots of the proximal femoral bone are acquired, transferred to the navigation system and the C-arm fluoroscope is removed from the patient (see Fig. 24.3).

The entrance point and axis of the guidewire is simulated and thus can be corrected simultaneously in both fluoroscopic image planes (see Fig. 24.4). Correct guidewire placement was verified fluoroscopically prior to implant insertion.

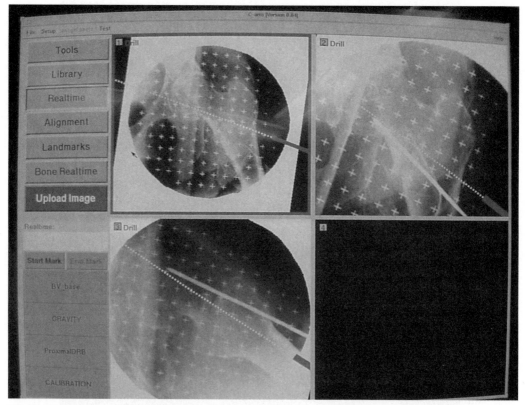

Fig. 24.4 Virtual fluoroscopy for guidewire placement for DHS osteosynthesis of a pertrochanteric femoral fracture. A Kirschner wire was inserted for temporary fracture fixation. Position of the central guidewire is simulated as a red bar and dotted line in an anterior-posterior and axial view simultaneously. See Plate 8.

24.2.4 **Laboratory test series**

Prior to clinical application of virtual fluoroscopy, the method was assessed in laboratory tests series. Sixty interlocking procedures of intramedullary implants were performed with an artificial bone model in an operating room setting. For simulation of distal interlocking, we made use of plastic models of human femora (Synbone, Davos, Switzerland) and the original proximal femoral nail (PFN[R], Stratec, Oberdorf, Switzerland) as the implant. We observed a 100% hit rate in the laboratory test series. Slight contact between the drill and the implant was reported in three out of 60 interlocking procedures. These test series demonstrated superior accuracy of the SurgiGATE system from a technical point of view.

A second laboratory study evaluated virtual fluoroscopy in the application for guidewire placement. 120 guidewires were placed in 40 artificial bone models simulating a femoral neck fracture. Sixty guidewires were placed in 20 bone models with computer guidance by virtual fluoroscopy and 60 guidewires were placed in 20 bone models with fluoroscopic guidance. The bone model was fixed and for computer guidance, a DRB was attached. Fluoroscopic shots showing the femoral neck in anterior-posterior and axial views were generated and were transferred to the navigation system. The guidewires were placed with continuous biplanar guidance.

For guidewire placement with fluoroscopic guidance, the C-arm fluoroscope was positioned in an anterior-posterior projection and the guidewire was correctly aligned in this projection plane. As the second step, guidewire alignment was checked and adapted in the second axial plane. As a third step correct position in the anterior-posterior plane had to be verified. After correct alignment had been achieved in both planes with this iterative procedure, the guidewire was inserted in the bone. The procedure was repeated with the second and third guidewire.

The procedure time needed to place three guidewires was similar with both methods (14.2 min fluoroscopic guidance versus 15.3 minutes virtual fluroscopy) but the fluroscopy time needed was significantly reduced with virtual fluoroscopy (0.43 min fluoroscopic guidance versus 0 min virtual fluoroscopy). All bone models were subject of CT imaging and three-dimensional reconstruction. Precision of guidewire placement was rated to be equivalent with both methods by a blind observer.

The test series described above simulate the intra-operative procedure but they fail to simulate the effects of soft tissues. It has to be clearly stated there is a very important difference between a system for virtual fluoroscopy being applied in a laboratory setup and clinical application of such system. The laboratory test series report on application of the method under optimized conditions. The main goal of the test series is to identify improvements that increase the accuracy achieved. In routine clinical practice, surgical navigation is applied under nonstandardized conditions, for example limited visibility of the DRB or poor image quality. Clinical evaluation requires to determine how accurate the input has to be to ensure success of this technique.

24.2.5 **Comparison with traditional techniques**

Application of virtual fluoroscopy for intra-operative guidance does require very few changes of the traditional surgical technique. This may be looked upon as the most important advantage of virtual fluoroscopy against other surgical navigation techniques.

In both applications exact preoperative planning of the intra-operative setup was useful to ensure good visibility of all reference bases at any step of the procedure.

Secure attachment of a DRB to the object to target at is uniquely required.

Additional steps have to be performed if surgical tools with variable geometry are applied with virtual fluoroscopy. For example variable length of the drill bit was calibrated prior to drilling the distal locking holes.

24.3 **Clinical trials**

24.3.1 **Pilot study with virtual fluoroscopy applied for guidewire placement**

The applications described above are subject of clinical evaluation within defined studies. In a pilot study computer guidance was successfully applied for guidewire placement in 11 patients with proximal femoral fractures. In seven patients the guidewire for a Dynamic Hip Screw (DHS, Stratec, Oberdorf, Switzerland) could be placed exactly within the femoral neck during osteosynthesis of pertrochanteric femoral fractures (see Fig. 24.3, 24.4). In four patients guidewires were placed for fixation of femoral neck fractures with canulated screws. No intra-operative problems occurred during these early clinical applications.

24.3.2 **Controlled prospective clinical study on guidance methods for distal interlocking**

Computer assisted distal locking was evaluated in a controlled clinical study with two branches. Patients in both branches were divided into control group and study group. For patients diagnosed with pertrochanteric femoral fractures (study branch 1) distal locking was performed with mechanical guidance in the control group and with virtual fluoroscopy in the study group. For patients diagnosed with diaphyseal fractures of the lower extremity (study branch 2) distal locking was performed with fluoroscopic guidance in the control group and with virtual fluoroscopy in the study group.

Virtual fluoroscopy required significantly shorter fluoroscopy time than fluoroscopic guidance ($p < 0.0001$) but in both branches caused a significant increase of the procedure time (virtual fluoroscopy versus mechanical guidance: $p < 0.0001$; virtual fluoroscopy versus fluoroscopic guidance: $p = 0.029$) and in the number of intra-operative problems compared with the standard guidance techniques. The learning curve indicates these problems are due to the novelty of virtual fluoroscopy: all problems observed with computer guidance occurred within the first 23 patients treated. The procedure time needed with virtual fluoroscopy approached to the procedure time needed with fluoroscopic guidance (see Table 24.1).

Table 24.1 Results of the controlled prospective clinical study on guidance methods for distal locking. In study branch 1 (grey) virtual fluoroscopy was compared with mechanical guidance. In study branch 2 virtual fluoroscopy was compared with fluoroscopic guidance. The accuracy achieved while drilling the interlocking holes was rated as misplaced interlocking hole/drilling the hole with contact to the implant/drilling the hole without contact to the implant

Guidance method	Virtual fluoroscopy	Mechanical guidance	Virtual fluoroscopy	Fluoroscopy
Patients (N)	26	24	25	19
Procedure time (min)	38	6.5	17	12.5
Fluoroscopy time (s)	6	6	6	107
Intra-operative Problems	4	2	3	1
Accuracy	(2 / 8 / 35)	(1 / 13 / 31)	(2 / 11 / 28)	(1 / 9 / 31)

24.4 **Discussion**

1. The goal of virtual fluoroscopy is to provide intra-operative guidance in order to improve efficiency of image guided orthopedic procedures while minimizing radiation exposure to both patient and surgeon.

2. Virtual fluoroscopy has to be evaluated with controlled clinical studies. The principles of evidence based medicine require a clear statement a new method improves therapy before it is applied in routine clinical practice. Duration of the follow up period needed for proper evaluation depends on the specific application. All parameters describing the effect of intra-operative guidance by virtual fluoroscopy for distal locking of intramedullary implants can be protocolled intra-operatively. Therefore follow up visits were not necessary to obtain final results in our controlled study on guidance methods for distal locking. Virtual fluoroscopy applied for guidewire placement in percutaneous screw fixation of femoral neck fractures needs a long term follow up, e.g. to evaluate the rate of post-operative femoral head necrosis as a relevant parameter to describe the success.

3. Our controlled clinical study on computer guidance by virtual fluoroscopy for distal locking demonstrated that this new technique significantly reduces fluoroscopy times. As distal locking of intramedullary implants requires guidance in a single plane, this clinical model is not able to demonstrate all the advantages offered by virtual fluoroscopy such as simultaneous multiplanar guidance. Virtual fluoroscopy applied for guidewire placement in a laboratory setup demonstrated the potential of the method to reduce procedure times, and the potential to increase precision of implant placement with decreased fluoroscopy times.

4. Virtual fluoroscopy is well adapted to standard techniques in orthopedic surgery. Without need for additional imaging or intra-operative registration it allows the surgeons to navigate the bony structures as if they were getting multiplanar continuous fluoroscopic feedback, without the X-ray exposure or the multiple C-arms. However, as fluoroscopic views are used for visualization, problems related to lack of soft tissue visualization and to limited three-dimensional modeling remain unsolved.

   There have been attempts to apply CT based surgical navigation methods to long bone trauma. From a clinical point of view preoperative CT evaluation of long bone fractures is justified for complex and intra-articular fractures. As CT-based systems use a preoperative CT study to create a 3D anatomical model these systems require an intra-operative registration procedure. The FRACAS system[8] uses intra-operative fluoroscopic images to register the preoperative CT model to the intra-operative situation based on the bone surface model and its projection in the fluoroscopic images.

   The option for intra-operative generation of three-dimensional image data sets is available with the latest generation of C-arm fluoroscopes. Integration of such data sets into the concept of virtual fluoroscopy will supply three-dimensional bone models from the fracture site without the need for preoperative CT studies.

   In order to address the increasing awareness about the important role of soft tissues in fracture healing, further imaging modalities have to be evaluated for intra-operative use. NMR might be the technology to allow online intra-operative guidance in three-dimensional anatomic models with visualization of bony structures and concomitant nerve or vascular lesions.

5. Virtual fluoroscopy and other systems for surgical navigation add new equipment into an already crowded operating theater. Nowadays navigation systems fail to integrate preexisting technologies and to offer the surgeon a single interface for communication with all equipment in the operating room.

   For example virtual fluoroscopy establishes only unidirectional communication with the C-arm fluoroscope to generate input image data. To become clinically useful the submillimetric precision we achieve with navigation in these fluoroscopic images requires similar precision for projection plane definition. But the C-arm fluoroscope is still moved manually within the operating room for any projection adjustment. This is time consuming as the radiologic technician acts as an interface between surgeon and C-arm fluoroscope.

6. Future work will have to integrate the C-arm fluoroscope as part of the navigation system by establishing bidirectional communication with the imaging unit. The MEPUC (Motorized Exact Positioning Unit for C-Bow, pat. pend.) concept allows the surgeon control on motorized movements of the C-arm along all axis of motion. Exact position data are generated with the tracking unit and are used for automatic motorized precision alignment of the C-arm fluoroscope. Thus the localization ability of the tracking unit becomes useful for positioning the C-arm fluoroscope and for acquisition of precise projections. The MEPUC adapts the C-arm to modern image guided orthopedic procedures, as it enables the surgeon to independently manipulate the imaged region.

Technical development of the existing virtual fluoroscopy modules will allow application for intraoperative guidance during minimal invasive plate osteosynthesis and for fracture reduction.

From a clinical point of view controlled clinical studies have to be initiated to evaluate virtual fluoroscopy in various applications. Multicenter studies will be helpful to acquire the numbers of patients needed for significant data.

24.5 **Summary**

Virtual fluoroscopy may be regarded as a first step to adapt the C-arm fluoroscope to the needs of image guided orthopedic surgery. Integration of three-dimensional fluoroscopic image data and improving the interface between C-arm fluoroscope and surgeon with the MEPUC concept will provide a system perfectly adapted to image guided fracture treatment.

References

1 Baumgaertel F, Buhl M, Rahn BA. Fracture healing in biological plate osteosynthesis. *Injury* 1998;29 (Suppl. 3):C3–6.

2 Sanders R, Koval KJ, DiPasquale T, Schmelling G, Stenzler S, Ross E. Exposure of the orthopaedic surgeon to radiation. *J Bone Joint Surg* 1993;75-A:326–30.

3 Suhm N, Jacob AL, Nolte LP, Regazzoni P, Messmer P. Surgical navigation reduces radiation doses during closed intramedullary nailing. In: Lemke HU, Vannier MW, Inamura K, Farman AG, Doi K, eds. *Computer assisted radiology and surgery. Proceedings of the 14th International Congress and Exhibition.* 2000:262–6. Amsterdam: Elsevier.

4 Laine T, Schlenzka D, Mäkitalo K, Tallroth K, Nolte LP, Visarius H. Improved accuracy of pedicle screw insertion with computer-assisted surgery. *Spine* 1997;22(11):1254–8.

5 Langlotz F, Bächler R, Berlemann U, Nolte LP, Ganz R. Computer assistance for pelvic osteotomies. *Clin Orthop Rel Res* 1998;354:92–102.

6 Hofstetter R, Slomczykowski M, Sati M, Nolte LP. Fluoroscopy as an imaging means for computer-assisted surgical navigation. *Comput Aided Surg* 1999;4:65–76.

7 Suhm N, Jacob AL, Nolte LP, Regazzoni P, Messmer P. Surgical navigation based on fluoroscopy— clinical application for computer-assisted distal locking of intramedullary implants. *Comput Aided Surg* 2000;5:391–400.

8 Joskowicz L, Milgrom C, Simkin A, Tockus L, Yaniv Z. FRACAS: a system for computer-aided image-guided long bone fracture surgery. *Comput Aided Surg* 1998;1998(3):271–88.

Chapter 25

Accuracy and validation

Andrew B. Mor, Branislav Jaramaz, and
Anthony M. DiGioia III

25.1 Introduction

Validation of a system's performance is very important to users of CAOS systems, and is an area in which no standardization has yet occurred. While all CAOS systems promise increased accuracy, and the possibility of less invasive surgery, the surgeon's reliance on the system, especially when coupled with reduced exposure, requires that the CAOS system be thoroughly characterized and tested to ensure that it achieves its advertised accuracy under operating room conditions. The characterization of system performance must be tested at all steps of a procedure in which the CAOS system is utilized, from preoperative imaging to surgical intervention.

Although no standard methodology or minimum accuracy thresholds exist for the testing of CAOS systems, researchers and developers have performed tests and reported results on system level and subsystem level accuracy testing. These tests have ranged from detailed testing of passive tracking systems to end-to-end tests of complete systems, with results reported in a variety of formats and reference frames.

Individual subsystem tests examine a particular component or methodology and determine the distribution of errors present in the results generated by that subsystem. They normally cover the wide range of variation in conditions and inputs that could conceivably be encountered in use, and ideally, variation beyond that which would typically be seen. The testing of the individual subsystems provides a very detailed examination of the characteristics of some components of a CAOS system, and can aid the developer of the system, as well as other researchers and clinicians who wish to use only a portion of a CAOS system for another procedure. Statistical results, if in similar reference frames, can also be combined to provide a rough estimate of the overall accuracy of the complete system, although there are likely to be unmodeled effects in the complete system that aren't represented in the subsystem testing.

End-to-end, or overall, testing of a complete CAOS system will yield accuracy results that will encompass the sum of the individual subsystems of the overall system, and any user interactions that may not be accounted for by individual subsystem testing. Testing results would include values on how close to the desired ideal result was the navigated result, expressed both in absolute terms and a statistical distribution of test results. The end result of this type of testing would be the variation a surgeon might expect to see in clinical practice, a very important consideration when selecting a CAOS system. The outcome of these accuracy tests will provide surgeons and researchers with the data needed to evaluate the differences between systems and their suitability for meeting the requirements of a particular application.

While individual subsystem tests are important for evaluating relative performance and highlighting the location of deficiencies in the system, they are not sufficient to fully characterize a system. Similarly, while end-to-end tests that validate the overall performance of a CAOS system are necessary, they are also insufficient for determining areas of decreased performance within a system that could be improved or where a more careful interaction is needed. A combination of the two testing methodologies, subsystem and end-to-end, in addition to post-operative evaluations, is necessary to fully characterize a system and provide surgeons with the information they need to determine the best system for their use and the proper way to use that system.

25.2 Subsystem testing

Multiple groups have looked into the accuracy of position tracking systems used in CAOS systems. Chassat et al.[1] examined four optical tracking systems using a set of four tests. The tests include an intrinsic accuracy test, which measures absolute accuracy across a 1 m^3 cube; a relative rigid body accuracy test, where two trackers are mounted a fixed distance apart, and their relative positions are tracked through a variety of actions; a pivot repeatability test, in which a point probe with a tracker is repeatedly calibrated, and the variation in the geometric parameters of the calibration is examined; and lastly, a surface digitization accuracy test, in which a calibrated point probe locates 100 points on a stabilized surface, and the distances of the points from the defined surface are reported. Schmerber et al.[2] extend this work with an extrapolation algorithm to improve results for the Polaris system with active trackers. He also described his group's use of the Flashpoint 5000 tracking system in a custom system for performing functional endoscopic sinus surgery. The clinical results reported were based on the surgeon's estimate of the difference in position between a landmark visible through the endoscope and its tracked location viewed on CT images. Almost 90% of the landmarks were estimated to be within 1.5 mm of the tracked position, with the remaining 10% within 2.5 mm.

Wagner et al.[3] report results on testing optical and electromagnetic tracking systems under real clinical conditions. Additionally, they compared serial and multi-slice CT scans, concluding that serial scans provide better results. Three optical and one electromagnetic system were tested in the following ways: with operating rooms lights on or off, with ferromagnetic items in the workspace, and with changes in the angle of the point probe. They found that OR lights did not cause problems with the trackers, unless the light was shining directly into the camera. The instruments also did not affect the results, possibly due to the small size of the instruments introduced into the field. Inclination of the point probe did cause variation in the reported distance, although they did not describe their calibration routine for the point probe. While the numerical results of this study are not conclusive, they do show a strong understanding of some of the issues that need to be identified and examined when determining the accuracy capabilities of a CAOS system.

Li et al.[4] described their tests on tracker accuracy within the context of frameless stereotactic neurosurgery. They utilized implantable fiducials randomly distributed around a phantom skull surface. CT scans of the phantom skull were acquired and used as the ground-truth for characterizing three different tracking systems. In addition to testing the three systems with markers randomly distributed around the skull, they also tested the systems with the markers mounted within a 7 × 7 cm area. This tested the assumption that a wide baseline for the markers would provide more accurate results. For the randomly distributed points, the three systems were not significantly different, statistically. Only one of the systems showed a significant difference between markers distributed across the whole surface of the skull and markers mounted only around the region of interest. In this chapter, Li et al. not only tested the tracking system, but the areas on the skull which are used to generate the transformation between the image space and the patient's anatomy.

Lindseth et al.[5] describe work on testing a neuronavigation system utilizing tracked ultrasound. Although intended for neurosurgery work, tracked ultrasound can also be used in CAOS systems.

They thoroughly characterized the accuracy of a 3D ultrasound probe, tracked with a Polaris position tracking system, for detecting the locations of wire crosses in a phantom model. The researchers varied different parameters during testing, including orientation of the ultrasound probe with respect to the phantom, distance and orientation of the Polaris camera with respect to the phantom, and the scan protocol of the ultrasound probe. They performed a statistical analysis, and looked at compounding factors where the interaction between variables influenced the outcome of the tests. In their analysis, they determined that calibration of the ultrasound probe in their tracking body reference frame was the largest source of error in the laboratory setting. They also looked at sources of error in a complete neuronavigation system, and estimated the overall accuracy of the system in clinical use.

25.3 End-to-end system testing

Hagelauer *et al.*[6] looked at the use of navigation systems for the treatment of orthopaedic diseases using shock wave lithotripters. Using an isocenter C-arm fluoroscope, the shock wave treatment is normally targeted at the isocenter of the C-arm, with the surgeon positioning the patient such that the diseased tissue is centered within the C-arm. Therefore, by mounting the tracking camera directly to the C-arm frame, only the therapy head is tracked. They described one test of the tracking system, where a test-bed was built that pivots a tracker around a single point. With the tracker calibrated to the pivot center, they looked at variation in the position reported over a 15° arc. While this did test the basic accuracy of the tracking setup, it did not address accuracy outside that arc, which could be used in practice, and the positions reported when the head is aimed away from the isocenter of the C-arm. The authors did discuss the accuracy values achieved with respect to the requirements of the surgical procedure, demonstrating the tradeoff of the necessary accuracy for the procedure instead of an absolute threshold of accuracy for a CAOS system.

Jacob *et al.*[7] described thier group's work on a registration-free system utilizing a CT scanner with an optical tracking system. The bed of the CT scanner has a calibration target on it for the optical tracker to allow the system to determine the location of any surgical tools within the reference frame of the CT scan. They tested differing values of base-edge lengths, the distance between LEDs in a tracker; repetitive accuracy of different commercial trackers; repetitive accuracy of their CT bed calibration target; and freehand accuracy for locating points in space. A strong statistical analysis was performed on the resultant data, showing the errors generated by this type of tool tracking with respect to a patient imaging device. The authors also describe some of the trade-offs of this type of navigation, but do not fully explore the issue of patient motion after the scan is acquired. During some procedures, patient motion can be quite subtle, but still large enough to destroy any correspondence between the acquired scan and the assumed reference frame.

Herring *et al.*[8] described the results from a sensitivity analysis for registration errors when the error where point data is collected from the patient's anatomy, in this case a vertebra, is varied. Five areas on the vertebra were identified as surface patches, and points on those surfaces were obtained with an optical tracking system, ultrasound images, and directly from CT images with added noise. For the points generated by the optical tracking system, a ground truth registration was determined based on fiducial locations. They also compared the effects of different CT scan protocols. By testing registration using different regions of the vertebral surface, they were able to determine the most cost-effective, in time, area to collect position data for registration. In testing the CT-scan protocol, they also showed the effects on the registration accuracy when the scan resolution was decreased.

Sugano *et al.*[9] described their work in characterizing the accuracy of a system combining a CT-scan of a cadaveric femur and pelvis, surface model generation, and registration when using an optical tracking system. They tested CT-scan protocols, segmentation thresholds, and the area of surface point collection. They also varied the number of surface points collected, to find the most cost-effective number of points to collect for each bone. In this way, they tested end-to-end accuracy while varying a few different parameters, to determine which would generate the best result, with the least amount of trade-offs. Statistical results were reported, with 20 sets of data for each test used.

Gaggl et al.[10] published work on navigated drilling of dental phantoms, looking for breaches of the maxillary sinus floor. After 60 drillings, the thickness of the resultant section was measured, with a mean distance of 0.11 mm to the floor wall and 13 perforations. They also followed up the basic drilling test by placing implant in another 60 navigated drill holes. In this second test, 47 of the 60 implants breached the sinus floor. By testing not only the navigation, but also the final result, the authors established the fact that while it is important to not breach the sinus floor during drilling, the implant can still breach the wall during insertion. Therefore, the authors suggest that ideal placement of the navigated drill does not ensure ideal placement of the implant, and that one method of ensuring that the sinus wall is not breached is to accurately leave a 1 mm security distance between the bottom of the drill hole and the sinus floor. Absolute accuracy of the navigation is not the only issue in this case, and the authors examined other contributing factors.

Hassfeld et al.[11] described a study where they contrasted the accuracy of a mechanical spatial tracking system with an optical tracking system. CT and magnetic resonance tomography (MRT) protocols were varied, and spatial tracking was tested on a plastic phantom. The authors found an inverse relationship between accuracy and slice thickness, with CT scans generating more accurate results than MRT scans. They also tested the accuracy of a paired point registration, finding that increasing the number of points and their distance from each other increased tracking accuracy.

Viant et al.[12] described a graph-based method to model the error propagation through a CAOS system, based on statistical models of errors characterized with a normal distribution. By graphing the connections between different steps in a CAOS system, such as measurement, registration, transformation, and reconstruction, Viant developed a theoretic framework that can model overall accuracies of a system based on individual component and action error distributions.

Simon et al.[13] described work looking at accuracy validation for image guided orthopaedic surgery. They identified sources of error for prototypical CT-based systems, and suggested techniques to minimize the effects of some of the sources. The results of an accuracy validation of the registration routine, and a description of a fiducial design were presented. They also identified the need for application specific error metrics, showing how the same measurement errors could be described with drastically different numerical values, based on the coordinate system used.

Plaskos et al.[14] performed a study aimed at identifying the errors generated by bone cutting during total knee arthroplasty. Using an optical tracking system commonly used in CAOS systems, the authors tracked the position of the saw guide before and after the cut was performed and the final orientation of the cut plane on the tibia or femur. They determined that cutting can be a significant source of error for knee implant alignment, and that guide movement during cutting aggravates other contributions to bone cutting errors. Therefore, they conclude that bone cutting errors may be a factor in some of the poor results reported for computer assisted total knee replacements.

25.4 Accuracy testing methodology

While the end to end accuracy of a computer assisted surgery system is of vital importance to its overall usefulness and safety, a better, additional understanding of the contributions that different components of the system and surgical actions make to the overall accuracy will allow the developers to identify, and improve, the areas which have disproportionate contributions. After the different components and actions are identified, their contributions to the accuracy of the system can be quantified and compared to a minimum level of accuracy determined for the surgical application.

Identification and determination of a minimally acceptable level of accuracy is the first step in determining if a CAOS system will satisfy the surgical requirements. This minimum level of accuracy will not necessarily be the same for different procedures, as patient outcomes are not equally sensitive to similar error distributions. For instance, for hip replacement surgery, positive outcomes will not be significantly affected if the acetabular implant is placed within 5° of the ideal orientation. But with total knee replacement surgery, where surgical outcomes have been shown to be more sensitive to implant alignment, if the implant is placed in valgus or varus orientation, the likelihood of a poor result increases. Therefore, a maximum error of 3° might be better suited for total knee arthroplasty. A system that could be used for both hips and knees would have to be able to achieve a maximum angular error of 3° in this case to satisfy the requirements of both procedures. By setting the maximum error appropriately for the procedure in question, a developer or researcher will not spend extra time and effort towards achieving an accuracy threshold that will not yield a corresponding improvement in patient outcomes.

To identify and quantify the contributions of different components and actions, the entire CAOS process and system needs to be examined to identify all possible contributors to the overall accuracy of the system. A chart tracking the flow of information through the procedure will help identify the sources of error, and assist in the identification of any missed terms. Each item in the flow chart will have an error value associated with it, allowing the summation of the error terms into a maximum possible error for the system. Different labels are used for different categories of error contributions, with rectangular boxes describing system components and round components describing user or patient actions. There may be multiple contributions to the accuracy of the system for an individual component; these are listed under each item in the flow chart. A basic outline of the chart is shown in Fig. 25.1, for a CAOS system that first builds a model of the patient's anatomy, places the implant at a surgeon defined location with respect to the model, and then navigates the tools for insertion of an implant.

After the flow chart has been created, and all sources of error identified, the amount of error for each term must be determined. Some terms may not be able to be quantified, such as patient motion during a CT or MRI, but they should still be included in the flow chart to alert users to the presence of

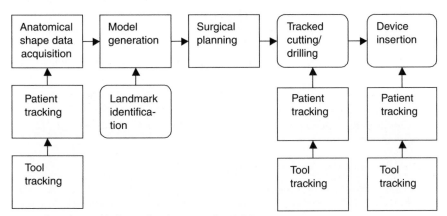

Fig. 25.1 Basic flowchart of information in a generic CAOS system.

the error term. For terms that can be quantified, an accurately characterized phantom model of the relevant anatomy is invaluable for acquiring test data. An anatomical phantom will not only test the subsystems in the manner in which they will be used, but may also uncover sources of unexpected error, such as OR lights confusing an optical tracking system. While a phantom model of the anatomy may not be able to accurately model soft tissue, it will allow the developers to examine the system at each step and possibly find unexpected errors. A well-constructed and characterized phantom model will also aid in application specific error measurements, which can be different than general error terms using an artificial construct, such as a calibration table.

The satisfactory phantom will contain either landmarks or fiducials that are easily locatable at all stages of a practice procedure, so that their positions can be recorded and assessed. The positions of the fiducials, and also the shape of the entire model if feasible, are then accurately determined. One method of determining fiducial positions is to locate them using a coordinate measuring machine (CMM), with accuracies on the order of 0.005 mm. An example of a pelvis phantom with fiducials and acetabular implants being measured b a CMM is shown in Fig. 25.2. For each item in the data flow chart of the CAOS system, the actual fiducial values can be compared to the measured values. By utilizing this accurately measured ground truth model, we can characterize all error terms that are based on patient anatomy.

For each term that can be quantified, a test should be devised that will characterize its error distribution under realistic conditions, including operating room lights, sterile drapes, and other tools in the area, which may effect the accuracy of the component being tested. A statistically sufficient number of data points should be collected for each term, such that the results are truly representative of the underlying error distribution. Once the data are collected, the mean or RMS error, the maximum error, and the variance should be calculated. These values can be individually compared to the maximum allowable error described previously, and can also be combined to determine the maximum

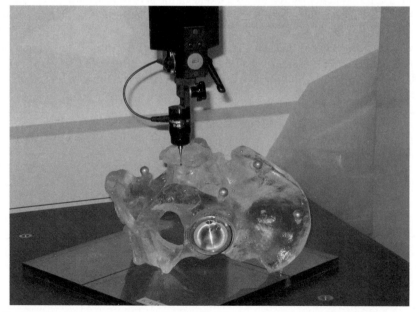

Fig. 25.2 Characterization of pelvic phantom with coordinate measuring machine (CMM).

potential error for the system. Position errors and orientation errors can be summed separately, but if the two types of error are to be combined, a suitable reference frame must be defined and the values transformed into the appropriate type. It is important to realize, however, that the component errors do not simply add up, and while some can propagate through the system with a cascading effect, others may partially cancel out during the procedure. The sum of the error values generated through these tests will likely be larger than values generated by an end-to-end test, due to the fact that during an end-to-end test, errors from different steps can partially cancel each other if their directions are opposite. For instance, if one step causes an error of 3 mm to the right, and the following step has an error of 2 mm to the left, the sum will be an error of 1 mm to the right, while the sum of the individual error terms would show a potential error of 5 mm. For this reason, individual component testing is most useful for determining where a system may be causing unnecessarily large errors.

After the component testing is completed, end-to-end testing with the well characterized anatomical phantom should be completed. This will show the effects of error terms canceling each other out, and will encode any error terms that may have been missed. It may also uncover any unexpected effects from actual conditions that the system will be used in. As before, a sufficient number of tests should be performed to characterize the underlying error distribution, and the error statistics computed. These statistical error values are then compared to the maximum error values determined for the surgical procedure. The overall system can then be described as meeting or not meeting the accuracy goal set for it. The complete process is diagramed in Fig. 25.3.

25.4.1 Clinical validation

After the accuracy of the CAOS system has been quantified in a laboratory setting with phantom models, clinical results must be validated, not only for patient outcomes but also for numerical accuracy results to show that the system is generating the accuracy it claims to deliver. The results generated during clinical testing will be representative of the actual end-to-end results a surgeon may achieve when using the system. However, additional care must be taken to acquire accurate post-operative results. For example, standard standing X-rays to measure knee implant orientation will not provide accurate angles, due to the distortion generated by a single source of radiation. Additionally, only orientation in the coronal plane is available in the standard X-ray, so any twist of the implant components will not be measurable by standard means. New techniques to generate orientation data by comparing X-rays with digitally reconstructed radiographs from CT data and calculated projections of implant CAD models,

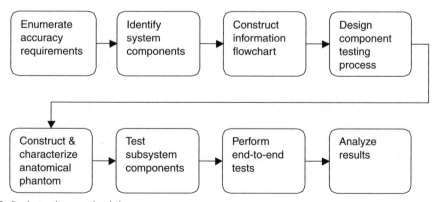

Fig. 25.3 Basic testing methodology process.

for example, may provide accurate measurements that can be used for post-operative evaluation of the surgical result. No matter what technique is used, though, clinical validation must be performed to ensure that post-operative results are in line with laboratory accuracy tests. Furthermore, the tools used in post-operative evaluation should be of comparable accuracy to those used in the preoperative planning and surgical intervention phases.

Through the combination of the three testing methods using the standard methodology described above, component testing, end-to-end testing, and validation of the accuracy of clinical results, CAOS systems can be thoroughly characterized and validated. A standard process of validating and reporting system accuracy will provide researchers and surgeons with the information needed to be able to objectively compare different CAOS systems and determine which one will best meet their needs.

25.4.2 **Case study**

To test the methodology described above, we applied the general framework to the HipNav system. HipNav is an image based computer assisted orthopaedic surgery system, and consists of a preoperative planner and an intra-operative navigation system. Surface models of the patient's pelvis and femur, built from a CT scan, are used by a surgeon to help plan the placement of the acetabular cup and femoral stem implant components. Given the component positions, a range of motion simulation test is done using typical leg motions, such as crossing one's leg and squatting. Depending on the feedback from the range of motion simulator, the surgeon can then alter the implant size and placement to maximize range of motion, instead of relying on a standard orientation. In this manner, implant placement is based on actual patient anatomy instead of an idealized assumption of their anatomy. During the surgical procedure, the patient and the surgical tools are tracked using a Polaris optical tracking system. The surgical tools are calibrated at the beginning of each case, and a tracker is attached to the patient's pelvis. After dislocation and the femoral osteotomy, a series of points is located on the pelvis with a tracked point probe tool. Registration between the point cloud and the surface model built preoperatively is then performed. Registration accuracy is verified by placing the point probe on the surface of the pelvis and ensuring that the tracked location, rendered onto both the CT and the surface model, also lies along the surface. The acetabulam is reamed, and the acetabular implant test fit. The final implant, mounted onto a tracked cup tool, is then inserted into the pelvis with the same orientation that the surgeon determined preoperatively during the planning stage. The surgery is then completed in a conventional fashion.

The accuracy threshold for HipNav was set to be 2° of rotation and 2 mm of translation. The translational component represents the error generated by the system between the point cloud collected from the patient's pelvis and the actual position of the pelvis, and the rotational component is the error between the actual placed orientation of the acetabular cup and the reported orientation. These thresholds are much better than the results obtainable using the mechanical guides provided by the implant manufacturers, which were shown to often be off by more than 15° in version.[15]

Two phantom models of the pelvis were constructed to facilitate the tests of the HipNav system. The model is based on a clear plastic Sawbones pelvis, rigidly mounted to a Lexan base defining the anterior pelvic (AP) plane. The AP plane is used by the HipNav system for reporting the acetabular cup implant orientation. Acetabular cup implants and spherical fiducials were mounted into both halves of the pelvis, to provide multiple data points for testing. The locations of the fiducials and the orientations of the mounted cups were then measured with a CMM, using the Lexan base as the AP plane when measuring cup orientation. The fiducial locations help test the tracking system, and the cup orientations can be used to test the end-to-end accuracy of the HipNav system.

The main actions within the HipNav system are: patient CT scanning, model building, preoperative planning, tool and patient tracking, and intra-operative registration. The main subsystems of the HipNav system, therefore, are: anatomical model builder, preoperative planner, tracking, and registration. Identification of these major subsystems is the first part of the accuracy validation framework.

The next portion of the validation framework was to examine each major subsystem and determine individual contributors to the system's accuracy. The model building stage of HipNav consists of the CT scan, segmentation, and then surface reconstruction. A chart similar to that shown in Fig. 25.1 was then created, with the items to be tested including: CT scan protocol and calibration, model construction, anatomical landmark identification, tracker accuracy, tool calibration (for point probe and cup impaction tool) and tool tracking, and registration accuracy.

Tests were designed to characterize each of these components of the HipNav system, and the data gathered was analyzed to determine the average error, standard deviation, and maximum error. End-to-end tests were also performed, using the phantom anatomical models, and were analyzed in a similar fashion. The end-to-end results are shown in Table 25.1. Figure 25.4 shows the distribution of orientation errors from the CMM measured orientations. The mean errors shown, which are not centered at zero, are probably due to the fact that the anterior pelvic (AP) plane used with the CMM is not guaranteed to be coincident with the AP plane identified the preoperative planner. The planner used fiducials mounted in the phantom. These fiducials were centered in grooves in the baseplate,

Table 25.1 End-to-end errors in acetabular cup implant alignment.

Errors	Abduction		Anteversion		Combined	
	RMS	Std. Dev.	RMS	Std. Dev.	RMS	Std. Dev.
Model 1 L	1.20°	0.34°	0.35°	0.23°	1.25°	0.36°
Model 1 R	0.80°	0.31°	0.27°	0.27°	0.84°	0.30°
Model 2 L	0.77°	0.16°	0.26°	0.27°	0.81°	0.16°
Model 2 R	0.59°	0.28°	0.85°	0.32°	1.04°	0.28°

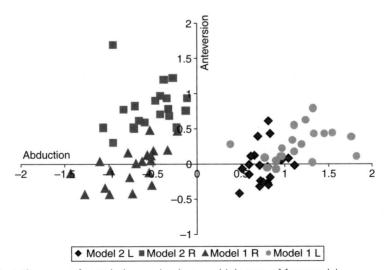

Fig. 25.4 Orientation error of acetabular cup implant: multiple tests of four models.

which determined the AP plane for the CMM. If the fiducials were not at all the same depth with respect to the plate, that could generate a small angular deflection, as could small errors when identifying the spheres in the planning process. Since the mean errors are scattered randomly between models, but are not scattered randomly about zero, we see that this error is not systemic. The significant component of the error at this point is the variance, which has a maximum at around 0.30°. This demonstrates that the system can guide the cup placement to an orientation less than 2.0° away from the plan generated by the surgeon, providing the surgeon with a tool to accurately place acetabular cup implants where he or she desires.

References

1 Chassat F, Lavallee S. Experimental protocol of accuracy evaluation of 6-D localizers for computer-integrated surgery: application to four optical localizers. *Medical Image Computing and Computer-Assisted Intervention – MICCAI'98. Proceedings of the First International Conference*, 1998:277–84. xxii + 1256.

2 Schmerber S, Chassat F. Accuracy evaluation of a CAS system: laboratory protocol and results with 6D localizers, and clinical experiences in otorhinolaryngology. *Comput Aided Surg* 2001;6(1):1–13.

3 Wagner A, Schicho K, Birkfellner W, Figl M, Seemann R, Konig F, Kainberger F, Ewers R. Quantitative analysis of factors affecting intra-operative precision and stability of optoelectronic and electromagnetic tracking systems. *Med Phys* 2002;29(5):905–12.

4 Li Q, Zamorano L, Jiang Z, Gong JX, Pandya A, Perez R, Diaz F. Effect of optical digitizer selection on the application accuracy of a surgical localization system-a quantitative comparison between the OPTOTRAK and flashpoint tracking systems. *Comput Aided Surg* 1999;4(6):314–21.

5 Lindseth F, Langø T, Bang J, Hagelhus Hernes T, Accuracy evaluation of a 3D ultrasound-based neuronavigation system. *Comput Aided Surg* 2002;7:197–222.

6 Hagelauer U, Russo S, Gigliotti S, de Durante C, Corrado EM. Interactive navigation system for shock wave applications. *Comput Aided Surg* 2001;6(1):22–31.

7 Jacob AL, Messmer P, Kaim A, Suhm N, Regazzoni P, Baumann B. A whole-body registration-free navigation system for image-guided surgery and interventional radiology. *Invest Radiol* 2000;35(5):279–88.

8 Herring JL, Dawant BM, Maurer CR Jr, Muratore DM, Galloway RL, Fitzpatrick JM. Surface-based registration of CT images to physical space for image-guided surgery of the spine: a sensitivity study. *IEEE Trans Med Imaging* 1998;17(5):743–52.

9 Sugano N, Sasama T, Sato Y, Nakajima Y, Nishii T, Yonenobu K, Tamura S, Ochi T. Accuracy evaluation of surface-based registration methods in a computer navigation system for hip surgery performed through a posterolateral approach. *Comput Aided Surg* 2001;6(4):195–203.

10 Gaggl A, Schultes G. Assessment of accuracy of navigated implant placement in the maxilla. *Int J Oral Maxillofac Implants* 2002;17(2):263–70.

11 Hassfeld S, Muhling J. Comparative examination of the accuracy of a mechanical and an optical system in CT and MRT based instrument navigation. *Int J Oral Maxillofac Surg* 2000;29(6):400–7.

12 Viant WJ. The development of an evaluation framework for the quantitative assessment of computer-assisted surgery and augmented reality accuracy performance. *Stud Health Technol Inform* 2001;81:534–40.

13 Simon D, O'Toole RV, Blackwell M, Morgan F, DiGioia AM III, Kanade T. Accuracy validation in image-guided orthopaedic surgery. *Proceedings of the Second International Symposium on Medical Robotics and Computer Assisted Surgery*, 1995:185–92.

14 Plaskos C, Hodgson AJ, Inkpen K, McGraw RW. Bone cutting errors in total knee arthroplasty. *J Arthroplasty* 2002;17(6):698–705.

15 DiGioia AM, Jaramaz B, Blackwell M, *et al*. The Otto Aufranc Award. Image guided navigation system to measure intra-operatively acetabular implant alignment. *Clin Orthop* 1998, Oct;(355):8–22.

Chapter 26

Future challenges

Jocelyne Troccaz and Philippe Merloz

26.1 Introduction

Two major populations of patients use orthopaedic surgery: those who have suffered trauma, and those who require correction of mechanical disorders. Orthopaedic surgery is a real public health issue: for instance, in Europe it concerns about 1,000,000 patients a year, and costs about 3,000,000,000 Euros. These populations are mostly young people (the average age is 40 and the median is 50), who will live for many years following the intervention. Any negative consequences of an intervention therefore represent a major factor in the patient's quality of life, as well as in the economy of the country due to the cost of the after care that becomes necessary and because of the consequences for the economic activity of victims (in 1994, an estimated 50,000,000 work days were lost in Europe after orthopaedic intervention). This tendency becomes more dramatic each year as life expectancy lengthens and since prosthesis implantation now is often considered indicated for younger and younger patients (the average age for hip prostheses in 1970 was 75, in 1980 it was 70, and in 1994 it was 65).

The age where the intervention is performed is a key parameter indicative of different types of problems to be faced. Trauma concerns mostly young people and the chief issue is to correct as precisely as possible the consequences of a trauma, knowing that the patient will have an active life for decades afterwards. But when elderly people are concerned, the first objective is to do an intervention that is as minimal as possible especially when post-operative consequences are considered: the revolution caused by total hip prosthesis in the 1970s is a model in this domain. Interventions for mechanical disorders typically occur at two stages of life: at under 20 years to correct abnormalities in skeletal development, or after 50 to correct the consequences of osteoarthritis. Scoliosis is a typical instance of the former case. The latter is illustrated by Total Knee Arthroplasty (TKA), which is also a good instance of the tendency to perform this sort of intervention on younger and younger people (the average age for TKA went from 75 in 1980, to 65 in 1994).

In the domain of orthopaedic surgery the above mentioned objectives of decreasing costs and improvement of the quality of the care delivered result in four major issues: development of new techniques, evaluation of these techniques, establishment of standards for the indications and implementation of these techniques and development of educational systems.

Two challenges are suggested for physicians and engineers: a *technical challenge* and a *clinical challenge*.

26.2 Clinical challenges

For hip and knee surgery these two challenges concern three major surgical applications: total hip arthroplasty (and revision) (THA); total knee arthroplasty (TKA) and anterior cruciate ligament replacement (ACLR).

Computer Assisted Surgery (CAS) systems exist. Most of them are passive systems. Some of them are active systems. Actually for hip and knee surgery four kinds of computer assisted surgery systems are available:

—CT based system with active navigation (robot)
—CT based system with passive navigation
—Virtual fluoroscopic systems (passive navigation)
—Non-CT and nonfluoroscopic systems.

These new techniques should offer solutions for minimally invasive surgery and for improvement of the accuracy and safety of interventions. Their implementation should take place in properly equipped operating rooms (OR) where design of adapted operating tables is of particular importance.

26.2.1 Minimally invasive surgery

Endoscopic surgery has proven its clinical interest: the interventions that can be performed using this technique present fewer post-operative complications since the patient can return to normal life much more quickly. This technique has already been applied in knee surgery. The limitation in developing such techniques is the difficulty of accurate control of the surgical act since the surgeon's perception is limited by a narrow visual field. These techniques emphasize the need for user-friendly access to preoperative data (Computer Tomography or CT, Magnetic Resonance Images or MRI, X-rays, etc). Making them available intra-operatively by registration with intra-operative data and tracking the position of instruments provides the surgeon with means to merge the real world he discloses with his knife with this virtual world.

26.2.2 Improvement of accuracy

Improved accuracy of orthopaedic interventions also limits complications from surgical interventions. In some cases, this can be observed during the intervention itself. It happens too often that an insufficiently precise evaluation of this effect ruins the result of the intervention and a follow up intervention is required. More often, however, the importance of accuracy is seen in the long term. In the case of hip prosthesis, accurate preparation of the medullar cavity of the femur allows use of a cementless prosthesis when there is a perfect fit of the cortical bone with the shank of the prosthesis. This improved accuracy could result in the long run in a decrease of the ratio of prostheses which break or get out of position, an estimated 40% after 10 years. Finally, precise definition of the tunnel for a ligamentoplasty in ACL reconstruction, or precise definition of the position of a TKA will result in an improved lifetime for the ligament, or in longer delay before the appearance of osteoarthritis. It also has to be borne in mind that mathematical accuracy alone will not equate with better outcome in every case. There are cases where an exact fit is a hindrance to good clinical outcome as it inhibits the natural process of acceptance of the prosthesis as a part of the body.

These instances clearly demonstrate the fact that accuracy is both a problem of selection of an optimal strategy, based on pre and intra-operative data, and of guiding the performance of this strategy. The first part of this problem corresponds to an enhancement of the capacity of sensing and decision for the surgeon, while the second part aims at improving his capacity in accurately manipulating his surgical tools.

26.2.3 Improvement of safety

Safety should be considered from the viewpoint of the patient, but also that of the surgical team. Vital issues are not very frequent in orthopaedic surgery but they do occur, particularly in spinal surgery. Omitting cement also may present interesting possibilities since it would eliminate untoward effects due to the cement itself (mostly embolism, which occurs in up to 10% of classical hip prosthesis cases, or 100,000 patients per year in Europe).

Safety critical systems, which in this context are those where a patient could be physically damaged or even killed as a result of software initiated actions (or absence of action), are currently the subject of much work by governments. Guidelines do exist on the choice of programming languages, the documentation required, the protocols to be followed, etc. The medical world has so far not been fully engaged in these activities.

26.2.4 Operating room enhancement

The classical OR is not always suitable for introducing the new sensors and information technology devices that are necessary to make the best use of the data gathered preoperatively and intra-operatively, nor are they always adapted to the introduction of new effectors that can prove necessary to accurately carry out the indicated action.

26.2.5 Hip surgery

Hip surgery is considered by many surgeons to be quite easy in most cases. However, difficult cases still raise a lot of geometrical and biomechanical problems. A large variety of implants exist, and the choice between cemented and non-cemented techniques still raises very controversial discussions. Significant patient pain is also frequently a problem. Finally, there is a great need to improve the life of hip prostheses because an increasing number of patients are younger than in the past. For difficult cases only, CT images are used in order to design individual implants that best fit the patient's bone morphology. It is assumed that the CT-based planning of the optimal position of standard implants, and accurate drilling of the femoral cavity in order to provide an optimal bone for implant fitting, will improve life of prostheses in all cases. To achieve such an objective, two solutions have been proposed recently.

- The first method is based on a ISS product named Robodoc that uses a robot that drills a cavity inside the femur. Robodoc is probably the most spectacular and famous system in the domain of computer assisted orthopaedics surgery. It was originally developed at IBM T.J. Watson Centre (New York). In this domain the spreading out of small robots (not bigger than a coffee self-dispenser) like CRIGOS (compact Robot for Image Guided Orthopaedic Surgery; Aachen University, Germany; J. Fourier University, France) is probably very attractive.

- The second method uses individual templates which are used for surface-based registration and which act like copying devices that allow the surgeon to drill the cavity himself although the system constrains the action to remain in the optimal region.

Future challenges for hip surgery are based on the use of statistical models (with registration between intra-operative bone morphing data and statistical models); on the use of registration between preoperative CT images and intra-operative ultrasound images and the use of the next generation of 3D fluoroscopic devices.

26.2.6 **Knee surgery**

Knee surgery is considered to be difficult mainly because of the complexity of the kinematics and dynamics of knee functioning that are to be restored during an operation. Therefore, several techniques have been proposed to optimize some geometric or biomechanical criteria. Computer assisted techniques in this domain mostly rely on the use of geometric information acquired from preoperative CT images or per-operative kinematic data.

26.2.6.1 Total knee arthroplasty (TKA)

The total knee prosthesis intervention consists in cutting extremities of the femoral and tibial bones, in order to render regular surfaces ready to admit the prosthesis. The difficulty of such an operation is to define the orientation of the bone cuts so that the defined tibial and femoral axes will be aligned. To solve this problem, three approaches have been proposed.

—First it is possible to use preoperative images (CT based) in order to define optimal cut locations, followed by registration techniques (paired points; four points; surface points matching or ultrasound matching) and completed by the use of robotic active systems or passive navigation systems to make the optimal cuts. In this domain we think that the use of micro-robots will be very helpful for the surgeon.

—A second approach is still relying on CT-based planning, but it uses individual templates instead of robotics systems in order to help the surgeon to make the optimal cuts.

—A third possible strategy consists in using only intra-operative kinematic (Aesculap orthopilot system) and geometric data (statistical models; J. Fourier University, Grenoble, France) acquired during the operation using a 3D optical localizer.

26.2.6.2 Anterior cruciate ligament (LCA) reconstruction

The treatment of an anterior cruciate ligament deficient knee appears to be rather difficult. When the broken ligament has to be replaced, the surgery consists (for most surgeons) in making two tunnels: one in the femur notch and one in the tibia, and then to insert a graft inside these tunnels which is usually taken on the patellar tendon. The main difficulty of this surgery is to find the optimal sites where the ligament graft should be inserted in the femur and in the tibia. Many different criteria, systems, and techniques have been proposed and no consensus exists. At the Grenoble hospital, a computer assisted technique has been developed in order to provide quantitative and referenced measurements that should help to gain some consensus on criteria. Unlike existing mechanical guiding systems that impose following a specific protocol on surgeons, the Grenoble computer-assisted method only provides accurate information for the surgeon's use in performing the intervention. To give a general idea of the technique, after preliminary geometric and kinematic data acquisition obtained using a 3D optical localizer, the surgeon has the possibility to examine the predicted variation of the length of the ligament graft during a flexion/extension of the knee (the so-called anisometry profile). The system indicates the location of the optimal anisometry profiles, but the surgeon can also decide to select a slightly different position, still having access to the predicted behavior of the graft. The comparison between recorded data and clinical outcomes will enable quantified prospective studies, that will probably lead to a major breakthrough in this difficult area.

26.3 **Technical challenges**

Over the last two decades, many systems have entered the operating theaters. Among them, a large number of prototypes taking advantage of the surgeons' enthusiasm demonstrated the clinical feasibility of CAS especially in the orthopaedics domain. Whist the success of some of these systems cannot be discussed, the routine use of CAS systems still raises a number of practical questions often related to more fundamental issues. In the following paragraphs, based on the state of the art, we will discuss some of these issues related to the main components of CAS systems, namely data acquisition and fusion, simulation and learning, and guiding systems.

26.3.1 **Data acquisition and processing**

26.3.1.1 Data acquisition

Data acquisition in CAOS systems is still very conservative, relying on a large part on traditional X-ray imaging and CT. CAOS would certainly benefit from the introduction of new digital X-ray sensors developed by the major imaging companies. Flat panel X-ray detectors offer new perspectives for X-ray interventional imaging. Commercial static imaging systems including digital detector of large size (up to 43×43 cm^2), high resolution (pixel size up to 143×143 mm^2) and good dynamic (14 bits) are now available. Dynamic detectors will be soon available in mobile fluoroscopic systems with a very good resolution (close to 200×200 mm^2) and a rate close to 30 images per seconds. These detectors do not suffer from geometric distortion as IIs (image intensifiers) therefore avoiding complex position dependant calibration procedures in the OR. They usually allow one to reduce the dose to the patient compared to IIs and are more ergonomic because they are flat. 3D reconstruction from X-ray projections on a 2D flat panel could improve the navigation during bone surgery compared to the traditional fluoro-navigation based on a couple of X-ray projections on II. The main problems for a wider use of 3D X-ray interventional reconstruction are the dose reduction and patient movement. How can we perform sufficiently good bone reconstruction from a set of few 2D X-ray projections? A priori information must be introduced to compensate for the low number of projections (see, e.g. Fleute00). Safe mechanical systems must be designed for interventional imaging and the movement of the patient must be tracked.

Arthroscopy is already widely used but as mentioned in the previous paragraphs, endoscopic surgery could be improved through augmentation of the endoscopic images. Developed for other specialties such as ENT surgery, augmented endoscopy consisting of tracking the instruments and adding to the endoscopic images preoperative or planning data would probably make this minimally invasive surgery easier and safer and would enlarge the range of clinical applications.

Echography (2.5D or 3D) which is mostly used for soft tissues, could be a very nice noninvasive, irradiationless sensor allowing intra-operative data acquisition for registration to preoperative data. Experimental studies[1,2] have demonstrated the feasibility of this technique for pelvis surgery. Similar approaches should be developed for other orthopaedic applications as an interesting alternative to methods using X-ray imaging or surface palpation of bones.

Finally, clinical performances could be probably improved by integrating micro-sensors (position, force, etc.) to the surgical instruments and to the surgical instrumentation.

26.3.1.2 Data processing

Data segmentation is still an issue especially concerning intra-operative images (X-ray, echography, endoscopy). Whilst preoperative image processing may be partly or fully automated in particular for

CT acquisition of bony structures, or may require the participation of the user in semi-interactive systems for instance for MRI data, intra-operative conditions require that the segmentation methods are automatic, fast, accurate and robust. This still remains a technical challenge even if major progress has been made over the last few years in particular using methods taking benefit of a priori models (statistical models or preoperative data for instance). Similarly, whilst many registration techniques have been developed worldwide, their clinical use is still an issue. Registration raises fundamental issues related to robustness and also more practical questions such as man/machine interface design. Depending on data acquisition and preprocessing and also depending on the initial transformation parameters fed to the algorithms, the performances of the different existing methods may vary a lot. Moreover, a difficult problem is the quality assessment of the computed transform; however accurate they could be, numbers are not information that the clinician can easily interpret.

26.3.2 Simulation and learning

Quality in orthopaedic surgery implies learning and following commonly agreed standard surgical procedures. This major public health issue turns into a scientific and pedagogic challenge: establishing and teaching surgical standards. Today, the specialist skills of orthopaedics are learned by the traditional qualitative apprenticeship system. An experienced surgeon supervises his junior, passing on practical experience. There are major issues with such an educational system, accounting for the great variation in orthopaedic practice throughout the world. These include:

- *Absence of consensual and quantitatively based 'gold standard'.* Each teaching senior surgeon performs clinical research to evaluate the clinical outcome of the surgical procedures that he uses. Yet the review mechanism of surgical journals has no tool to compare these results on a quantitative, multicentric and permanent basis. The same pathology can be treated by very different techniques, though they may have very different clinical outcomes.

- *'Chapel effect'.* The junior surgeon usually interacts with a limited set of senior surgeons, and can only partially compensate for this 'geographic' limitation by using pedagogic material. The learning 'material' is indeed limited to anatomical specimens and patients: books and journals provide reference information for the assimilation of declarative knowledge. Their format is inadequate to meet the requirements of the procedural learning process, where relevant information is highly multimodal since *visual and tactile information plays a major role.*

- *Variance of surgeons' skills.* The skill acquired by a junior surgeon can be evaluated only in a qualitative way: no mechanism exists to quantify the 'learning curve'. Clinical outcome critically depends on the skill of the surgeon and on his or her practice of the procedures.

- *Limited surgical influence upon the introduction of CAOS techniques.* The introduction Computer Aided Orthopaedic Surgery (CAOS) depends on the experience of pioneer surgeons, who contribute to the development of these tools. However these experts cannot share their expertise directly and widely. They are dependant upon industrial partners, who organize training sessions where teachers are usually engineers and not surgeons. Commercial and public health interests may diverge, and the control of medical education by university established bodies in orthopaedics is an essential issue.

Therefore there is a very strong need for developing systems that may modify these learning methods. Recent advances in information technologies should enable this revolution. The purpose is to learn diseases, surgical procedures but also existing CAOS systems. This requires the development of models of courses, multicentric multimodal databases and simulators and to provide any user with easy remote access to such material. Concerning simulators, most of them, developed worldwide, are very interesting research tools demonstrating the ability to render realistic haptic and visual feedback in real time. Very few of them have been thought of for actual clinical educational use and are integrated into a package which would enable students to learn and to simulate a given surgical procedure and then to quantitatively evaluate students of different levels in a quantitative way. Orthopaedics is a domain where modelling may be a little bit simpler than for other soft tissue surgery; this should encourage researchers and engineers to develop such simulators.

26.3.3 Guiding systems

26.3.3.1 Human/computer interface (HCI) design

Computer aided surgery most often requires a strong interaction between the user, a surgeon or an assistant, and a computerized system. The man-machine interface has to be considered not only on a development level but with a methodological approach. Information has to be rendered to the human operator in a usable way that should allow him to evaluate the correctness of the process; this may be, in some cases (for example registration), a very difficult task. A well-designed user interface probably increases the chance of wide clinical use of CAS systems by augmenting the usability and appropriateness of the system for the surgeon. Little attention has been paid to these considerations in the CAS domain[3,4] while several studies in many domains have largely demonstrated that the HCI may have some severe impact on task realization especially for critical applications. A certain number of choices have to be made as for instance: Which information is rendered? What type of device is used to render this information? What representation of the information is used? etc. In order to make these interaction choices more rational, suitable formalisms (see for instance)[5] have to be used in order to describe the surgical procedures from the information point of view and the man-machine interactions and their characteristics. These formalisms allow the predictive analysis, thus the design, or the evaluation of CAOS systems. Moreover, the design of new man-machine interface devices is necessary. Some have to be invented. Others such as haptic devices and see-through displays (screens and helmets) have to be made more adapted to the application domain.

26.3.3.2 Robots

As already mentioned, Robodoc[6] is certainly the most famous robotic medical assistant. Despite the fact that it was a very pioneering work, robots have not invaded the orthopedics operating rooms. A question is still not correctly answered in the domain of orthopedics: is a robot really necessary for CAOS? This question has been made more and more prevalent as navigation has been developed and has demonstrated its potentiality. Two types of questions are raised by robots:

—The first one is quasi-philosophical as it is related to the fact that the surgeon may reject the idea of being replaced by the robot at least for a subpart of the intervention. On a more rational level, it is true that robots are still far from being able to integrate sensing as the human being is and from reacting correctly and intelligently to unexpected and nonmodeled events.

—The second type of questions is related to the ability for clinicians to use such systems. On one hand, robots remain very cumbersome machines which integration in the OR and use may be difficult and long. On the other hand, cost remains a critical issue.

These open questions may be answered in different ways. Concerning automation issues, alternative techniques such as tele-operation and synergistic devices (cf.[7]) have to be evaluated. To our knowledge,

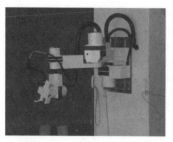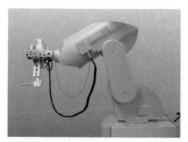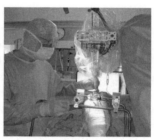

Fig. 26.1 Synergistic systems (left); PADyC (middle and right) ACROBOT (by courtesy of Pr B.Davies, Imperial College of Science, Technology and Medicine, London, GB).

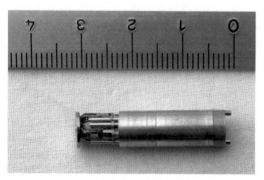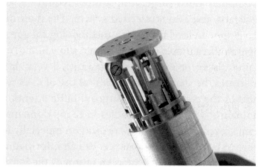

Fig. 26.2 MIPS system (by courtesy of Dr J.P. Merlet, INRIA, Sophia Antipolis, France).

medical tele-robotics, initially developed for microsurgery (neurosurgery, ophthalmologic surgery) and then applied to minimally invasive surgery (see for instance the DaVinci system from Intuitive Surgical Devices)[8,9] has never been applied to orthopedics.[1] Synergistic devices have been developed to compromise between the automation approach of active robots adapted to rather generic applications and the more cooperative approach related to semi-active systems but generally limited to a single type of action (for instance, linear motion or planar motion). A synergistic device is a robot supporting the surgical instrument, held by a human operator and with which control is shared between the operator and the machine. ACROBOT,[10,11] PADyC[12,13] and Cobot[14,15] are examples of such systems. ACROBOT is a motorized robot whilst Cobot and PADyC are nonactuated mechanical structures. ACROBOT has been demonstrated for total knee arthroplasty procedures. Figure 26.1 presents PADyC and ACROBOT prototypes. These types of systems have received a very good reaction from the clinicians. Such collaborative approaches have certainly to be encouraged.

Concerning, the second type of question, miniaturization and integration of robotic devices is a crucial issue. Medical robotics has very slightly moved from the adaptation of industrial robots to the OR, to a more specific service robotics dedicated to clinical use. New types of systems are on the way: we can cite[16] and.[17] This last system, developed to assist colonoscopy, is a miniature disposable robot. Merlet also

----

[1] Or perhaps for demonstrations of remote surgery, independently from any other considerations (motion scaling, filtering, extra dofs) traditionally discussed for micro-surgery and endoscopic applications.

developed a miniature robot. This three degrees of freedom parallel robot (cf. Fig. 26.2) is designed to be integrated to endoscopic instruments. This type of integrated technology is probably the future of medical robotics.

26.3.4 OR of the future: towards the invisible technology …

Over the ten past years, the way computers are integrated into everyday life has evolved a lot. Computers have moved from office desks to homes. Nowadays, many very common objects (TV, cars, refrigerators, washing machines, etc.) integrate some 'intelligence' and connectivity functions. Informatics has been made simultaneously more and more present but invisible to the users. In most cases, using these augmented common use objects does not require any computer science or technical special abilities. We may hope that a similar (r)evolution will happen in operating rooms. Indeed, the existing CAOS systems, even if they have evolved a lot, still require the OR and its staff to adapt to them. Often, technicians or engineers have to assist surgeons in using the systems. We may dream that the OR of the future will be wireless, screenless, and that all the technology will be integrated enough in the instruments, instrumentation and ancillaries to be transparent to the users. This is a major technical challenge considering clinical constraints such as sterilization among others.

References

1 Tonetti J, Cloppet O, Clerc M, Pittet L, Troccaz J, Merloz P, Chirossel J. Implantation of iliosacral screws. Simulation of optimal placement by 3-dimensional X-ray computed tomography. *Rev Chir Orthop Reparatrice Appar Mot* 2000;86(4):360–9.

2 Carrat L, Tonetti J, Merloz P, Troccaz J. Percutaneous computer-assisted iliosacral screwing: clinical validation. MICCAI'2000. In: Delp, DiGioia, Jaramaz, eds. *Lecture notes in computer science series*, vol. 1935. 1229–1237, Springer Verlag, 2000:1229–37.

3 Radermacher K, Zimolong A, Anton M, Thull B. Recommendation for ergonomic analysis Deliverable 04 of IGOS European project. Aachen: Helmholtz Institute, 1996.

4 Dubois E, Nigay L, Troccaz J, Carrat L, Chavanon O. A methodological tool for computer-assisted surgery interface design: its application to computer-assisted pericardial puncture. In: *Medicine meets virtual reality*. Westwood JD ed. IOS Press, 2001:136–9.

5 Jannin P, Raimbault M, Morandi X, Seigneuret E, Gibaud B. Design of a neurosurgical procedure model for multimodal image-guided surgery. In: Lemke, *et al*, eds. CARS'2001. Elsevier Science, 2001.

6 Paul H, Bargar W, Mittlestadt B, Musit B, Taylor R, Kazanzides P, Williamson B, Hanson W. Development of a surgical robot for cementless total hip arthroplasty. *Clini Orthop Rel Res* 1992;(285):57–66.

7 Troccaz J, Peshkin M, Davies B. Guiding systems for computer-assisted surgery (CAS): introducing synergistic devices and discussing the different approaches. *Med Image Anal* 1998;2(2):101–19.

8 Loulmet D, Carpentier A, d'Attelis N, Mill F, Rosa D, Guthart G, Berrebi A, Cardon C, Ponzio O, Aupecle B. First endoscopic coronary artery bypass grafting using computer-assisted instruments. *J Thoracic Cardiovasc Surg* 1999;118(1):4–10.

9 Guthart GS, Salisbury JK. The Intuitive™ telesurgery system: overview and application. *Proceedings of IEEE Robotics and Automation Conference*, April 2000. San Francisco.

10 Davies B, Harris S, Jakopec M, Cobb J. A novel hands-on robot for knee replacement surgery. *Proceedings of the CAOS USA '99 Conference on Computer Assisted Orthopaedic Surgery*, June 1999; 70–4. UPMC, Shadyside Hospital, PA, USA.

11 Davies BL, Harris S, Jakopec M, Fan KL, Cobb J. Intra-operative application of a robotic knee surgery system. MICCAI'99, *Lecture notes in computer science*, September 1999, vol. 1679, 1116–24. Springer Verlag.

12 Troccaz J, Delnondedieu Y. Semi-active guiding systems in surgery. A two-dof prototype of the passive arm with dynamic constraints (PADyC). *Mechatronics* 1996;6(4):399–421.

13 Schneider O, Troccaz J, Chavanon O, Blin D. PADyC: a synergistic robot for cardiac puncturing. *Proceedings of the IEEE Conference on Robotics and Automation*, 2000. San Francisco.

14 Colgate JE, Peshkin M, Moore C. Passive robots and haptic displays based on nonholonomic elements. *Proceedings of the IEEE International Conference on Robotics and Automation*, 1996.

15 Peshkin MA, Colgate JE, Wannasuphoprasit. Nonholonomic haptic displays. *IEEE International Conference on Robotics and Automation*, 1996.

16 Stoianovici D, Whitcomb LL, Anderson JH, Taylor RH, Kavoussi LR. A modular surgical robotic system for image guided percutaneous procedures. *Proceedings of Medical Image Computing and Computer-Assisted Intervention - MICCAI'98, LNCS Series*, 1998, vol. 1496. Springer Verlag.

17 Carrozza MC, Lencioni L, Magnani B, D'Attanasio S, Dario P. The development of a microrobot system for colonoscopy. *Proceedings of the CVRMed-MRCAS'97*, 1997; LNCS, vol. 1205, 779–88. Springer Verlag.

Index